Image Analysis
and Modeling
in Ophthalmology

Image Analysis and Modeling in Ophthalmology

Edited by

E. Y. K. Ng
U. Rajendra Acharya
Aurélio Campilho
Jasjit S. Suri

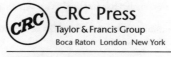

CRC Press
Taylor & Francis Group
Boca Raton London New York

CRC Press is an imprint of the
Taylor & Francis Group, an **informa** business

CRC Press
Taylor & Francis Group
6000 Broken Sound Parkway NW, Suite 300
Boca Raton, FL 33487-2742

First issued in paperback 2017

© 2014 by Taylor & Francis Group, LLC
CRC Press is an imprint of Taylor & Francis Group, an Informa business

No claim to original U.S. Government works

ISBN-13: 978-1-4665-5930-1 (hbk)
ISBN-13: 978-1-138-07175-9 (pbk)

Visit the Taylor & Francis Web site at
http://www.taylorandfrancis.com

and the CRC Press Web site at
http://www.crcpress.com

Contents

Preface

The human eye is a complex and important organ that works similarly to the conventional camera. Many advanced image-processing algorithms have been proposed to analyze the subtle changes in the eye to diagnose eye abnormalities efficiently. Digital fundus images have been used efficiently for the diagnosis of diabetes retinopathy and glaucoma. Infrared imaging provides a temperature profile that depicts changes in the vascular tissues, which helps to study the ocular surface temperature (OST) and ocular diseases like dry eye and cataracts. This book covers the detection of diabetes retinopathy, glaucoma, and anterior segment eye abnormalities; instruments for the detection of glaucoma; and the development of a human eye model using computational fluid dynamics and heat transfer principles to predict inner temperatures of the eye from its surface temperature.

Ultrasound biomicroscopy (UBM) is one of the imaging systems that allow visualization of the anatomy and pathology of the anterior segment. It is particularly beneficial in evaluating regions of the eye behind the iris such as the ciliary body, lens zonular attachment, and lens periphery, which are obscured in other anterior scanning systems. In glaucoma imaging, UBM plays a significant role in objective assessment of peripheral anterior chamber angle morphology, which is useful in angle closure glaucoma diagnosis and management. Chapter 1 presents a UBM system for anterior chamber angle imaging.

Chapter 2 describes both the formal design and development of an automated anterior segment eye disease classification system. The proposed system can be used for early disease diagnosis and treatment management. The classification is done with a two-step processing model. The first processing step extracts nine features from optical eye image data using higher-order spectra, discrete wavelet transform, and texture techniques. The processing step feeds these clinically significant features to a support vector machine (SVM) algorithm for automated classification. The authors have obtained classification accuracy of 90%, sensitivity of 93.8%, and specificity of 100%.

The segmentation and structural properties of the blood vessels of the retina such as width, length, branching pattern, and angles are important features during the screening of diabetes, eye diseases, and cardiovascular diseases. An efficacious retinal vessel segmentation methodology is presented in Chapter 3, which is founded on supervised classification using an ensemble classifier of boosted and bagged decision trees. In this chapter, a more detailed theoretical background, experimental evaluation, and analysis of results are presented.

In Chapter 4, a detailed review, analysis, and categorization of retinal vessel segmentation and caliber measurement techniques are presented. The objective is to provide a detailed resource of the algorithms employed for vessel segmentation and width measurement as a ready reference. The key points are highlighted, the differences and performance measures are illustrated, and the advantages and disadvantages of various approaches are discussed.

Chapter 5 focuses on the segmentation of the blood vessels in high-resolution retinal images. Very recent methods (from the last two to three years) for retinal image analysis are outlined first, by surveying some papers in the segmentation methodologies and their clinical applications. In the next sections, methodology for blood vessel retinal segmentation, with special emphasis on the segmentation of high-resolution fundus images and its validation for the arteriovenous ratio (AVR) calculation, is discussed.

An automated procedure for the location of microaneurysms from retinal images as well as a methodology for lesion registration in order to compute the microaneurysm turnover is proposed in Chapter 6. This chapter also describes the integration of the image-processing methodologies in a web-based framework aimed at retinal analysis. The web framework simplifies data management and provides a user-friendly interface to interact with the image-processing algorithms.

To boost the performance of the level set algorithm, the A-Levelset algorithm, which cascades the level set and active shape model, is proposed in Chapter 7. The A-Levelset-based ARGALI system is built to automatically segment the optic cup and optic disc from 2D digital fundus images. The ARGALI system further calculates the cup-to-disc ratio (CDR), which is an important indicator for glaucoma assessment and diagnosis. It paves the way for automatic objective glaucoma diagnosis and screening using widely available fundus images.

Chapter 8 describes a holistic tool, the Singapore Eye Vessel Assessment (SIVA) system, which brings together various technologies from image processing and artificial intelligence to construct vascular models from retinal images. Subsequently, these models of blood vessels can be queried for a variety of measurements. Incorporating automated techniques reduces manual intervention, allowing a large number of retinal images to be used for population studies. A number of these measurements of vascular morphology have already been shown to be correlated with certain diseases, while others are under active study.

Diabetic retinopathy is a common complication that results in impaired visual function. Low-cost automated detection and assessment of diabetic retinopathy is an invaluable tool to encourage regular screenings. Chapter 9 discusses a methodology for assessing the severity of diabetic retinopathy using digital fundus images. The methodology uses the foveal region and exudates in order to quantify the severity of diabetic retinopathy. Results from sample digital fundus images were used to demonstrate the behavior of the methodology as well as its potential role as a complement to the standard ophthalmological assessment.

Glaucoma (repeated) is typically a silent but progressive illness that increases the intraocular pressure causing damage to the optic nerve. Chapter 10 reviews the use of mechanical and optical instruments for the diagnosis and health-care administration of glaucoma. The working principles of these instruments are furnished.

Glaucoma cannot be cured but when early detected and treated, blindness due to glaucoma can be prevented. Chapter 11 reviews state-of-the-art CDR calculation and its research application in detail. Finally, a discussion on the existing methods and databases that facilitate the research and comparison of results among researchers and future lines of research is presented.

Chapter 12 describes the stages involved in the computation of the AVR and explains how it can be implemented using image-processing techniques. The problems related to each stage are analyzed and the solutions proposed to overcome the limitations are discussed. Moreover, different approaches proposed in the literature with the aim of providing alternatives for developing an automatic methodology for the AVR computation are analyzed.

Chapter 13 discusses the research efforts and existing techniques on iris segmentation, normalization, and the corresponding phases of iris recognition and their limitations. It explains clearly the need to develop new algorithms in segmentation and matching phases of iris recognition.

Glaucoma is one of the most common causes of blindness. Robust mass screening may help to extend the symptom-free life of affected patients. In Chapter 14, a novel automated glaucoma diagnosis system based on texture features and data-mining techniques is proposed. Various texture features are extracted from the digital fundus images and fed to the SVM classifier. The SVM classifier with kernel functions of polynomial order 1 and radial basis function (RBF) correctly identified the glaucoma and normal images with an accuracy of 93.33%, and sensitivity and specificity of 86.7% and 100%, respectively.

Chapter 15 concentrates on the investigation of thermally induced threshold damage to the cornea and retina. It describes the fundaments of physics-based models intended for this specific laser–tissue interaction and for reproducing experimental threshold values. Also, it briefly reviews the optics of the eye and of layered tissues, and discusses setting up the bioheat equation and modeling the occurrence of macroscopic damage.

Dry eye is a symptomatic disease that affects activities of daily living, adversely affecting important tasks such as computer use and driving. In practice, there are several clinical tests to diagnose this syndrome by means of analyzing the tear film quality. Chapter 16 describes automatic image-processing methodologies to perform two clinical tests: the analysis of the interference lipid pattern and the tear film breakup time test.

Chapter 17 explains the calculation of numerical OST distributions for different age groups and conditions and compares them with measurements. It was shown that, in agreement with experimental results, computational eye models, which consider the physiological and anatomical changes with ageing and are constructed accordingly, could predict the decrease in the minimum temperature of the cornea with age, as well as the approach of its location to the geometric corneal center (GCC). Moreover, based on the numerical simulations, the authors have proposed that the changes in the aqueous humor (AH) flow that occur with age inside the anterior chamber, as a result of anatomical changes, could be another possible mechanism explaining the above effect, in addition to reduced blood flow and the blinking rate of the older eye.

Optical microscopy is a vital tool in life science investigations with the aim of imaging at subcellular resolution. Confocal microscopy is used for obtaining three-dimensional images of thick objects. Chapter 18 discusses how detailed imaging of the ocular surface structures and associated cell types can be performed using *in vivo* confocal microscopy. This technology will enable in-depth understanding of ocular surface physiology and pathology without the necessity of tissue excisions.

The efficiency of melanoma treatment by transpupillary thermotherapy (TTT) depends largely on the amount of energy absorbed by the tumor and surrounding tissues. The calculation of the amount of energy in heterogeneous tissues represents a very complex task due to a lack of accurate information on the coefficients of absorption, on scattering of the laser radiation, and on the tissues' thermophysical properties. In Chapter 19, a model is proposed for calculating the value of thermal damage at various depths within the melanoma. The methodology presented here can be improved by considering correlations that take into account the variation of the physical properties with the temperature, mainly in melanotic tissues.

Many authors have contributed immensely and made this book possible with their hard work and precious time. We thank them heartily for their valuable contributions. In no particular order, they are Maria Cecilia Aquino, Paul Chew, Muthu Rama Krishnan Mookiah, Chandan Chakraborty, Lim Choo Min, Muhammad Moazam Fraz, Sarah A. Barman, Ana Maria Mendonça, Behdad Dashtbozorg, Noelia Barreira, Manuel G. Penedo, Sonia González, Lucía Ramos, Brais Cancela, Ana González, Jiang Liu, Fengshou Yin, Damon Wing Kee Wong, Zhuo Zhang, Ngan Meng Tan, Carol Cheung, Mani Baskaran,

Tin Aung, Tien Yin Wong, Qiangfeng Peter Lau, Mong Li Lee, Wynne Hsu, Hasan Mir, Hasan Al-Nashash, Teik-Cheng Lim, Subhagata Chattopadhyay, Irene Fondón, Carmen Serrano, Begoña Acha, Soledad Jiménez, Marc Saez, Antonio Pose-Reino, María Rodríguez-Blanco, Nagarajan Malmurugan, Shanmugam Selvamuthukumaran, Sugadev Shanmugaprabha, Oliver Faust, Chan Wei Yan, Wenwei Yu, Mathieu Jean, Karl Schulmeister, Beatriz Remeseiro, Carlos García-Resúa, Eva Yebra-Pimentel, Antonio Mosquera, Anastasios Papaioannou, Theodoros Samaras, Sze-Yee Lee, Andrea Petznick, Shakil Rehman, Louis Tong, José Duarte da Silva, Alcides Fernandes, Paulo Roberto Maciel Lyra, and Rita de Cássia Fernandes de Lima.

**Eddie Y.K. Ng, U. Rajendra Acharya,
Aurélio Campilho, and Jasjit S. Suri**

MATLAB® is a registered trademark of The MathWorks, Inc. For product information, please contact:

The MathWorks, Inc.
3 Apple Hill Drive
Natick, MA 01760-2098 USA
Tel: 508 647 7000
Fax: 508-647-7001
E-mail: info@mathworks.com
Web: www.mathworks.com

Editors

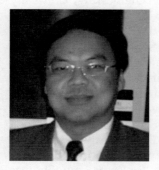

Eddie Y. K. Ng received a PhD from Cambridge University with a Cambridge Commonwealth Scholarship. His main areas of research are thermal imaging, biomedical engineering, and computational methods of fluid dynamics and heat transfer. He is a faculty member at the Nanyang Technological University in the School of Mechanical and Aerospace Engineering. He has published more than 320 papers in Science Citation Information journals (210) and Science Citation Information conference proceedings (25); textbook chapters (82); and others. Professor Ng is editor-in-chief for the *Journal of Mechanics in Medicine and Biology* and *Journal of Medical Imaging and Health Informatics*; associate editor for the *International Journal of Rotating Machinery, Computational Fluid Dynamics Journal, International Journal of Breast Cancer, Chinese Journal of Medicine, The Open Medical Informatics Journal, The Open Numerical Methods Journal*, and *Journal of Healthcare Engineering*; and strategy associate editor-in-chief for the *World Journal of Clinical Oncology*. Professor Ng has been an invited speaker at many international scientific conferences and workshops. Recently, he has coedited nine books; *Cardiac Perfusion and Pumping Engineering* published by World Scientific Press (2007); *Image Modelling of the Human Eye* published by Artech House (2008); *Distributed Diagnosis and Home Healthcare*, Volumes 1 and 3, published by American Scientific Publishers (2009 and 2011); *Performance Evaluation in Breast Cancer: Screening, Diagnosis and Treatment*, published by American Scientific Publishers (2010); *Computational Analysis of the Human Eye with Applications*, published by World Scientific Press (2011); *Human Eye Imaging and Modeling*, published by CRC Press (2011); *Multimodality Breast Cancer Imaging*, published by SPIE (2013); and *Ophthalmology Imaging and Applications*, published by CRC (in press). He also coauthored a textbook: *Compressor Instability with Integral Methods*, published by Springer (2007). More details are available upon request and at the URL http://www.researcherid.com/rid/A-1375-2011.

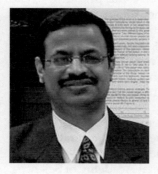

U. Rajendra Acharya is a visiting faculty member at Ngee Ann Polytechnic, Singapore. He is also adjunct professor at the University of Malaya, Malaysia; adjunct faculty member at the Singapore Institute of Technology–University of Glasgow, Singapore; associate faculty member at in SIM University, Singapore; and adjunct faculty member at the Manipal Institute of Technology, Manipal, India. He received his PhD from the National Institute of Technology Karnataka, Surathkal, India, and doctor of engineering from Chiba University, Japan. He has had more than 275 pieces published, including papers in refereed international Science Citation Information journals (176), papers in international conference proceedings (48), textbook chapters (62), and books (16 including in those in press), with an h-index of 25 without self-citations in SCOPUS. He has worked on various funded projects with grants worth more than 2 million SGD. He is on the editorial board of many journals and has served as guest editor for many journals. His major interests are in biomedical signal processing, bioimaging, data mining, visualization, and biophysics for better health-care design, delivery, and therapy. Please visit http://urajen-draacharya.webs.com/ for more details.

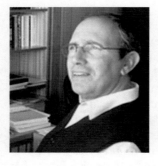

Aurélio Campilho is a full professor in the Department of Electrical and Computer Engineering, Faculty of Engineering, University of Porto, Porto, Portugal. From 1994 to 2000, he served as chair of the Institute for Biomedical Engineering. For several years, he also served as president of the Portuguese Association for Pattern Recognition, which is a member of the International Association of Pattern Recognition. He served as director of the doctoral program in electrical and computer engineering at the Faculty of Engineering, University of Porto and as a member of the scientific committee of the master's degree in bioengineering offered at the University of Porto. He is the coordinator of the Institute for Biomedical Engineering Bioimaging Group. His current research interests include the areas of medical image analysis, image processing, and computer vision. Professor Campilho has served as the organizer of several special issues and conferences. He served as associate editor of the journals *IEEE Transactions on Biomedical Engineering* and the *Machine Vision Applications Journal*. He is chair of the International Conference on Image Analysis and Recognition series of conferences. For more details and a publication list, please visit http://www.fe.up.pt/~campilho.

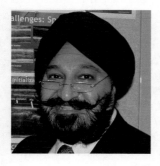

Jasjit S. Suri is an innovator, scientist, visionary, industrialist, and internationally known world leader in biomedical devices and biomedical imaging sciences—applied to diagnostics and therapeutics. He has worked as a scientist, manager, senior director, vice president, and chief technology officer and chief executive officer during his professional career in several million-dollar industries such as IBM, Siemens Medical, Philips Medical Systems, Fisher Imaging, Eigen, Global Biomedical Technologies, and AtheroPoint.

He has written over 400 publications, 70 innovations (patents and trademarks), 4 Food and Drug Administration clearances, and over 30 books in medical imaging and biotechnologies (diagnostic and therapeutic), and has had a leadership role in releasing products in the men's and women's markets applied to the fields of cardiology, neurology (image-guided brain surgery and spinal surgery), urology (image-guided prostate biopsy and high-intensity focused ultrasound for benign prostatic hyperplasia), vascular disease management (atherosclerosis: magnetic resonance and ultrasound), ophthalmology (thermal imaging), and breast cancer (magnetic resonance, x-ray–ultrasound fusion guidance).

He received his master of science in neurological magnetic resonance imaging from the University of Illinois, Chicago, his PhD in cardiac imaging from the University of Washington, Seattle, and his master of business administration from the Ivy League Weatherhead School of Management, Case Western Reserve University, Cleveland. He was awarded the Director General's Gold Model and became one of the youngest Fellows of the American Institute of Medical and Biological Engineering (National Academy of Sciences, Washington, DC). He has won over 50 awards during his career. Dr. Suri is also a strategic advisory board member for over half a dozen industries and international journals in biomedical imaging and technologies.

His main interests are commercialization of cancer imaging for diagnosis and therapeutic applications for men's and women's markets.

Contributors

Begoña Acha
Signal Theory and Communications
    Department
University of Seville
Seville, Spain

U. Rajendra Acharya
Department of Electronics and Computer
    Engineering
Ngee Ann Polytechnic
Singapore

Hasan Al-Nashash
Department of Electrical Engineering
American University of Sharjah
Sharjah, United Arab Emirates

Maria Cecilia Aquino
Department of Ophthalmology
National University Hospital
Singapore

Tin Aung
Singapore Eye Research Institute
Singapore

Sarah A. Barman
Faculty of Science, Engineering and
    Computing
Kingston University
London, United Kingdom

Noelia Barreira
Department of Computer Science
University of A Coruña
A Coruña, Spain

Mani Baskaran
Singapore Eye Research Institute
Singapore

Aurélio Campilho
Biomedical Engineering Institute and
    Faculty of Engineering
University of Porto
Porto, Portugal

Brais Cancela
Department of Computer Science
University of A Coruña
A Coruña, Spain

Chandan Chakraborty
School of Medical Science and
    Technology
Indian Institute of Technology
    Kharagpur
Kharagpur, India

Subhagata Chattopadhyay
National Institute of Science and
    Technology
Berhampur, India

Carol Cheung
Singapore Eye Research Institute
Singapore

Paul Chew
Department of Ophthalmology
National University Hospital
Singapore

Behdad Dashtbozorg
Biomedical Engineering Institute
and
Faculty of Engineering
University of Porto
Porto, Portugal

Oliver Faust
Department of Electrical and Computer
   Engineering
Ngee Ann Polytechnic
Singapore

Alcides Fernandes
Department of Ophthalmology
Emory University School of Medicine
Atlanta, Georgia

Irene Fondón
Signal Theory and Communications
   Department
University of Seville
Seville, Spain

Muhammad Moazam Fraz
Faculty of Science, Engineering and
   Computing
Kingston University
London, United Kingdom

Carlos García-Resúa
Faculty of Optics and Optometry
University of Santiago de Compostela
Santiago de Compostela, Spain

Ana González
Department of Computer Science
University of A Coruña
A Coruña, Spain

Sonia González
Department of Computer Science
University of A Coruña
A Coruña, Spain

Wynne Hsu
Department of Computer Science
National University of Singapore
Singapore

Mathieu Jean
Seibersdorf Labor GmbH
Seibersdorf, Austria

Soledad Jiménez
Puerta del Mar University Hospital
Hospital Universitario Puerta del Mar
Cádiz, Spain

Qiangfeng Peter Lau
Department of Computer Science
National University of Singapore
Singapore

Mong Li Lee
Department of Computer Science
National University of Singapore
Singapore

Sze-Yee Lee
Singapore Eye Research Institute
Singapore

Rita de Cássia Fernandes de Lima
Mechanical Engineering Department
Federal University of Pernambuco
Recife, Brazil

Teik-Cheng Lim
School of Science and Technology
SIM University
Singapore

Jiang Liu
Institute for Infocomm Research
Singapore

Paulo Roberto Maciel Lyra
Department of Mechanical Engineering
Federal University of Pernambuco
Recife, Brazil

Nagarajan Malmurugan
Satyam Computer Services Limited
Singapore

Ana Maria Mendonça
Biomedical Engineering Institute
and
Faculty of Engineering
University of Porto
Porto, Portugal

Lim Choo Min
School of Engineering
Ngee Ann Polytechnic
Singapore

Hasan Mir
Department of Electrical Engineering
American University of Sharjah
Sharjah, United Arab Emirates

Muthu Rama Krishnan Mookiah
Department of Electronics and Computer
    Engineering
Ngee Ann Polytechnic
Singapore

Antonio Mosquera
Computer Vision Group
University of Santiago de Compostela
Santiago de Compostela, Spain

Eddie Y. K. Ng
School of Mechanical and Aerospace
    Engineering
Nanyang Technological University
Nanyang, Singapore

Anastasios Papaioannou
Department of Physics
Aristotle University of Thessaloniki
Thessaloniki, Greece

Manuel G. Penedo
Department of Computer Science
University of A Coruña
A Coruña, Spain

Andrea Petznick
Singapore Eye Research Institute
Singapore

Antonio Pose-Reino
Internal Medicine
University Hospital Complex
Santiago de Compostela, Spain

Lucía Ramos
Department of Computer Science
University of A Coruña
A Coruña, Spain

Shakil Rehman
Singapore Eye Research Institute
and
Singapore-MIT Alliance for Research and
    Technology
Singapore

Beatriz Remeseiro
Department of Computer Science
University of A Coruña
A Coruña, Spain

María Rodríguez-Blanco
Ophthalmology Department
University Hospital Complex
Santiago de Compostela, Spain

Marc Saez
GRECS Group
University of Girona
Girona, Spain

Theodoros Samaras
Department of Physics
Aristotle University of Thessaloniki
Thessaloniki, Greece

Karl Schulmeister
Seibersdorf Labor GmbH
Seibersdorf, Austria

Shanmugam Selvamuthukumaran
A.V.C. College of Engineering
Mayiladuthurai, India

Carmen Serrano
Signal Theory and Communications
    Department
University of Seville
Seville, Spain

Sugadev Shanmugaprabha
Sri Ranganathar Institute of Engineering
    and Technology
Coimbatore, India

José Duarte da Silva
Department of Industrial Controls
Federal Institute of Education, Science and
    Technology of Pernambuco
Recife, Brazil

Jasjit S. Suri
Department of Biomedical Engineering
Idaho State University
Pocatello, Idaho

and

Global Biomedical Technologies, Inc.
and
Atheropoint, LLC
Roseville, California

Ngan Meng Tan
Institute for Infocomm Research
Singapore

Louis Tong
Singapore Eye Research Institute
and
Duke-NUS Graduate Medical School
Singapore

Damon Wing Kee Wong
Institute for Infocomm Research
Singapore

Tien Yin Wong
Singapore Eye Research Institute
Singapore

Chan Wei Yan
Department of Electronics and
    Communication
Ngee Ann Polytechnic
Singapore

Eva Yebra-Pimentel
Faculty of Optics and Optometry
University of Santiago de Compostela
Santiago de Compostela, Spain

Fengshou Yin
Institute for Infocomm Research
Singapore

Wenwei Yu
School of Engineering
Chiba University
Chiba, Japan

Zhuo Zhang
Institute for Infocomm Research
Singapore

1

Ultrasound Biomicroscopic Imaging of the Anterior Chamber Angle

Maria Cecilia Aquino and Paul Chew

CONTENTS

1.1 Introduction

A number of modalities are now available to assess not only the posterior, but also the anterior parts of the eye. Ultrasound biomicroscopy (UBM) is one of the imaging systems that allow visualization of the anatomy and pathology of the anterior segment. It is particularly beneficial in evaluating regions of the eye behind the iris such as the ciliary body, lens zonular attachment, and the lens periphery that are obscured in other anterior scanning systems. In glaucoma imaging, UBM plays a significant role in the objective assessment of peripheral anterior chamber (AC) angle morphology, which is useful in angle closure glaucoma diagnosis and management. This chapter presents an ultrasound biomicroscopy system for AC angle imaging.

1.2 Principles and Technology

Ultrasound biomicroscopy is an imaging technique that utilizes high-frequency acoustic pulses to create eye images of microscopic resolution. Stuart Foster and Charles Pavlin first developed this system in 1979 in research laboratories in Toronto, Canada. It started from the development of transducers for very-high-frequency ultrasound imaging based on the polymer polyvinylidene difluoride.[1] By 1984, 13 MHz polymer devices were being used to map the acoustical properties of human tissues.[2] The continued development of these probes culminated in a 1987 publication by Sherar et al. which showed the enormous potential of ultrasound imaging of tissue in the frequency range from 40 to 100 MHz.[3] A microscopic (15 μm) subsurface resolution in living tissue was demonstrated by this high-frequency system that was never achieved by any other noninvasive approach.[4] The success of the technique rapidly led to the development by Sherar et al. of the first real-time

B-scan imaging systems for microscopic imaging.[5] This system was further refined for ocular imaging by collaboration between Foster and Pavlin, and in 1990 they came up with the first practical UBM system for the eye.[6,7]

Knowledge of the background principles of ultrasound is key to understanding the clinical utility and limitations of this system. Ultrasound consists of waves of compression and rarefaction which propagate through a medium. Wavelength and frequency are defined by the relation $c = \upsilon\lambda$, where c is the speed of sound, λ is wavelength, and υ is frequency.[8]

The speed of sound is related to the medium's composition and temperature, but is largely independent of frequency. Wavelength is a crucial element in image resolution and is linearly proportional to both frequency and speed of sound.

The three basic tissue properties that are of significance in ultrasound imaging are attenuation, reflectivity, and speed of sound. Attenuation describes the loss of energy in the ultrasound beam resulting from absorption and reflectivity as it propagates through tissue.[4] As a result of absorption, acoustic energy is converted to heat. Acoustic reflection occurs at interfaces between regions of different acoustic impedance (density × speed of sound).[8] The absorbed ultrasound energy that has been converted to heat is lost, while the reflected component is either scattered or undergoes specular reflection or backscattering. Scattering occurs where these discontinuities are smaller than a wavelength.[8] Only backscatter and near-normal incidence specular reflection are eventually converted into image formation.[4]

Real-time image acquisition of the anterior and posterior chambers of the eye by UBM occurs as follows. Inside an ultrasound probe is a piezoelectric material called a transducer. The transducer is mounted on a vibration-free mechanism, the scanhead/probe, which allows precise placement over the cornea or sclera. This piezoelectric transducer, coupled to a microprocessor-controlled radio frequency signal generator, converts electrical signals into ultrasonic sound waves of specific high frequency. Higher frequency transducers provide finer resolution of more superficial structures, whereas lower frequency transducers provide greater depth of penetration with less resolution.[9] The commercially available units operate at 50 MHz and provide lateral and axial physical resolutions of approximately 50 and 25 μm, respectively, with approximately 4–5 mm tissue penetration.[9] The transducer delivers continuous ultrasonic waves to the eye through saline solution or methylcellulose, held in a reservoir within an eye cup or inside the probe itself placed on the cornea. These waves are propagated through the various ocular tissues at different speeds and reflected back at different intervals, depending on the acoustic impedance (density) of the tissues. The reflected signals are received back by the transducer and these reflected sound waves are collected and assembled by the computer. The scanner produces a 5 × 5 mm field with 256 vertical image lines (or A-scans) at a scan rate of 8 frames per second, whereby each A-scan is mapped onto oversampled 1024 points, with 256 grayscale levels representing the logged amplitude of reflection, and then the number of points is downsized to 432 pixels to fit on the UBM monitor.[9] The resulting image is a real-time, magnified, high-resolution sectional B-scan image displayed on a video monitor.

1.3 Clinical Application

AC angle imaging by ultrasound biomicroscopy gives a two-dimensional cross-section of the globe in a radial orientation at the region of the corneoscleral junction. This image is optimal for AC angle analysis. But the key to analysis and interpretation of an AC angle UBM scan is identification of the scleral spur, a constant landmark where trabecular meshwork meets the interface line between the sclera and the ciliary body. Using the said reference point, the relationship of different anterior segment structures, such as iris to trabecular meshwork to ciliary body to lens, provides significant clinical insight into the underlying pathophysiologic mechanisms useful in making accurate disease diagnosis. The scan in Figure 1.1 shows all of the anterior segment structures of a wide-open AC angle.

Pavlin et al. showed the utility of UBM in characterizing several forms of glaucoma, including plateau iris syndrome[10] and pupillary block,[11] which together constitute the most common forms of primary angle closure glaucoma.[12]

Pupil block mechanism of angle closure is illustrated in Figures 1.2 and 1.3. Pressure in the posterior chamber is elevated relative to that in the AC owing to impairment of the flow of aqueous through the pupil.[8] This results in forward bowing of the iris from the root to the pupil margin in the presence of a formed posterior chamber.[8]

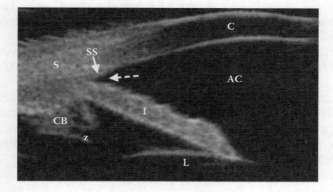

FIGURE 1.1
Radial image of an open peripheral AC angle showing all anterior segment structures. C, cornea; AC, anterior chamber; I, iris; S, sclera; SS, scleral spur; CB, ciliary body; L, lens; Z, zonule (*broken arrow* points to open angle).

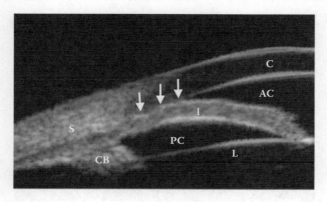

FIGURE 1.2
Radial image of a closed peripheral AC angle: iridotrabecular contact (*white arrows*); C, cornea; AC, anterior chamber; I, iris; PC, posterior chamber; L, lens; CB, ciliary body; S, sclera.

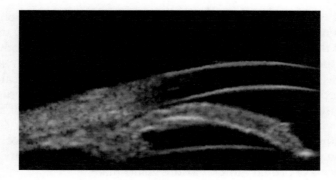

FIGURE 1.3
Pupil block mechanism of angle closure. Convex iris profile, shallow peripheral AC, and a very small zone of iris–lens contact.

Plateau iris (Figure 1.4) is a nonpupil block type of angle closure. The mechanism shows the peripheral iris rising from its root in apposition to or very near to the angle wall and then turning sharply away from the angle toward the visual axis. This configuration results from the anterior rotation or position of the ciliary body. The central AC depth is deep but the periphery is shallow.

Pseudoplateau iris (Figure 1.5) is a nonpupil block angle closure resulting from iris or iridociliary cysts underneath the peripheral iris, pushing the peripheral iris against the angle wall.

Malignant glaucoma (Figure 1.6), also known as aqueous misdirection, has a typical appearance on UBM. All anterior segment structures are pushed anteriorly.

Differentiating a cystic (Figure 1.5) from a solid *tumor* (Figure 1.7) involving the ciliary body is one of the indispensable clinical applications of UBM. Tumors involving the ciliary body may cause iris bulging similar to that caused by retroiridal cysts.[8]

Ocular trauma often presents a challenge due to poor visibility of the damaged ocular structure in the presence of hyphema. Accurate assessment of the structural damage and locating small foreign bodies can be a difficult task when clear direct visualization is not achieved.[9] UBM can be performed over a plano soft contact lens to minimize the risk of further injury with eyecups or with infection in a micro-open wound.[9] With the help of UBM, angle recession can be plainly differentiated from cyclodialysis.[13,14] In eyes with

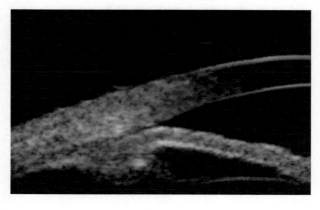

FIGURE 1.4
Plateau iris mechanism of angle closure.

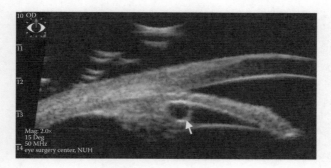

FIGURE 1.5
Pseudoplateau iris showing iridociliary cyst.

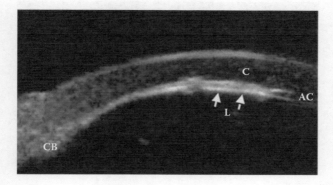

FIGURE 1.6
Malignant glaucoma.

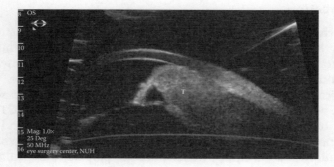

FIGURE 1.7
Metastatic solid tumor involving ciliary body (T-tumor).

angle recession (Figure 1.8) the ciliary body face is torn at the iris insertion, resulting in a wide-angle appearance with no disruption of the interface in-between the sclera and ciliary body.[9] In contrast, in *cyclodialysis* (Figure 1.9) the ciliary body is detached from its normal location at the scleral spur, creating a direct pathway from the AC to the supraciliary space.[9]

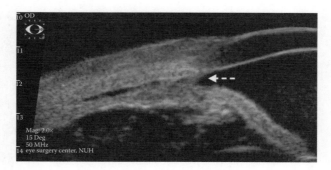

FIGURE 1.8
Angle recession (*broken arrow*).

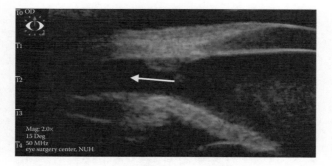

FIGURE 1.9
Cyclodialysis (*solid white arrow*).

1.4 Future Directions

New imaging technologies are continuously being developed and existing ones such as the UBM system are constantly being improved. High-frequency annular arrays have been developed for improved sensitivity and depth of field.[15] Linear arrays have also been developed, enabling scanning without mechanical motion of the probe.[16] Current single-element mechanically scanned UBM systems are being upgraded to increase their relative speed in order to be comparable to that of Fourier over time-domain OCT systems.[17]

We may see a merging of ultrasound with optics so that ultrasound can be used to increase OCT penetration via photon–phonon interaction.[8,18] It may also be possible to use the acoustic radiation force emitted by a transducer to "palpate" thin ocular tissues such as the retina or cornea to image their elastic properties. This technique, called *acoustic radiation force imaging*,[8,19] is now used in nonophthalmic clinical specialties.

References

1. Brown LF. Ferroelectric polymers: Current and future applications. In: *Proceedings of the IEEE Ultrasonics Symposium*, pp. 539–545. IEEE, New York, 1992.

2. Foster FS, Strban M, Austin G. The ultrasound macroscope. *Ultrasonic Imaging* 1984;6:243–261.
3. Sherar MD, Noss MB, Foster FS. Ultrasound backscatter microscopy images the internal structure of living tumour spheroids multicellular tumour spheroids. *Nature* 1987;330:493–495.
4. Pavlin CJ, Foster FS. *Ultrasound Biomicroscopy of the Eye*, 1st edn. Springer, New York, 1994.
5. Sherar MD, Starkoski BG, Taylor WB, Foster FS. A 100 MHz B-scan ultrasound backscatter microscope. *Ultrasonic Imaging* 1989;11:95–105.
6. Pavlin CJ, Sherar MD, Foster FS. Subsurface ultrasound microscopic imaging of the intact eye. *Ophthalmology* 1990;97:244–250.
7. Pavlin CJ, Harasiewicz K, Sherar MD, Foster FS. Clinical use of ultrasound biomicroscopy. *Ophthalmology* 1991;98:287–295.
8. Silverman RH. High-resolution ultrasound imaging of the eye: A review. *Clin Exp Ophthalmol* 2009;37(1):54–67.
9. Ishikawa H, Schuman JS. Anterior segment imaging: Ultrasound biomicroscopy. *Ophthalmol Clin North Am* 2004;17(1):7–20.
10. Pavlin CJ, Ritch R, Foster FS. Ultrasound biomicroscopy in plateau iris syndrome. *Am J Ophthalmol* 1992;113:390–395.
11. Aslanides IM, Libre PE, Silverman RH, et al. High frequency ultrasound imaging in papillary block glaucoma. *Br J Ophthalmol* 1995;79:972–976.
12. Mandell MA, Pavlin CJ, Weisbrod DJ, Simpson ER. Anterior chamber depth in plateau iris syndrome and papillary block as measured by ultrasound biomicroscopy. *Am J Ophthalmol* 2003;136:900–903.
13. Berinstein DM, Gentile RC, Sidoti PA, et al. Ultrasound biomicroscopy in anterior ocular trauma. *Ophthalmic Surg Las* 1997;28:201–207.
14. Park M, Kondo T. Ultrasound biomicroscopic findings in a case of cyclodialysis. *Ophthalmologica* 1998;212:194–197.
15. Silverman RH, Ketterling JA, Coleman DJ. High-frequency ultrasonic imaging of the anterior segment using an annular array transducer. *Ophthalmology* 2007;114:816–822.
16. Hu CH, Xu XC, Cannata JM, et al. Development of a real-time, high-frequency ultrasound digital beamformer for high-frequency linear array transducers. *IEEE Trans Ultrason Ferroelectr Freq Control* 2006;53:317–323.
17. Ursea R, Silverman RH. Anterior segment imaging for assessment of glaucoma. *Expert Rev Ophthalmol* 2010;5(1):59–74.
18. Huang C, Liu B, Brezinski ME. Ultrasound-enhanced optical coherence tomography: Improved penetration and resolution. *J Opt Soc Am A Opt Image Sci Vis* 2008;25:938–946.
19. Nightingale KR, Palmeri ML, Nightingale RW, Trahey GE. On the feasibility of remote palpation using acoustic radiation force. *J Acoust Soc Am* 2001;110:625–634.

2

Automated Glaucoma Identification Using Retinal Fundus Images: A Hybrid Texture Feature Extraction Paradigm

Muthu Rama Krishnan Mookiah, U. Rajendra Acharya, Chandan Chakraborty, Lim Choo Min, Eddie Y. K. Ng, and Jasjit S. Suri

CONTENTS

2.1 Introduction

An increase in the pressure inside the eye causes blockage of the aqueous humor flow and damage to the optic nerve, which carries information to the brain. This results in glaucoma, which, in many cases, can occur without any symptoms [1].

Glaucoma causes irreversible damage to the eye. Hence, its early diagnosis may prevent permanent damage to the vision. In Figure 2.1, the optic nerve head (ONH) clearly reflects the degeneration of the optic nerve fibers and the astrocytes. Additionally, there will be a steady decline in the retinal nerve fibers (RNF) [17].

Compared with other eye diseases, the mean occurrence of glaucoma is about 4.7% for individuals over 75 years of age and about 2.4% for all other age groups [2]. According to a recent glaucoma report, in the United States about 9%–12% of blindness is due to glaucoma. Within these percentages, about 2% are aged between 40 and 50 years and 8% are aged over 70 years [3]. An examination of the ONH and measurements of the visual field defects help to detect glaucoma [4–6]. Various parameters, such as area, diameter,

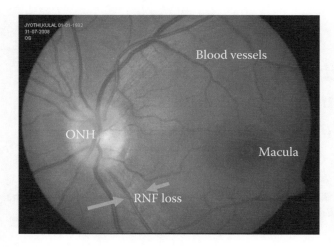

FIGURE 2.1
The main features of the glaucoma fundus image.

and volume, can be used to detect the deformation of the optic disc and hence evaluate glaucoma [7].

The performance of ONH stereophotographs (ONHPs), confocal scanning laser ophthalmoscopy (CSLO), scanning laser polarimetry (SLP), and optical coherence tomography (OCT) to distinguish normal and early to moderate glaucomatous visual field defects has been studied [8]. Greany et al. reported that a combination of these imaging methods significantly improved this distinguishing ability.

A combination of the optic disc parameters measured by Heidelberg retinal tomography (HRT) and the neural network performed better in classifying normal and glaucoma images [9]. The morphological changes in glaucoma were studied using HRT images [10,11].

Nowadays, textural features are increasingly used to detect subtle changes in medical images [5,6,12–14,23]. A texture-based method was used to automatically detect moderate and severe peripapillary chorioretinal atrophy (PPA) of glaucoma with a sensitivity and specificity of 73% and 95%, respectively [15]. PPA features, optic disc values, and support vector machines (SVMs) were used to automatically detect glaucoma [16]. Similarly, a combination of textural changes in the RNF, power spectral changes, and an SVM classifier was used to classify normal and glaucoma classes with an accuracy of 74% [17]. Texture features, fast Fourier transform (FFT) coefficients, and principle component analysis (PCA) coefficients coupled with an SVM classifier yielded an accuracy of 86% [18].

In this chapter, we propose a screening system that is fast and robust, and helps to detect glaucomatous changes in the fundus image. Such a system can help to diagnose suspected glaucomatous cases and to control the progression of the disease.

Figure 2.2 depicts a block diagram of the proposed automated system. Robust texture features, namely, a local binary pattern (LBP), Laws' texture energy (LTE), a trace transform (TT), a fuzzy gray-level co-occurrence matrix (FGLCM), and fuzzy run-length matrices (FRLMs) were extracted from the image. An independent sample "*t*" was used to select the clinically significant features. Finally, these features were fed to an SVM classifier for an automated diagnosis.

The outline of this chapter is as follows. Section 2.2 explains the image acquisition process. The preprocessing and the extraction of the features using the different texture

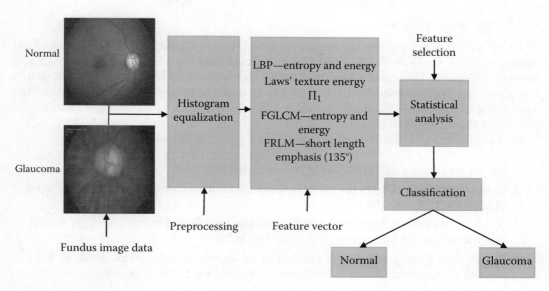

FIGURE 2.2
Block diagram of the proposed automated glaucoma detection system.

methods are discussed in Section 2.3. Section 2.3.6 discusses the feature selection using an independent sample *t*-test. A brief description of the SVM classifier is given in Section 2.3.7. Section 2.4 introduces a new integrated index called the glaucoma risk index (GRI). Sections 2.5 and 2.6 present and discuss the results of the proposed method, respectively. Section 2.7 concludes the chapter.

2.2 Image Acquisition

In this study, uncompressed bitmap format images of 560×720 resolution were obtained from the Kasturba Medical College, Manipal, India. We used 60 fundus images: 30 normal and 30 open-angle glaucoma images. Subjects aged 20–70 years were recruited for this study (both normal and glaucoma classes). The hospital ethics committee, composed of senior doctors, approved this study and certified the image classes.

2.3 Preprocessing and Feature Extraction

Feature extraction is an important step in the classification process. In this study, the features were extracted from the preprocessed images. A contrast enhancement of the retinal fundus image by histogram equalization was performed to improve the image quality. First, the color (red-green-blue [RGB]) fundus images were converted into grayscale images. This increased the dynamic range of the image histogram [19], resulting in a uniform distribution of the intensities in the output image. Then, five types of texture features were extracted: (1) LBP energy and entropy, (2) LTE, (3) TT, (4) FGLCM energy and entropy, and (5) fuzzy short run-length emphasis. A brief explanation of these features is given in the following sections.

2.3.1 Local Binary Pattern

The LBP is a powerful texture feature that is widely used for computer vision and medical imaging [27,28]. Ojala et al. [20] proposed and developed the LBP, which is rotation and contrast invariant. This method helps to detect subtle changes in an image and to define the edges and borders more accurately [21,22]. In order to understand the working of the LBP, we need to assume the mask of radius 1 (8 pixels), radius 2 (16 pixels), or radius 3 (24 pixels), as shown in Figure 2.3.

The steps of the LBP feature computation (see Figure 2.4) are as follows [20]:

1. Let us assume a mask of radius $(R) = 1$ and pixels $(P) = 8$.
2. In the mask, each pixel in the circle is compared with its center pixel in a clockwise or counterclockwise direction.
3. If the value of the neighboring pixel is greater than that of the center pixel, then it is recorded as "1." Otherwise, it is recorded as "0."
4. The 8-digit binary number is converted to grayscale value. The mask is then shifted by one column and the process is repeated for all rows and columns in the image.
5. This procedure is repeated for radii 2 and 3.
6. As a result, we get the LBP image of radii 1, 2, and 3.
7. The entropy and energy are evaluated on this LBP image. Thus, we have evaluated six LBP features from each LBP image.

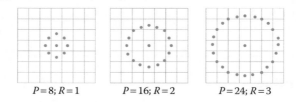

$$P = 8; R = 1 \qquad P = 16; R = 2 \qquad P = 24; R = 3$$

FIGURE 2.3
Circularly symmetric neighbor sets for different P and R. (From Ojala, T., Pietikäinen, M., and Maenpaa, T., *IEEE Transactions on Pattern Analysis and Machine Intelligence*, 24, 971–987, 2002.)

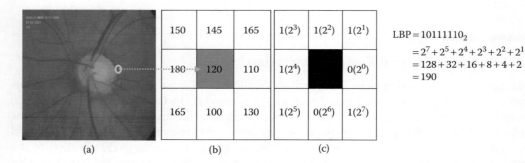

$$\begin{aligned}
LBP &= 10111110_2 \\
&= 2^7 + 2^5 + 2^4 + 2^3 + 2^2 + 2^1 \\
&= 128 + 32 + 16 + 8 + 4 + 2 \\
&= 190
\end{aligned}$$

(a)   (b)   (c)

FIGURE 2.4
Computation of the LBP code. (a) Glaucoma image; (b) image mask; and (c) weighted threshold values.

2.3.2 Laws' Mask Energy (LME)

LME is another texture feature that is able to capture the uniformity, density, coarseness, roughness, regularity, linearity, directionality, direction, frequency, and phase information in a grayscale image [23,24]. Various masks of appropriate sizes have been proposed to evaluate subtle variations in a grayscale image. The masks are applied to the images to estimate the amount of energy that passes within the region of filters.

One-dimensional (1D) vectors of three pixels describing the level, edge, and spot, respectively: *L3* [1 2 1], *E3* [–1 0 1], and *S3* [–1 2 –1], constitute the mask. Nine two-dimensional (2D) matrices (3 × 3) *L3L3*, *L3E3*, *L3S3*, *E3E3*, *E3L3*, *E3S3*, *S3S3*, *S3L3*, and *S3E3* were generated by convolving the 1D vectors with a horizontal vector.

$$\underbrace{\begin{pmatrix} 1 \\ 2 \\ 1 \end{pmatrix}}_{L3} \times \underbrace{\begin{pmatrix} -1 & 0 & 1 \end{pmatrix}}_{E3} = \underbrace{\begin{pmatrix} -1 & 0 & 1 \\ -2 & 0 & 2 \\ -1 & 0 & 1 \end{pmatrix}}_{L3E3}$$

In order to extract the texture information from an image $I(i, j)$, the image is first convolved with each 2D mask. For example, if we used *L3E3* to filter the image $I(i, j)$, the result would be a texture image, TI_{L3E3}, as shown in Equation 2.1.

$$TI_{L3E3} = I(i, j) \times L3E3 \tag{2.1}$$

In order to make the resultant images independent of contrast, the texture image TI_{L3L3} is used to normalize the contrast of all other texture images as given in Equation 2.2.

$$\text{Normalize}\left(TI_{\text{mask}}\right) = \frac{TI_{(i,j)^{\text{mask}}}}{TI_{(i,j)^{L3L3}}} \tag{2.2}$$

The resultant normalized *TI*s are passed to texture energy measurement (TEM) filters, which consist of a moving nonlinear window average of absolute values, as shown in the following equation:

$$\text{TEM}_{(i,j)} = \sum_{u=-3}^{3} \sum_{v=-3}^{3} \left| TI_{(i+u, j+v)} \right| \tag{2.3}$$

Therefore, by using this feature extraction method, images are filtered and their energies are used as feature descriptors.

2.3.3 Trace Transform

A TT is similar to a Radon transform, which calculates the functionals of an image along lines that crisscross its domain. The radon transform evaluates the integral of the function and hence it is a special case of a TT. The purpose of a functional is to characterize a function with a number. Various functionals are used for representing the rotation, translation, and scaling invariant features of an image [25–27].

With TT, a given image is transformed to another 2D function (image) depending on the parameters (ϕ, p), which characterize each line. In this work, we have used Π_1 and Π_2 TT features, which are rotation, scale, and translation invariant texture features.

2.3.4 Fuzzy Gray-Level Co-Occurrence Matrix

A gray-level co-occurrence matrix (GLCM) is a second-order texture moment, and it is constructed by the frequency variations of a gray-level image. The FGLCM [28] of an image I of size $L \times L$ is given by

$$F_d(m, n) = [F_{mn}]_{L \times L} \tag{2.4}$$

where F_{mn} corresponds to the occurrence of a gray value "around m" separated from another pixel with a gray value "around n," with a distance d in a definite direction θ. It is represented as $F = f(I, d, \theta)$.

In this work, the rotational invariant co-occurrence matrix F', obtained by averaging the four symmetrical fuzzy co-occurrence matrices computed with $\theta = 0°$, $45°$, $90°$, and $135°$, and $d = 20$, to find the texture feature value was used. The pyramidal membership function $\mu_{\tilde{m}l(x,y),\tilde{n}l(x,y\pm d)}$ that is used to build these matrices has a support of 11×11 pixels. Here, μ represents the fuzzy membership distribution of the gray values around m and n. Given F', it is normalized to obtain F'_{norm}, which gives the joint probability of the occurrence of one pixel having a gray value around m with another pixel separated by a defined spatial relationship and having a gray value around n. The FGLCM-based features used are

$$\text{Energy: } E_{\text{fuzzy}} = \sum_m \sum_n \left[F_d(m, n) \right]^2 \tag{2.5}$$

$$\text{Entropy: } H_{\text{fuzzy}} = -\sum_m \sum_n F_d(m, n) \cdot \ln F_d(m, n) \tag{2.6}$$

The homogeneity feature depicts the similarity between two pixels and the contrast feature indicates the local variation between those two pixels. The energy and entropy highlight the uniformity and the degree of randomness in the image.

2.3.5 Fuzzy Run-Length Matrices

The run-length matrix, $F_\theta(m, n)$, consists of a number of elements where the gray-level value i has the run length j continuous in the direction θ [29,30]. Often, the direction θ is set as $0°$, $45°$, $90°$, and $135°$ [29]. The feature listed in Equation 2.7 was computed for analysis and classification.

Short run emphasis (SRE):

$$\text{SRE}_{\text{fuzzy}} = \frac{\displaystyle\sum_m \sum_n \frac{F_\theta(m, n)}{n^2}}{\displaystyle\sum_m \sum_n F_\theta(m, n)} \tag{2.7}$$

2.3.6 Statistical Analysis Using Independent Sample *t*-Test

Before classification, we need to test whether the extracted features possess the ability to discriminate the two classes (normal and glaucoma). In this work, we have used the Student's *t*-test, which compares the *means* of two classes. It yields good results for large samples [31] and provides a high confidence interval for the two different *means*.

2.3.7 Support Vector Machine Classification

The SVM classifier is a supervised learning method that aims to determine a separating hyperplane that maximizes the margin between the input data classes in an *n*-dimensional space, where *n* stands for the number of features used as inputs. It calculates the margin by constructing two parallel hyperplanes on each side of the separating hyperplane. Using nonlinear kernel functions, the input data are often transformed to a high-dimensional space to make them more separable from the original input data [32–34]. The radial basis function (RBF), and linear, quadratic, and polynomial degree 1–3 kernel functions [38] are used in this work.

2.4 Glaucoma Risk Index

In this study, we have proposed a GRI using the significant texture features listed in Table 2.1. The novel approach [33] of the GRI using the extracted features was used to discriminate the two classes (normal and glaucoma) using one value. We propose Equation 2.8 to distinguish eye fundus images into two groups.

$$GRI = \frac{(\alpha \times \gamma)}{(\beta) \times 10^{-41}} \tag{2.8}$$

TABLE 2.1

Summary of Texture Features Used in This Study

Features	Normal	Glaucoma	*p*-Value
$LBP_{Energy\,(8,1)}$	0.15 ± 0.01	0.15 ± 0.01	.0054
$LBP_{Entropy\,(16,2)}$	2.76 ± 0.51	3.23 ± 0.30	<.0001
$LBP_{Energy\,(16,2)}$	0.29 ± 0.11	0.19 ± 0.07	<.0001
$LBP_{Entropy\,(24,3)}$	2.80 ± 0.59	3.28 ± 0.34	.0002
$LBP_{Energy\,(24,3)}$	0.33 ± 0.12	0.23 ± 0.07	<.0001
LTE4	$(1.04 \pm 1.16) \times 10^{07}$	$(6.11 \pm 2.48) \times 10^{07}$	<.0001
LTE5	$(1.69 \pm 2.64) \times 10^{07}$	$1.54 \times 10^{08} \pm 6.59 \times 10^{07}$	<.0001
LTE6	$(1.99 \pm 2.75) \times 10^{09}$	$(7.07 \pm 2.80) \times 10^{08}$	.0138
LTE7	$(1.65 \pm 1.80) \times 10^{07}$	$1.28 \times 10^{08} \pm 5.20 \times 10^{07}$	<.0001
LTE8	$(3.36 \pm 4.89) \times 10^{07}$	$(3.39 \pm 1.40) \times 10^{08}$	<.0001
TT1	2.67 ± 0.51	2.45 ± 0.21	.0319
$FGLCM_{Energy}$	$1.96 \times 10^{06} \pm 202768.2$	$2.15 \times 10^{06} \pm 154070.3$	<.0001
$FGLCM_{Entropy}$	1.12 ± 0.10	1.03 ± 0.07	<.0001
$SRE_{fuzzy}\,(135°)$	0.84 ± 0.04	0.86 ± 0.02	.0042

where:

$$\alpha = \text{LBP}_{\text{Energy (8,1)}} \times \text{LBP}_{\text{Energy (16,2)}} \times \text{LBP}_{\text{Energy (24,3)}} \times \text{LTE4} \times \text{LTE5} \times \text{LTE6} \times \text{LTE7} \times \text{LTE8} \times \text{FGLCM}_{\text{Energy}}$$

$$\beta = \text{LBP}_{\text{Entropy (16,2)}} \times \text{LBP}_{\text{Entropy (24,3)}} \times \text{FGLCM}_{\text{Entropy}}$$

$$\gamma = \text{fuzzy short length emphasis}$$

2.5 Results

In this study, we have extracted 15 clinically significant texture features from digital fundus images. Table 2.1 shows the texture features (mean ± standard deviation) and the corresponding *p*-values for the two classes (normal and glaucoma). The independent sample *t*-test was used to estimate whether the *mean* of each texture feature was significantly different for normal and glaucoma subjects. It can be observed from Table 2.1 that all the features show low *p*-values (<.05), indicating that the features are significant.

Except for LBP energies, FGLCM energy, and entropy, all the features show a higher value for glaucoma than the normal class. This is because there is a more subtle variation in the glaucoma images as compared with the normal class. These features contribute significantly to the automatic classification.

Figure 2.5a and d show a 3D scatterplot for the LBP and LTE energy features. Figure 2.5b shows a 2D scatterplot for the LBP entropy features, and Figure 2.5c shows a box plot for the LTE feature, which implies that the median of the features is noticeably different for the two groups. We can infer from these plots that these features are distinct and can be used to distinguish the normal and glaucoma subjects with a higher accuracy.

Table 2.2 shows the range of GRI values (mean and standard deviation) for the two groups. From Table 2.2 it can be inferred that the GRI can be efficiently employed to distinguish the normal and glaucoma subjects. Figure 2.6 shows the distribution plot of an integrated index for the normal and glaucoma classes. This plot graphically shows the spread of the integrated index values for the two classes (normal and glaucoma).

The GRI equation was computed using the LBP, LTE, TT, FGLCM, and FRLM features. For the energy values of Laws' mask, the FGLCM was high and the LBP energy was low (Table 2.1) especially for glaucoma, which gives α. The entropy values of the LBP and the FGLCM were low especially for glaucoma, which gives β, and γ was determined based on the FRLM feature, which was high particularly for glaucoma. The higher values of the LTE and the FGLCM energy features and the lower values of the LBP energy feature for glaucoma indicate that it has a coarser textural variation than that of the normal class. Physiologically, during an optic nerve hemorrhage, the blood typically collects along the individual nerve fibers that radiate outward from the nerve. Such physiological changes were manifested in the fundus images, and our experiments show that the texture features were able to capture and quantify such differences in the eye physiology [5].

In this work, we used a threefold stratified cross-validation method to evaluate the performance of the classifier. Forty images were used to train the classifier and 20 images were used to test the performance of the classifier. We repeated this procedure three times and took the average as the performance measure. The average of the accuracy (Acc), sensitivity (Sn), specificity (Sp), and positive predictive value (PPV) was used to report the overall performance of the proposed system. The results of the classification using the texture features reported in Table 2.2 were fed to the SVM classifier as shown in Table 2.3. It can

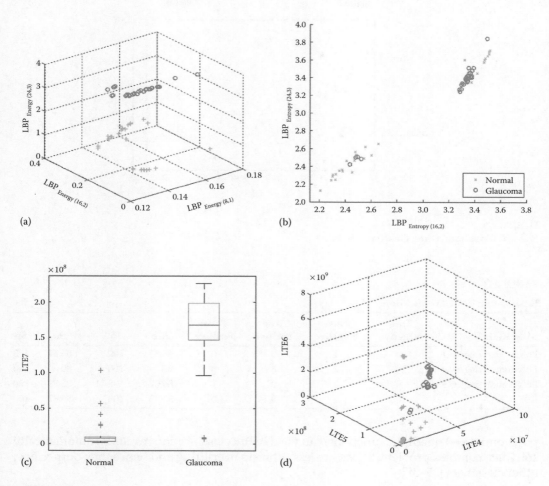

FIGURE 2.5
Plots showing how the features are distinctly different for the normal and glaucoma classes. (a) 3D plot for LBP energy features; (b) scatterplot for LBP entropy features; (c) box plot for feature LTE7; and (d) 3D plot for LTE features.

TABLE 2.2

Range of Glaucoma Risk Index for Normal and Glaucoma Data Set

Feature	Normal	Glaucoma	*p*-Value
GRI	33.16 ± 0.01	4.70 ± 0.01	$<.0001$

be seen from Table 2.3 that the polynomial kernel (degree 1) and the RBF kernel performed better than the other kernels with an accuracy of 93.33%, and a sensitivity and specificity of 86.67% and 100%, respectively.

The advantage of the SVM classifier is that it has a simple geometric interpretation and it yields a sparse solution. The solution to this classifier is global and unique, and it uses structural risk minimization. SVMs with various kernel functions, such as the RBF and the

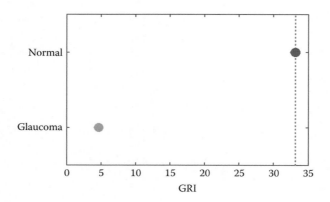

FIGURE 2.6
Plot of GRI for normal and glaucoma classes.

TABLE 2.3

Results of SVM Classification

SVM Kernels	True Negative	False Negative	True Positive	False Positive	Acc	PPV	Sn	Sp
Polynomial degree 1	10	1	9	0	93.33	100	86.67	100
Polynomial degree 2	10	2	8	0	90	100	80	100
Polynomial degree 3	9	2	8	1	86.67	92.31	83.33	90
RBF	10	1	9	0	93.33	100	86.67	100

polynomial and quadratic functions, can yield better classification results by automatically solving a complex problem. SVMs are less prone to overfitting and hence they outperform other classifiers [35–37].

2.6 Discussion

In this work, we have used textures from digital fundus images as features. These features can pick out the subtle changes (pixel intensities) in the images, which helps in the classification. Table 2.4 summarizes the classification accuracies of the automated detection of the normal and glaucoma classes. Retinal image variations, such as nonuniform illumination, image size differences, and blood vessels, were removed from the fundus images [7]. Then, a principal component analysis (PCA) was applied to the extracted features, such as the pixel intensities, FFT coefficients, and B-spline coefficients. These PCA coefficients combined with the classifier were able to achieve an accuracy of 80% for detecting glaucomatous retina fundus images.

An artificial neural network (ANN) model coupled with multifocal visual evoked potential (M-VEP) data was able to classify glaucoma with a high sensitivity of 95% [39].

An ANN was used to recognize glaucomatous visual field defects and its diagnostic accuracy was compared with other algorithms proposed for the detection of visual field loss [40].

TABLE 2.4

Summary of Automated Glaucoma Detection Techniques Used in This Study

Authors	Features	Classifier	Performance Measure
Classification Using Morphological Features of the Retinal Fundus Images			
Nagarajan et al. [39]	Multifocal visual evoked potential	ANN	Sensitivity 95%
Bizios et al. [40]	Optic nerve head parameters	ANN	Sensitivity 93% Specificity 94%
		Cluster algorithm	Sensitivity 95% Specificity 82%
Nayak et al. [41]	Optic disc parameters Blood vessel parameters	ANN	Sensitivity 100% Specificity 80%
Balasubramanian et al. [42]	Optic nerve head parameters	Proper orthogonal decomposition	AROC 0.94
Huang et al. [43]	Retinal nerve fiber thickness	LDA	AROC 0.95
		ANN	AROC 0.97
Chisako et al. [16]	GLCM features	LDA	Sensitivity 73% Specificity 95%
Kolar and Jan [17]	Fractal dimension of RNF	SVM	Accuracy 74%
Nyul [7]	Pixel intensities, FFT, and B-spline	SVM	Accuracy 80%
Acharya et al. [5]	Higher-order spectra and GLCM	Random forest	Accuracy 91%
Dua et al. [44]	Wavelet energy features	Sequential minimal optimization	Accuracy 93%
Mookiah et al. [45]	HOS and wavelet energy features	SVM	Accuracy 95%
Mookiah et al. [46]	HOS, trace transform, and discrete wavelet transform	SVM	Accuracy 91.67%
This study	LBP, LTE, TT, F GLCM, FRLM	SVM	Sensitivity 86.67% Specificity 100% Accuracy 93.33%

It yielded a sensitivity of 93%, a specificity of 94%, and an area under the receiver operating characteristic (AROC) curve of 0.984. The glaucoma hemifield test yielded a sensitivity of 92% and a specificity of 91%. The pattern standard deviation showed a sensitivity of 89% and a specificity of 93%. The cluster algorithm obtained a sensitivity of 95% and a specificity of 82%.

Various features, such as the cup-to-disc (c/d) ratio, the ratio of the distance between the optic disc center and the ONH to the diameter of the optic disc, and the ratio of the blood vessels area in the inferior–superior side to the blood vessels area in the nasal–temporal side were extracted from the fundus image using morphological techniques [41]. This system was able to classify glaucoma with a sensitivity and a specificity of 100% and 80%, respectively.

Changes in the ONH were quantified using a proper orthogonal decomposition, which was proposed by Balasubramanian et al. [42] to detect glaucoma. The changes in the ONH during a follow-up study were predicted by comparing the follow-up ONH topography with a sub-space representation of a topography that had been constructed earlier. ONH topography was quantified using the image correspondence measures L1-norm and L2-norm, correlation, and image Euclidean distance (IMED). Using the L2-norm and IMED in the new framework, good AROC curves of 0.94 at 10° field of imaging and 0.91 at 15° field of imaging were obtained.

A linear discriminant analysis (LDA) and an ANN were used to improve the classification of glaucomatous and normal eyes in a Taiwanese Chinese population based on the RNF layer thickness measurement data from an SLP variable corneal compensation [43].

The results showed that the nerve fiber thickness (NFT) produced the higher AROC of 0.932 in differentiating between a normal and a glaucomatous eye. The AROC curves for the LDA and ANN methods were 0.950 and 0.970, respectively. Hence, the NFT, ANN, and LDA methods demonstrated equal diagnostic power in glaucoma detection.

A combination of higher-order spectra (HOS) and GLCM features was extracted from fundus images and fed to the random forest classifier for automatic detection [5]. This system was able to classify the two classes with an accuracy of greater than 91%.

Wavelet energy features were extracted from the fundus images and fed to the sequential minimum optimization for classification [44]. This system was able to correctly classify the two classes with an accuracy of 93%.

HOS and wavelet energy features were extracted from normal and glaucoma fundus images and these features were subjected to classification using SVM with polynomial degree 2 kernel function to discriminate the two classes. This system was able to discriminate normal and glaucoma classes with an accuracy of 95% [45].

HOS, trace transform and discrete wavelet transform based features were extracted from fundus images of normal and glaucoma for automated classification using SVM with polynomial degree 2 kernel function. This system was able to identify normal and glaucoma classes with an accuracy of 91.67% [46].

In this study, we were able to classify the normal and the glaucoma classes correctly with an average accuracy of 93.3%, a sensitivity of 86.7%, and a specificity of 100% using the SVM classifier with polynomial degree 1 and the RBF kernel. The novelty of this work is the GRI, which can be used to discriminate the two classes by accurately using just one number, as shown in Figure 2.6.

2.7 Conclusion

Nowadays, the number of subjects suffering from glaucoma is steadily increasing. In this chapter, we developed a novel computer-aided diagnosis (CAD) system to diagnose glaucoma using texture features. We extracted LBP, LTE, TT, and GLCM texture features from digital fundus images. These features were fed to the SVM classifier with various kernel functions. We obtained a highest average accuracy of 93.33%, a sensitivity of 86.67%, and a specificity of 100%. Additionally, we also developed a novel integrated index (Equation 2.8) using the extracted features to classify the two classes using just one number. We feel that this will help ophthalmologists during the mass screening of the eye.

References

1. R.A. Abdel Ghafar, T. Morris, T. Ritchings, I. Wood, Detection and characterisation of the optic disk in glaucoma and diabetic retinopathy, in: *Proceedings MIUA*, pp. 2–5. London, University of Birmingham, 2004.
2. R. Bock, J. Meier, L.G. Nyúl, J. Hornegger, G. Michelson, Glaucoma risk index: Automated glaucoma detection from color fundus images, *Medical Image Analysis*, 14 (2010) 471–481.
3. Glaucoma Research Foundation, Glaucoma facts and stats (2011), http://www.glaucoma.org/glaucoma/glaucoma-facts-and-stats.php.

4. S.C. Lin, K. Singh, H.D. Jampel, E.A. Hodapp, S.D. Smith, B.A. Francis, D.K. Dueker, et al., Optic nerve head and retinal nerve fiber layer analysis: A report by the american academy of ophthalmology, *Ophthalmology*, 114 (2007) 1937–1949.

5. U.R. Acharya, S. Dua, D. Xian, S. Vinitha Sree, C. Chua Kuang, Automated diagnosis of glaucoma using texture and higher order spectra features, *IEEE Transactions on Information Technology in Biomedicine*, 15 (2011) 449–455.

6. U.R. Acharya, O. Faust, F. Molinari, L. Saba, A. Nicolaides, J.S. Suri, An accurate and generalized approach to plaque characterization in 346 carotid ultrasound scans, *IEEE Transactions on Instrumentation and Measurement*, 61 (2012) 1045–1053.

7. L.G. Nyúl, Retinal image analysis for automated glaucoma risk evaluation, in: *Proceedings of the SPIE*, vol. 7497, pp. 1–9. October 30, SPIEDL 2009.

8. M.J. Greany, D.C. Hoffman, D.F. Garway-Heath, M. Nakla, A.L. Coleman, J. Caprioli, Comparisons of optic nerve imaging methods to distinguish normal eyes from those with glaucoma, *Investigative Ophthalmology and Visual Science*, 43 (2002) 140–145.

9. C. Bowd, K. Chan, M. Zangwill, M.H. Goldbaum, T.W. Lee, T.J. Sejnowski, R.N. Weinreb, Comparing neural networks and linear discriminant functions for glaucoma detection using confocal scanning laser ophthalmoscopy of the optic disc, *Investigative Ophthalmology and Visual Science*, 43 (2002) 3444–3454.

10. H. Uchida, L. Brigatti, J. Caprioli, Detection of structural damage from glaucoma with confocal laser image analysis, *Investigative Ophthalmology and Visual Science*, 37 (1996) 2393–2401.

11. M. Iester, N.V. Swindale, F.S. Mikelberg, Sector-based analysis of optic nerve head shape parameters and visual field indices in healthy and glaucomatous eyes, *Journal of Glaucoma*, 6 (1997) 370–376.

12. T.M.A. Basile, L. Caponetti, G. Castellano, G. Sforza, A texture-based image processing approach for the description of human oocyte cytoplasm, *IEEE Transactions on Instrumentation and Measurement*, 59 (2010) 2591–2601.

13. N. Szekely, N. Toth, B. Pataki, A hybrid system for detecting masses in mammographic images, *IEEE Transactions on Instrumentation and Measurement*, 55 (2006) 944–952.

14. J. Stoitsis, S. Golemati, K.S. Nikita, A modular software system to assist interpretation of medical images—Application to vascular ultrasound images, *IEEE Transactions on Instrumentation and Measurement*, 55 (2006) 1944–1952.

15. M. Chisako, H. Yuji, S. Akira, Y. Tetsuya, F. Hiroshi, Computerized detection of peripapillary chorioretinal atrophy by texture analysis, in: *Proceedings of the 33rd Annual International Conference of the IEEE EMBS*, pp. 5947–5950. Boston, MA, IEEE 2011.

16. L.M. Zangwill, K. Chan, C. Bowd, J. Hao, T.W. Lee, R.N. Weinreb, T.J. Sejnowski, M.H. Goldbaum, Heidelberg retina tomograph measurements of the optic disc and parapapillary retina for detecting glaucoma analyzed by machine learning classifiers, *Investigative Ophthalmology and Visual Science*, 45 (2004) 3144–3151.

17. R. Kolar, J. Jan, Detection of glaucomatous eye via color fundus images using fractal dimensions, *Radio Engineering*, 17 (2008) 109–114.

18. R. Bock, J. Meier, G. Michelson, L.G. Nyul, J. Hornegger, Classifying glaucoma with image-based features from fundus photographs, in: *Proceedings of the 29th DAGM Conference on Pattern Recognition*, pp. 355–364. Heidelberg: Springer-Verlag, 2007.

19. R. Gonzalez, R.E. Woods, *Digital Image Processing*, 2nd edn., New York: Prentice Hall, 2002.

20. T. Ojala, M. Pietikäinen, T. Maenpaa, Multiresolution gray-scale and rotation invariant texture classification with local binary patterns, *IEEE Transactions on Pattern Analysis and Machine Intelligence*, 24 (2002) 971–987.

21. S. Liao, M.W.K. Law, A.C.S. Chung, Dominant local binary patterns for texture classification, *IEEE Transactions on Image Processing*, 18 (2009) 1107–1118.

22. Z. Baochang, G. Yongsheng, Z. Sanqiang, L. Jianzhuang, Local derivative pattern versus local binary pattern: Face recognition with high-order local pattern descriptor, *IEEE Transactions on Image Processing*, 19 (2010) 533–544.

23. R. Gupta, P.E. Undrill, The use of texture analysis to delineate suspicious masses in mammography, *Physics in Medicine and Biology*, 40 (1995) 835–855.

24. K.I. Laws, Rapid texture identification, in: *Proceedings of the SPIE Conference Series*, pp. 376–380, SPIEDL 1980.

25. M. Petrou, P.G. Sevilla, *Image Processing: Dealing with Texture*, Chichester: Wiley, 2006.

26. A. Kadyrov, M. Petrou, The trace transform and its applications, *IEEE Transactions on Pattern Analysis and Machine Intelligence*, 23 (2001) 811–828.

27. M. Petrou, R. Piroddi, A. Talebpour, Texture recognition from sparsely and irregularly sampled data, *Computer Vision and Image Understanding*, 102 (2006) 95–104.

28. C.V. Jawahar, A.K. Ray, Incorporation of gray-level imprecision in representation and processing of digital images, *Pattern Recognition Letters*, 17 (1996) 541–546.

29. M.M. Galloway, Texture analysis using gray level run lengths, *Computer Graphics and Image Processing*, 4 (1975) 172–179.

30. K.V. Ramana, B. Ramamoorthy, Statistical methods to compare the texture features of machined surfaces, *Pattern Recognition* 29 (1996) 1447–1459.

31. A.M. Gun, M.K. Gupta, B. Dasgupta, *An Outline of Statistical Theory*, 3rd edn., Kolkata: World Press, 2005.

32. V. Vapnik, *Statistical Learning Theory*, New York: Wiley, 1998.

33. U.R. Acharya, O. Faust, V.S. Sree, F. Molinari, R. Garberoglio, J.S. Suri, Cost-effective and non-invasive automated benign and malignant thyroid lesion classification in 3D contrast-enhanced ultrasound using combination of wavelets and textures: A class of ThyroScan™ algorithms, *Technology in Cancer Research and Treatment*, 10 (2011) 371–380.

34. W. Chmielnicki, I. Roterman-Konieczna, K. Stąpor, An improved protein fold recognition with support vector machines, *Expert Systems*, 29 (2012) 200–211.

35. E.K.P. Chong, S.H. Zak, *An Introduction to Optimization*, 2nd edn., New York: Wiley Interscience, 2001.

36. A. Ravindran, K.M. Ragsdell, G.V. Reklaitis, *Engineering Optimization Methods and Applications*, 2nd edn., Wiley Interscience, New York 2006.

37. R.J. Martis, C. Chakraborty, Arrhythmia disease diagnosis using neural network, SVM and genetic algorithm optimized k-means clustering, *Journal of Mechanics in Medicine and Biology*, 11 (2011) 897–915.

38. N. Christianini, J.S. Taylor, *An Introduction to Support Vector Machines and Other Kernel Based Learning Methods*, Cambridge University Press, Cambridge, UK 2000.

39. R. Nagarajan, C. Balachandran, D. Gunaratnam, A. Klistorner, S. Graham, Neural network model for early detection of glaucoma using multi-focal visual evoked potential (M-VEP), *Investigative Ophthalmology and Visual Science*, 43, 12 (2002) 3902.

40. D. Bizios, A. Heijl, B. Bengtsson, Trained artificial neural network for glaucoma diagnosis using visual field data: A comparison with conventional algorithms, *Journal of Glaucoma*, 16 (2007) 20–28.

41. J. Nayak, U.R. Acharya, P.S. Bhat, A. Shetty, T.C. Lim, Automated diagnosis of glaucoma using digital fundus images, *Journal of Medical System*, 33 (2009) 337–346.

42. M. Balasubramanian, S. Zabic, C. Bowd, H.W. Thompson, P. Wolenski, S.S. Iyengar, B.B. Karki, L.M. Zangwill, A framework for detecting glaucomatous progression in the optic nerve head of an eye using proper orthogonal decomposition, *IEEE Transactions on Information Technology in Biomedicine*, 13 (2009) 781–793.

43. M.L. Huang, H.Y. Chen, W.C. Huang, Y.Y. Tsai, Linear discriminant analysis and artificial neural network for glaucoma diagnosis using scanning laser polarimetry-variable cornea compensation measurements in Taiwan Chinese population, *Graefe's Archive for Clinical and Experimental Ophthalmology*, 248 (2010) 435–441.

44. S. Dua, U.R. Acharya, P. Chowriappa, S. Vinitha Sree, Wavelet-based energy features for glaucomatous image classification, *IEEE Transactions on Information Technology in BioMedicine*, 16, 1 (2012) 80–87.

45. M.R.K. Mookiah, M.U.R. Acharya, C.M. Lim, A. Petznick, J.S. Suri. Data mining technique for automated diagnosis of glaucoma using higher order spectra and wavelet energy features, *Knowledge-Based Systems*, 33 (2012) 73–82.

46. M.R.K. Mookiah, O. Faust, Automated glaucoma detection using hybrid feature extraction in retinal fundus images. *Journal of Mechanics in Medicine and Biology*, 13, 1 (2013).

3

Ensemble Classification Applied to Retinal Blood Vessel Segmentation: Theory and Implementation

Muhammad Moazam Fraz and Sarah A. Barman

CONTENTS

3.1 Introduction

Retinal vessel segmentation and the quantification of morphological attributes of retinal blood vessels, such as length, width, tortuosity and branching pattern, and angles are utilized for diagnosis, screening, treatment, and evaluation of various cardiovascular [1] and ophthalmologic diseases [2] such as hypertension, arteriosclerosis, chorodial neovascularization, and diabetes [3]. Automatic detection and analysis of the vasculature can assist in the implementation of screening programs for diabetic retinopathy [4], evaluation of retinopathy of prematurity [5], arteriolar narrowing [6], the relationship between vessel tortuosity and hypertensive retinopathy [7], vessel diameter measurement in relation to diagnosis of hypertension [8], and computer-assisted laser surgery [9,10]. Automatic generation of retinal maps and extraction of branch points have been used for temporal or multimodal image registration [10], retinal image mosaic synthesis [11], optic disc identification [12], and fovea localization [13]. Moreover, besides the other widely used biometric methods which include face, fingerprint, hand palm, ear, gait, signature, voice, and iris, the retinal vascular tree can also be used for biometric identification [14].

The retinal vasculature is composed of arteries and veins appearing as piecewise linear structures, with their tributaries visible within the retinal image. The wide range of vessel widths ranges from one pixel to twenty pixels, depending on both the width of the vessel and the image resolution. Other structures appearing in retinal images include the retina boundary, the optic disc, and pathologies in the form of microaneurysms, cotton wool spots, bright and dark lesions, and exudates. These types of pathologies are particularly challenging for automatic vessel extraction because they may appear as a series of bright spots, sometimes with narrow, darker gaps in between, and may have similar attributes to vessels. The vessel cross-sectional intensity profiles approximate a Gaussian shape or a mixture of Gaussians in the case where a central vessel reflex is present. The orientation and gray level of a vessel does not change abruptly; they are locally linear and gradually change in intensity along their lengths. The vessels can be expected to be connected and, in the retina, form a binary tree-like structure. However, the shape, size, and local gray level of blood vessels can vary hugely and the central intensity of some vessels varies very little in comparison with the background gray level. Narrow vessels often have the lowest contrast.

Vessel crossing and branching can further complicate the profile model. As with the processing of most medical images, signal noise, drift in image intensity, and lack of image contrast pose significant challenges to the extraction of blood vessels. Retinal vessels also show evidence of a strong reflection along their centerline known as a central vessel reflex, which is more apparent in arterioles than venules, is stronger in images taken at longer wavelengths, and is typically found in the retinal images of younger patients.

Images acquired in a controlled environment are high quality and hence facilitate retinal image processing. However, the quality of retinal images acquired during large population-based studies and screening programs is frequently reduced due to a number of factors. This includes the pressure of taking retinal scans of a large number of patients within a stipulated time, which in turn increases subjective errors in image acquisition by the human operator. Moreover, there are specular reflections from the cornea and lens and the light is scattered due to ocular media turbidity, which causes large regional variations in the image intensity. This results in very dark and very bright regions within the same image, with widely different contrast between the blood vessels and the background. This degradation of image quality may significantly encumber visual inspection as well as cause automated retinal image processing to become more difficult.

The morphological characteristics of retinal images of premature infants and children are very different than those of the adult retina. Choroidal vessels are more visible alongside the retinal vessels in retinal images taken from premature infants [15]. Bright central reflexes on the vessels and illumination artifacts contribute to challenges in image processing when retinal images from school children are considered [16].

Manual segmentation of retinal blood vessels is a long and tedious task which also requires training and skill. It is commonly accepted by the medical community that automatic quantification of retinal vessels is the first step in the development of a computer-assisted diagnostic system for ophthalmic disorders [17]. The quantification of the width and morphology of blood vessels in the retina has been a heavily researched area in recent years and a detailed review can be found in Fraz et al. [18]. The accurate extraction of the retinal vascular tree forms the backbone of many automated computer-aided systems for screening and diagnosis of cardiovascular and ophthalmic diseases. Therefore it is important to have fast and robust vessel segmentation algorithms which are not critically dependent on several parameter configurations, so that these techniques can be used by health professionals. This is the motivation for using a supervised classification framework which depends only on the manually segmented images for training. The nonvessel region in the retina is not smooth due to the presence of the bright and dark lesions which include hemorrhages, exudates, drusen, and the optic disc boundary. Most of the existing retinal segmentation methodologies are evaluated on healthy retinal images free from pathologies; therefore, their performance can be considerably degraded in the presence of lesions. Moreover, many methods are founded on sets of rules for dealing with specific cases, which leads to parameter-dependent complex algorithms [19–21] and even with a large number of rules, cases such as central vessel reflex and branching/crossing points usually fail to be dealt with satisfactorily. In turn, the supervised classification approach is conceptually simpler and allows the classifier to take care of more specific cases, thus avoiding rule formulation and parameter adjustment.

The process of consulting multiple experts or seeking multiple opinions before making a final decision is almost second nature to humans. The extensive benefits of such a process in automated decision-making applications have also been discovered by the computational intelligence community which gives rise to the ensemble classification framework. In this chapter, a new supervised method for segmentation of blood vessels by using an ensemble classifier of boosted and bagged decision trees is presented. The feature vector is based on gradient orientation analysis, morphological transformation, line strength measures, and the Gabor filter response which encodes information to successfully handle both normal and pathological retinas with bright and dark lesions simultaneously. The classifier based on the bootstrapped and boosted decision trees is a classic ensemble classifier which has been widely used in many application areas of image analysis, but has not been applied within the framework of retinal vessel segmentation for automated retinal image analysis. The method is training-set robust as it offers a better performance even when it is trained on the DRIVE [22] database and tested on the STARE [23] database, thus making it suitable for images taken in different conditions without retraining. This attribute is particularly useful when implementing screening programs over a large multiethnic population where there is a large variability in the background pigmentation level of the acquired retinal images. Moreover, the algorithm is computationally fast in training and classification and needs fewer samples for training. The classification accuracy of the ensemble can be estimated during the training phase without supplying the test data. A new public database CHASE_DB1 [24] is also introduced for evaluation of the algorithm. This image database includes retinal images of 9- and 10-year-old children of different ethnic origin, along with the ground truths for annotated blood vessels. The database includes images with stark differences in background levels of retinal pigmentation (being more pigmented in South Asian and Afro-Caribbean people compared with white Europeans). The method and some of the results presented in this chapter were previously published in a journal paper [25]. In this chapter, a more detailed theoretical background, experimental evaluation, and analysis of the results is presented.

3.1.1 Ensemble Classification

Ensemble classification [26] is the process by which multiple classifiers are strategically generated and combined to solve a particular machine learning problem. Ensemble learning is primarily used to improve the classification or prediction performance of a model, or to reduce the likelihood of a poor or unfortunate selection. This approach is intuitively used in our daily lives when we seek the guidance of multiple experts and weigh and combine their views in order to make a more informed and optimized decision. In the same way the ensemble methods use multiple models or classifiers to obtain better predictive performance by combining the results from many weak learners into one high-quality ensemble predictor.

The primary benefit of using ensemble systems is the reduction of variance and an increase in confidence of the decision. In this approach, we have used decision trees as the component classifier of the ensemble system, which is created by using bootstrap aggregation, also known as bagging [27] and boosting [28] algorithms.

3.1.1.1 Bagging

Breiman's bagging [27], short for bootstrap aggregating, is one of the earliest ensemble-based algorithms. It is also one of the most intuitive and simplest to implement, with a surprisingly good performance [26]. In bagging, the component classifiers (in this case the decision trees) are grown on the bootstrap replicas of the training data set, which are generated by randomly selecting M observations out of N with replacement, where N is the training set size. The predicted responses of the individual component classifiers are then combined by taking a majority vote of their decisions. For any given instance the class chosen by most of the component classifiers is the ensemble decision. Traditionally, the component classifiers are of the same general form; for example, all hidden Markov model, all neural networks, or all decision trees, which is the case in this work.

Given the original training set D, multiple sets of training data D_m are created, where m ϵ {1,2, ..., N} by randomly sampling D with replacement. M is the number of component classifiers used in the ensemble system. On average, each training set D_m only contains two-thirds of the original samples. The bagging algorithm as explained in Polikar [29] is illustrated below:

Inputs for algorithm bagging

- Training data $D = \{x_1, x_2, ..., x_n\}$, $x_i \epsilon N$, with correct labels $w_i \in \Omega = \{w_1, ..., w_C\}$
- Weak learning algorithm WeakLearn
- Integer B, specifying number of iterations

Do $b = 1, ..., B$

1. Obtain bootstrap sample D_m by randomly drawing m instances, with replacement, from D.
2. Call WeakLearn with D_m and receive the hypothesis (classifier) $h_B: X \to \Omega$.
3. Add h_B to the ensemble, E.

End Do Loop

Test: Simple Majority Voting—given the unlabeled instance z

1. Evaluate the ensemble $E = \{h_1, ..., h_B\}$ on z
2. Let the vote given to class w_j by classifier h_B be

3. $v_{b,j} = \begin{cases} 1, & \text{if } h_b \text{ picks class } w_j \\ 0, & \text{otherwise} \end{cases}$

4. Obtain total vote received by each class

5. $V_j = \sum_{b=1}^{B} v_{b,j}, \quad j = 1, \ldots, C$

6. Choose the class that receives the highest total vote as the final classification

Therefore picking up the M out of N observations with replacement omits on average 37% of observations for each component classifier. These are "out-of-bag" observations and can be used to estimate the predictive power of the classifier as well as the importance of each individual feature from the feature vector in the decision-making process. The average out-of-bag error is estimated by comparing the out-of-bag predicted responses against the observed responses for all observations used for training, which is an unbiased estimator of the true ensemble error. The out-of-bag estimated feature of importance can be obtained by randomly permuting out-of-bag data across one variable or column at a time and estimating the increase in the out-of-bag error due to this permutation. The larger the increase, the more important is the feature in classification. Thus, an attractive feature of bagging is that the reliable estimates of predictive power and feature importance can be obtained during the training process without supplying the test data.

3.1.1.2 Boosting

Boosting also creates an ensemble of classifiers by resampling the data, which is then combined by majority voting, but it takes a different resampling approach than bagging, which maintains a constant probability of 1/N for selecting each individual example. For definiteness, consider creating a three-component classifier for a binary classification problem through boosting. Given training data set D of N instances, the first classifier C1 is trained on a training subset D1 obtained using a bootstrap sample of m < N instances. The training data subset D2 for the second classifier C2 is chosen such that exactly half of D2 is correctly classified by C1 and the other half is misclassified. The third classifier C3 is then trained with instances on which C1 and C2 disagree. The three classifiers are combined through a three-way majority vote. The altered distribution ensures that more informative instances are drawn into the next data set. This iterative distribution update makes the boosting algorithm a strong learner with an arbitrarily high accuracy that is obtained by combining weak learners.

The upper bound for the error of the boosting algorithm is shown by Schapire [30]. If the largest individual error of all three classifiers (as computed on D) is ε, then the error of the ensemble is bounded above by $f(\varepsilon) = 3\varepsilon^2 - 2\varepsilon^3$. Note that $f(\varepsilon) \leq \varepsilon$ for $\varepsilon < 1/2$. That is, as long as all classifiers can do at least better than random guessing, then the boosting ensemble will always outperform the best classifier in the ensemble. The performance can be further improved by repeated application of the boosting process [29].

A number of variants of boosting are available in the literature. We have used AdaBoostM1 and its variation LogitBoost [31] which are popular algorithms for binary classification. AdaboostM1 trains the learners in a sequential manner such that for every learner k, the weighted classification error is computed as,

$$\varepsilon_k = \sum_{n=1}^{N} d_n^k I\left(y_n = h_k(x_n)\right) \tag{3.1}$$

where:

x_n is the predictor values vector for n observations

y_n is the class label

h_k is the hypothesis

I is the indicator function

d_n^k is the weight of observation at step k

The algorithm then increases weights for observations misclassified by learner k and reduces weights for observations correctly classified by learner k. The next learner $k + 1$ is then trained on the data with updated weights d_n^{k+1}.

The trained classifier then computes the prediction for new data using

$$f(x) = \sum_{k=1}^{K} \alpha_k h_k(x) \tag{3.2}$$

such that $\alpha_k = 0.5 \log((1 - \varepsilon_k)/\varepsilon_k)$ are the weights for weak hypotheses in the ensemble.

LogitBoost works similarly to AdaBoostM1, except that AdaboostM1 iteratively minimizes the exponential loss as

$$\sum_{n=1}^{N} w_n \exp(-y_n f(x_n)) \tag{3.3}$$

whereas LogitBoost minimizes the binomial deviance, which can be expressed as

$$\sum_{n=1}^{N} w_n \log(1 + \exp(-2y_n f(x_n))) \tag{3.4}$$

where:

$y_n \in \{-1, +1\}$ is the true class label

w_n are observation weights normalized to add up to 1

$f(x_n) \in (-\infty, +\infty)$ is the predicted classification score

Binomial deviance assigns less weight to badly misclassified observations that have large negative values of $y_n f(x_n)$.

3.2 Feature Vector and Pixel Classification

The feature vector contains the quantifiable measurement for each pixel in such a way that the classifier successfully differentiates the blood vessels and the bright and dark lesions. We have used a 9-D feature vector which includes the orientation analysis of gradient vector field (one feature) for removal of bright and dark lesions with vessel enhancement, morphological transformation (one feature) for eradicating bright lesions, line strength measures (two features), and a Gabor filter response at multiple scales (four features) for eliminating the dark lesions. The intensity of each pixel in the inverted green channel is taken as one of the features. All of the features are extracted from the green plane of the RGB colored image without any preprocessing.

3.2.1 Orientation Analysis of Gradient Vector Field

The blood vessels are localized by analyzing the orientation of the gradient vector field. The unit gradient vectors of the image are highly discontinuous along the bilaterally symmetrical regions, that is, the linear structures which represent the blood vessels. Therefore the blood vessels are localized by finding the discontinuities in the gradient orientation. The feature extraction depends on the orientation of the gradient vector field not its magnitude; therefore it is robust against low contrast and nonuniform illumination [32].

The gradient vectors for the image $I(x, y)$ are approximated by the first order derivative operators in the horizontal (k_x) and vertical (k_y) directions.

$$
\begin{aligned}
g_x(x,y) &= I(x,y) \times k_x \\
g_y(x,y) &= I(x,y) \times k_y
\end{aligned}
\tag{3.5}
$$

The gradient vectors $g_x(x, y)$ and $g_y(x, y)$ are normalized by dividing with their magnitude to compute the unit gradient vectors $u_x(x, y)$ and $u_y(x, y)$.

$$
\begin{aligned}
u_x(x,y) &= \frac{g_x(x,y)}{\sqrt{g_x^2(x,y) + g_y^2(x,y)}} \\
u_y(x,y) &= \frac{g_y(x,y)}{\sqrt{g_x^2(x,y) + g_y^2(x,y)}}
\end{aligned}
\tag{3.6}
$$

The unit vectors are assigned to zero if the gradient magnitude is too small (<3 out of 255). The first derivatives of unit vectors are computed to find the discontinuities in gradient orientation, as:

$$
\begin{aligned}
d_{xx}(x,y) &= u_x(x,y) \times k_x \\
d_{xy}(x,y) &= u_x(x,y) \times k_y \\
d_{yx}(x,y) &= u_y(x,y) \times k_x \\
d_{yy}(x,y) &= u_y(x,y) \times k_y
\end{aligned}
\tag{3.7}
$$

The discontinuity magnitude in the gradient orientation $D(x, y)$ is expressed in terms of the first derivatives of unit vectors as

$$
D(x,y) = d_{xx}^2(x,y) + d_{xy}^2(x,y) + d_{yx}^2(x,y) + d_{yy}^2(x,y)
\tag{3.8}
$$

The $D(x, y)$ contains the gradient orientation analysis (GOA) map of enhanced blood vessels. There is a variance in vessel width as it travels radially from the optic disc. Therefore the first order derivative operator is employed at multiple scales $(\sigma = \{\sqrt{2}, 2\sqrt{2}, 4\})$ to generate the multiple GOA maps of blood vessels of different widths. The final GOA map, which also serves as one of the chosen feature vectors, is obtained by summing up the individual maps produced at multiple scales. The GOA maps containing the enhanced blood vessels are shown in Figure 3.1. It is observed that only the curvilinear-shaped blood vessels are enhanced despite the presence of irregular-shaped bright lesions in the first two images and dark lesions in the third image.

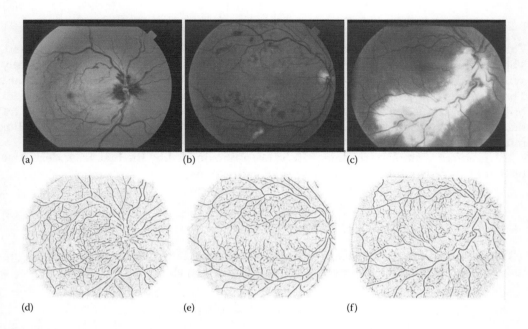

FIGURE 3.1

The inverted GOA map of blood vessels. (a,b) Retinal images with *dark* lesions; (c) retina with *bright* lesions; (d–f) GOA map of retinal images in a, b, and c respectively.

3.2.2 Multiscale Gabor Filter

A Gabor filter is a linear filter and has been broadly used for multiscale and multidirectional edge detection. The Gabor filter can be fine-tuned to particular frequencies, scales, and directions and therefore acts as a low-level feature extractor and background noise suppressor. The impulse response of a Gabor filter kernel is defined by the product of a Gaussian kernel and a complex sinusoid. It can be expressed as

$$g(x,y) = \exp\left\{-0.5\left(\frac{x'^2 + \gamma y'^2}{2\sigma^2}\right)\right\} \exp\left\{i\left(2\pi\frac{x'}{\lambda} + \psi\right)\right\} \tag{3.9}$$

where:
   λ is the wavelength of the sinusoidal factor
   θ is the orientation
   ψ is the phase offset
   σ is the scale of the Gaussian envelope
   γ is the spatial aspect ratio

$x' = x\cos\theta + y\sin\theta$

$y' = -x\sin\theta + y\cos\theta$

The Gabor filter response to the inverted green channel of the colored retinal image is obtained by a 2-D convolution operator and is computed in the frequency domain. The detailed procedure can be seen in Movellan [33] and Soares et al. [34]. The maximum filter response over the angle θ, spanning [0, π] in steps of π/18 is computed for each pixel in the image at different scales (σ = {2, 3, 4, 5}). The maximum response across the orientation at a scale is taken as the pixel feature vector. The feature space is normalized to zero mean and unit standard deviation by applying the normal transformation. The filter response of the image containing dark lesions is shown in Figure 3.2(a), illustrating the removal of dark lesions while enhancing the blood vessels.

3.2.3 Line Strength Features

The retinal vasculature appears as piecewise linear features, with variation in width and their tributaries visible within the retinal image. The concept of employing line operators for detection of linear structures in medical images is introduced in Zwiggelaar et al. [35], which is modified and extended in Ricci and Perfetti [36] to incorporate the morphological attributes of retinal blood vessels. The average gray level is measured along lines of a particular length passing through the pixel under consideration at 12 different orientations spaced by 15° each. The line with the highest average gray value is marked. The line strength of a pixel is calculated by computing the difference in the average gray values of a square sub-window centered at the target pixel with the average gray value of the marked line. The calculated line strength for each pixel is taken as the pixel feature vector. The line strength image can be observed in Figure 3.2(b), where the elimination of dark lesions can be observed with the enhanced blood vessel map.

3.2.4 Morphological Transformation

The morphological opening using a linear structuring element oriented at a particular angle will eradicate a vessel or part of it when the structuring element cannot be contained within the vessel. This happens when the vessel and the structuring element have orthogonal directions and the structuring element is longer than the vessel width.

$$I_{th}^\theta = I - (I \; o \; S_e^\theta) \tag{3.10a}$$

$$Is_{th} = \sum_{\theta \in A} I_{th}^\theta \tag{3.10b}$$

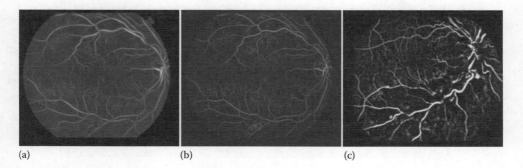

(a)   (b)   (c)

FIGURE 3.2
(a) The Gabor filter response (scale σ = 3) on image with *dark* lesions shown in Figure 3.1b. (b) The line strength image on image with *dark* lesions shown in Figure 3.1b. (c) Morphological transformation on retinal image with *bright* lesions shown in Figure 3.1c.

The morphological top-hat transformation is shown in (3.10a) where I_{th}^{θ} is the top-hat transformed image, I is the image to be processed, S_e are structuring elements for morphological opening o, and θ is the angular rotation of the structuring element. If the opening along a class of linear structuring elements is considered, a sum of top-hat along each direction will brighten the vessels regardless of their direction, provided that the length of the structuring element is large enough to extract the vessel with the largest diameter. Therefore, the chosen structuring element is 21 pixels long, 1 pixel wide, and is rotated at an angle spanning $[0, \pi]$ in steps of $\pi/8$. Its size is approximately in the range of the diameter of the largest vessels in the retinal image. The sum of top-hat Is_{th} is depicted in (3.10b), which is the summation of the top-hat transformation described in (3.10a). The set A consists of the angular orientations of structuring element and can be defined as $\{x \,|\, 0 \leq x \leq \pi \,\&\, x mod(\pi/8) = 0\}$. The sum of the top-hat on the retinal image will enhance all vessels whatever their direction, including small or tortuous vessels eliminating the bright zones as depicted in Figure 3.2(c).

3.2.5 Classification

Each pixel in the retinal image is characterized by a vector in 9-D feature space.

$$Fv(x, y) = \left[f_1(x, y), f_2(x, y), \ldots, f_9(x, y) \right] \tag{3.11}$$

A classification procedure assigns one of the classes Cv(vessel) or Cnv(nonvessels) to each candidate pixel when its representation in feature space $Fv(x,y)$ is known. One of the key advantages of ensemble-based bootstrap aggregation is that the predictive power can be evaluated by using out-of-bag observations and without employing the test data. More than one ensemble of 300 bagged trees are created and trained with the samples in the range of 1×10^4 and 3×10^4, in order to find the optimal number of training samples and the number of decision trees. The out-of-bag classification error is then computed for each of the ensemble classifiers. The relationship among the number of decision trees used to construct the ensemble, the number of training samples, and the respective out-of-bag classification error for the DRIVE database is illustrated in Figure 3.3.

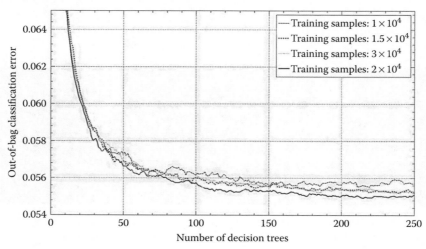

FIGURE 3.3
Out-of-bag classification error as a function of number of training samples and the weak learners.

There is a negligible difference in the out-of-bag classification error of ensembles trained with a range of samples between 1×10^4 and 3×10^4 but the predictive power of the ensemble trained with 2×10^4 samples is best. The almost straight line in the graph for the out-of-bag classification error after 150 weak learners suggests that there is a negligible increase in ensemble performance if the number of trees used to construct the ensemble is greater than 150, but at the cost of processing time. Therefore, we chose 200 decision trees for creating the ensemble classifiers.

3.3 Experimental Evaluation

3.3.1 Materials

The methodology has been evaluated using two established publicly available databases (DRIVE and STARE) and a new public database (CHASE_DB1).

The DRIVE [22] database contains 40 color images of the retina. The image set is divided into a test set and a training set and each one contains 20 images. The performance of the vessel segmentation algorithms is measured on the test set. The training of the classifier is performed on 20 training images using 2×10^4 samples such that 10000 pixels are chosen at random from each image.

The STARE [23] database contains 20 colored retinal images, out of which 10 images contain pathologies. The STARE database does not have separate test and training sets available. The classifier training for STARE is performed using 75000 manually segmented pixels randomly extracted from the 20 images (3750 pixels per image). Due to the small size of the training set (0.8% of the entire database), the performance is evaluated on the whole set of 20 images.

The CHASE_DB1 [24] is a new retinal vessel reference data set acquired from multiethnic school children. This database is a part of the Child Heart and Health Study in England (CHASE), a cardiovascular health survey in 200 primary schools in London, Birmingham, and Leicester [37]. The ocular imaging was carried out in 46 schools and demonstrated associations between retinal vessel tortuosity and early risk factors for cardiovascular disease in over 1000 British primary school children of different ethnic origin [38]. The images were captured at 30° FOV with a resolution of 1280×960 pixels. The data set of images are characterized by having nonuniform background illumination, poor contrast of blood vessels as compared with the background, and wider arteriolars that have a bright strip running down the center known as the central vessel reflex. This work is based on 14 children recruited from one of the 46 primary schools. The 28 images are divided such that 20 images are included in the test set and 8 images comprise the training set. The training of the classifier is performed on 8 training images using 2×10^5 samples such that 25000 pixels are randomly selected from each of the images. For CHASE_DB1, the Gabor features are calculated at scales ($\sigma = \{3,4,5,6\}$), the structuring element for morphological transformation is 25 pixels in length.

For each of the three databases, there are two manual segmentations available made by two independent human observers for each of the images. The manually segmented images in set A by the first human observer are used as a ground truth. The human observer performance is measured using the manual segmentations by the second human observer. The binary mask for the FOV for each of the DRIVE database images is available with the database. We have created the FOV binary mask for each of the images in the STARE and CHASE_DB1 databases as explained in Soares et al. [34].

3.3.2 Performance Measures

In the retinal vessel segmentation process any pixel is classified as either vessel or surrounding tissue. Consequently, there are four events: two classifications and two misclassifications, which are defined in Table 3.1.

The accuracy (Acc) is measured by the ratio of the total number of correctly classified pixels to the number of pixels in the image FOV. Sensitivity (SN) reflects the ability of an algorithm to detect the vessel pixels. Specificity (SP) is the ability to detect nonvessel pixels. The positive predictive value (PPV) or precision rate is the probability that an identified vessel pixel is a true positive. These metrics are defined in Table 3.2 based on the terms in Table 3.1. In our experiments, these metrics are calculated over all test images, considering only pixels inside the FOV.

In addition, the performance of the algorithm is also measured with the area under receiver operating characteristic (ROC) curve (AUC). An ROC curve is a plot of true-positive fractions (SN) versus false-positive fractions (1-SP) by varying the threshold on the probability map image.

3.3.3 Method Evaluation

The outcome the ensemble classifier is a vessel probability map, where each value corresponds to the confidence measure of each pixel to be a part of a vessel or not. The probability map is often considered as a grayscale image such that the bright pixels in this image indicate a higher probability of being a vessel pixel. The probability maps of image from each of the image databases are shown in Figure 3.4.

In order to evaluate the ensemble algorithms, we have created three ensemble classifiers: one using the bootstrap aggregation (bagging) and the other two by using two boosting algorithms, the AdaBoostM1 and its variation LogitBoost. These classifiers are then employed for vessel segmentation on DRIVE, STARE, and CHASE_DB1. A vector of

TABLE 3.1

Vessel Classification

	Vessel Present	Vessel Absent
Vessel detected	True positive (TP)	False positive (FP)
Vessel not detected	False negative (FN)	True negative (TN)

TABLE 3.2

Performance Measures for Retinal Vessel Segmentation

Measure	Description
SN	TP/(TP + FN)
SP	TN/(TN + FP)
Acc	(TP + TN)/(TP + FP + TN + FN)
PPV	TP/(TP + FP)
FDR	FP/(FP + TP)

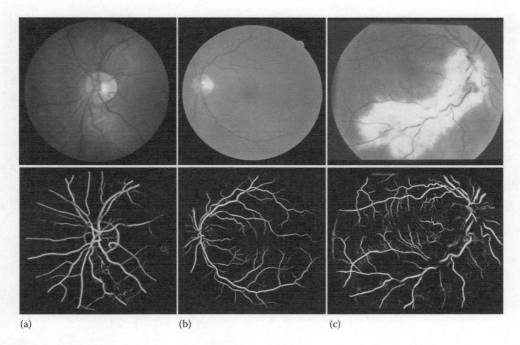

FIGURE 3.4
Probability map images (a) CHASE_DB1; (b) DRIVE; (c) STARE.

true-positive fractions (SN) and false-positive fractions (1-SP) is obtained for each of the images in the respective image databases by varying the threshold on the probability map image. The ROC is plotted (Figure 3.5) for each of the image databases and the aggregated area under the curve (AUC) is computed using these vectors, as summarized in Table 3.3.

There is a fractional difference in the values but results of the LogitBoost algorithm are the best for all of the three retinal image sets. Therefore, we have chosen the probability map image resulting from the LogitBoost ensemble to get the binary vessel segmentation image. In order to obtain a binary vessel segmentation, a thresholding scheme on the probability map is used to decide whether a particular pixel is part of a vessel or not. This procedure assigns one of the classes Cv or Cnv to each candidate pixel, depending on whether its associated probability is greater than a threshold Th. A resultant binary vessel image (Figure 3.8) is obtained by associating classes Cv and Cnv to the values 1 and 0 respectively. Mathematically,

$$I_{res}(x,y) = \begin{cases} 1(\equiv C_v), & \rho\big(C_v \mid Fv(x,y)\big) \geq T_h \\ 0(\equiv C_{nv}), & \text{otherwise} \end{cases} \tag{3.12}$$

where $\rho(C_v|Fv(x,y))$ is the probability that a pixel (x,y) belongs to class C_v given the feature vector $Fv(x,y)$.

Several threshold values Th are selected to produce the binary vessel image and the accuracy is computed for each of the particular threshold values. The final threshold value selected for a given database is the one which produced the binary vessel image with the greatest accuracy. Figure 3.6 shows the plot of accuracy versus threshold Th used for

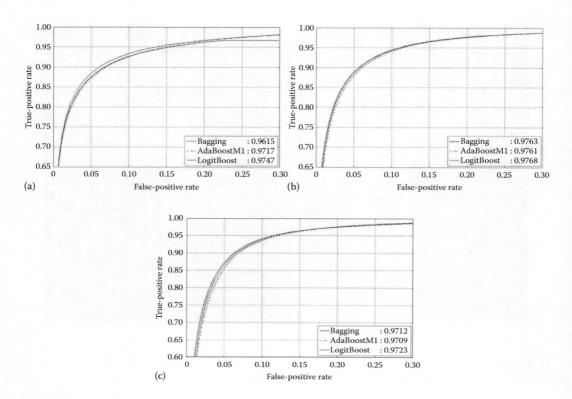

FIGURE 3.5
ROC plots with bagging and boosting for (a) DRIVE, (b) STARE, and (c) CHASE_DB1.

TABLE 3.3

Area under ROC with Different Ensembles

Database	Bootstrap Aggregation	AdaBoostM1	LogitBoost
DRIVE	0.9615	0.9717	0.9747
STARE	0.9763	0.9761	0.9768
CHASE_DB1	0.9712	0.9709	0.9723

producing I_{res} as defined in (Equation 3.12). The optimal threshold value for the DRIVE database is 0.55 and 0.64 for the STARE and CHASE_DB1 databases respectively.

3.3.3.1 Vessel Segmentation Results

The binary vessel segmentation image is obtained from the probability map image and the performance metrics are calculated by taking the first human observer as the ground truth. The average of the selected measures of performance for the DRIVE, STARE, and CHASE_DB1 databases is tabulated in Table 3.4.

The average accuracy values and precision rates incurred by the algorithm are more than those of the second human observer for the DRIVE and STARE databases. The specificity values for the algorithm are also higher than those of the second human observer for each of the three image databases, which indicates the low false-positive

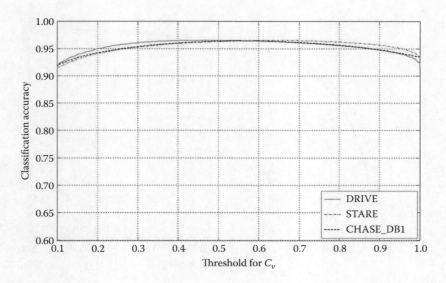

FIGURE 3.6
Accuracy as a function of threshold parameter for *Cv*.

TABLE 3.4

Performance Measures on DRIVE, STARE, and CHASE_DB1

Database	Segmentation	AUC	Acc	SN	SP	PPV	FDR
DRIVE	Second human observer	–	0.9464	0.7796	0.9717	0.8072	0.1927
	Ensemble classifier	0.9747	0.9480	0.7406	0.9807	0.8532	0.1467
STARE	Second human observer	–	0.9347	0.8955	0.9382	0.6432	0.3567
	Ensemble classifier	0.9768	0.9534	0.7548	0.9763	0.7956	0.2043
CHASE_DB1	Second human observer	–	0.9538	0.8092	0.9699	0.7492	0.2507
	Ensemble classifier	0.9712	0.9469	0.7224	0.9711	0.7415	0.2585

rate of the methodology as compared with the second human observer. This in turn indicates that the algorithm has identified less background pixels or pathological area pixels as part of a vessel than the second human observer. The AUC values produced by the method are more than 0.97 for each of the retinal image sets, as illustrated in Figure 3.7.

The segmented images with best case and worst case accuracy from the DRIVE, STARE, and CHASE_DB1 databases are illustrated in Figures 3.8 through 3.10, respectively.

The best case accuracy, sensitivity, specificity, and PPV for the DRIVE database are 0.9637, 0.8615, 0.9780, and 0.8471, respectively, and the worst case measures are 0.9360, 0.7475, 0.9688, and 0.8071, respectively. For the STARE database, the best case accuracy is 0.968, sensitivity is 0.8628, specificity is 0.9801, and PPV is 0.8322; the worst case accuracy is 0.9353, sensitivity is 0.4360, and specificity is 0.9924. The best case vessel segmentation result for the CHASE_DB1 database has an accuracy of 0.9524, a sensitivity of 0.7803, a specificity of 0.9720, and a PPV of 0.7600; the worst case accuracy is 0.9398, sensitivity is 0.5983, and specificity is 0.8011.

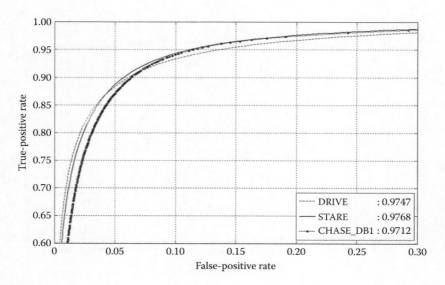

FIGURE 3.7
ROC plot for DRIVE, STARE, and CHASE_DB1.

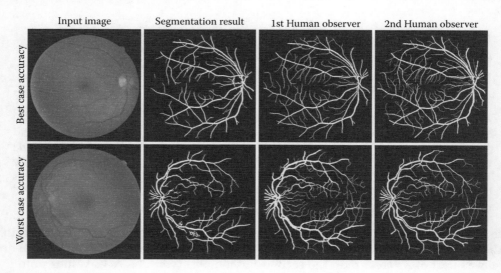

FIGURE 3.8
Segmentation results for DRIVE database.

3.3.3.2 Cross-Training of Classifier

The methodology is also tested for its dependency on training data and its suitability to be applied to any retinal image in a more realistic way, such that the classifier is trained on DRIVE and evaluated on STARE and vice versa. The performance metrics for cross-training are shown in Table 3.5. There is a slight decrease in performance as the AUC falls to 0.9697 from 0.9759 for DRIVE and to 0.9660 from 0.9797 for the STARE database. There is a fractional decrease in observed accuracy of 0.0008 for DRIVE and 0.0039 for the STARE database. The same pattern is observed in the specificity, sensitivity, and the precision rate of vessel segmentation.

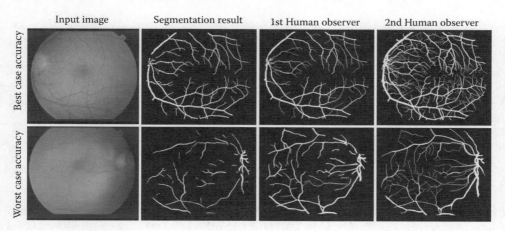

FIGURE 3.9
Segmentation results for STARE database.

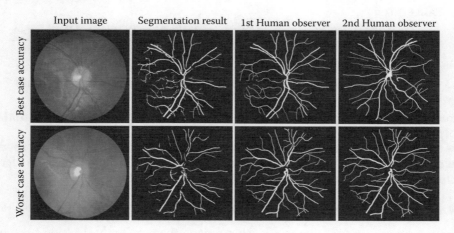

FIGURE 3.10
Segmentation results for CHASE_DB1 database.

3.3.3.3 Feature Importance

A graph to illustrate the importance of each feature in the feature vector in decision making for the LogitBoost-based ensemble classifier is shown in Figure 3.11(a). It indicates that a set of four features for DRIVE which includes one feature from the line strength measure, one feature from the Gabor filter response at scale 2, the GOA, and morphological transformation, are most highly ranked in decision making. The most important features for the STARE database are shown in Figure 3.11(b) which includes one feature from the

TABLE 3.5

Average Performance Measures on DRIVE and STARE with Cross-Training

Database	AUC	Acc	SN	SP	PPV	FDR
DRIVE (trained on STARE)	0.9697	0.9456	0.7242	0.9792	0.8478	0.1522
STARE (trained on DRIVE)	0.9660	0.9495	0.7010	0.9770	0.8123	0.1876

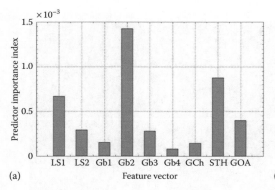
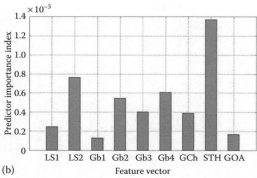

(a)   (b)

FIGURE 3.11

Predictor importance in classification: (a) for DRIVE; (b) for STARE. LS1–2 are line strength features; Gb1–4 are Gabor filter responses at four scales; GCh is green channel pixel values; STH is morphological transformation; and GOA is gradient orientation analysis feature.

TABLE 3.6

Average Performance Measures on DRIVE and STARE with Reduced Feature Set

Database	AUC	Acc	SN	SP	PPV	FDR
DRIVE (Reduced feature set)	0.9716	0.9468	0.7336	0.9789	0.8440	0.1560
STARE (Reduced feature set)	0.9755	0.9509	0.7528	0.9735	0.7810	0.2190

line strength measure, two features from the Gabor filter responses at scales 2 and 4, and the morphological transformation.

Table 3.6 shows the performance metrics when a reduced feature vector is used. This illustrates that even with dimensionality reduction the AUC achieved by the algorithm outperforms other segmentation algorithms mentioned in Tables 3.8 and 3.9.

3.3.3.4 Ensemble Classifier Parameters, Processing Time, and Performance

For demonstration purposes, the relationship among the number of decision trees used to construct the ensemble classifier, the number of pixels used to train the classifier, training time, segmentation time, and achieved area under ROC by the classifier on DRIVE database is tabulated in Table 3.7. It is observed that an ensemble created with bootstrap aggregation takes more time in training and classification as compared with AdaBoostM1 and LogitBoost, while the area under ROC achieved by the ensembles is approximately the same.

3.3.3.5 Comparison with Other Methods

The performance of the proposed methodology is compared with state of the art algorithms published in the last decade in Tables 3.8 and 3.9 for DRIVE and STARE, respectively. The SN, SP, Acc, and area under ROC of the proposed method are compared with the results of published methodologies reported in their respective publications. The performance measures of Hoover [23] and Soares [34] were calculated using the segmented images from their websites.[*][†] The results of Zana [20] and Jiang [39] are taken from the DRIVE database website.[‡]

---

* http://sourceforge.net/apps/mediawiki/retinal/index.php?title=Segmentation_results.

† http://www.parl.clemson.edu/~ahoover/stare/index.html.

‡ http://www.isi.uu.nl/Research/Databases/DRIVE/results.php.

TABLE 3.7

Comparative Analysis of Number of Decision Trees and Training Samples on Training Time, Segmentation Time, and Area under ROC

Training Samples (pixels)	Decision Trees	Training Time (seconds)			Segmentation Time (seconds)			Area under ROC		
		Bagging	AdaBoostM1	LogitBoost	Bagging	AdaBoostM1	LogitBoost	Bagging	AdaBoostM1	LogitBoost
2×10^5	100	485.26	66.48	47.03	27.53	13.51	10.24	0.9556	0.9556	0.9598
	150	732.70	98.84	68.69	41.20	20.17	15.30	0.9563	0.9590	0.9678
	200	980.47	131.25	90.85	62.62	26.86	20.37	0.9570	0.9618	0.9681
	250	1239.73	164.49	113.92	74.15	33.60	25.40	0.9578	0.9635	0.9680
	300	1501.84	196.56	137.20	86.10	40.38	30.44	0.9584	0.9646	0.9706
2.5×10^5	100	689.83	93.43	62.27	27.71	13.50	10.18	0.9580	0.9622	0.960418
	150	918.69	137.37	99.72	41.99	20.36	15.22	0.9594	0.9634	0.960379
	200	1240.81	166.00	116.71	56.15	27.13	20.28	0.9592	0.9660	0.960284
	250	1557.14	209.59	145.31	70.25	33.82	25.45	0.9586	0.9671	0.960221
	300	1879.79	247.30	173.50	85.46	40.43	30.41	0.9593	0.9678	0.960133
3×10^5	100	717.56	97.31	69.03	29.12	13.54	10.20	0.9558	0.9606	0.9656
	150	1078.83	147.92	102.71	43.65	20.36	15.23	0.9567	0.9628	0.9680
	200	1448.13	197.24	136.98	63.38	27.22	20.30	0.9572	0.9645	0.9699
	250	1817.36	248.44	177.30	74.06	33.92	25.46	0.9569	0.9654	0.9702
	300	2204.69	297.73	205.78	90.82	40.57	30.52	0.9588	0.9666	0.9700

TABLE 3.8

Performance Comparison of Vessel Segmentation Methods (DRIVE Images)

No.	Type	Methods	SN	SP	Acc	AUC
1		Second human observer	0.7796	0.9717	0.9470	NA
2	Unsupervised methods	Zana [20]	0.6971	NA	0.9377	0.8984
3		Jiang [39]	NA	NA	0.9212	0.9114
4		Mendonca [40]	0.7344	0.9764	0.9452	NA
5		Al-Diri [41]	0.7282	0.9551	NA	NA
6		Lam [42]	NA	NA	0.9472	0.9614
7		Miri [43]	0.7352	0.9795	0.9458	NA
8		Fraz [44]	0.7152	0.9759	0.9430	NA
9		You [45]	0.7410	0.9751	0.9434	NA
10	Supervised methods	Niemeijer [6]	NA	NA	0.9416	0.9294
11		Soares [34]	0.7332	0.9782	0.9461	0.9614
12		Staal [22]	NA	NA	0.9441	0.9520
13		Ricci [36]	NA	NA	0.9595	0.9558
14		Lupascu [46]	0.7200	NA	0.9597	0.9561
15		Marin [47]	0.7067	0.9801	0.9452	0.9588
16		**Proposed method**	**0.7406**	**0.9807**	**0.9480**	**0.9747**

Note: NA, not available.

A comparative analysis shows that the proposed method achieved better performance metrics than most of the other methods. The area under ROC and the true-positive rate achieved by the algorithm appears better than all the published methods for both the DRIVE and the STARE databases.

The methodologies presented by Ricci [36] and Marin [47] also reported the average accuracy in the case of cross-training of the classifier. The segmented images with the

TABLE 3.9

Performance Comparison of Vessel Segmentation Methods (STARE Images)

No.	Type	Methods	SN	SP	Acc	AUC
1		Second human observer	0.8951	0.9384	0.9348	–
2	Unsupervised methods	Hoover [23]	0.6747	0.9565	0.9264	NA
3		Jiang [39]	NA	NA	0.9009	NA
4		Mendonca [40]	0.6996	0.9730	0.9440	NA
5		Lam [19]	NA	NA	0.9474	0.9392
6		Al-Diri [41]	0.7521	0.9681	NA	NA
7		Lam [42]	NA	NA	0.9567	0.9739
8		Fraz [44]	0.7311	0.9680	0.9442	NA
9		You [45]	0.7260	0.9756	0.9497	NA
10	Supervised methods	Staal [22]	NA	NA	0.9516	0.9614
11		Soares [34]	0.7207	0.9747	0.9479	0.9671
12		Ricci [36]	NA	NA	0.9584	0.9602
13		Marin [47]	0.6944	0.9819	0.9526	0.9769
14		**Proposed method**	**0.7548**	**0.9763**	**0.9534**	**0.9768**

Note: NA, not available.

TABLE 3.10

Performance Comparison of Results with
Cross-Training in Terms of Average Accuracy

Method	DRIVE (Trained on STARE)	STARE (Trained on DRIVE)
Soares [34]	0.9397	0.9327
Ricci [36]	0.9266	0.9464
Marin [47]	0.9448	0.9528
Proposed method	**0.9456**	**0.9493**

TABLE 3.11

Performance Comparison of Results on
Abnormal Retinas (STARE Database)

Method	SN	SP	Acc
Second human observer	0.8719	0.9384	0.9324
Hoover [23]	0.6587	0.9565	0.9258
Soares [34]	0.7181	0.9765	0.9500
Proposed method	**0.7262**	**0.9764**	**0.9511**

cross-trained classifier for Soares' [34] method are also available on their website. We have downloaded and computed the average accuracy of these images. The results are summarized in Table 3.10 where we can observe that the proposed method performs better than Ricci and Soares for both DRIVE and STARE images, and better than Marin for DRIVE images.

The STARE database contains ten pathological images. In order to compare the performance of our method in pathological cases, the performance measures are computed on ten downloaded pathological segmented images of Hoover [23] and Soares [34], and compared with our results in Table 3.11.

Figure 3.12 shows the visual comparison between the vessel classification images of pathological and nonuniform illumination images resulting from our method and those downloaded from Soares' website. It is observed that the proposed method performs better in the removal of pathological artifacts and uneven illumination areas.

3.4 Discussion and Conclusion

In this chapter, we have presented an effective retinal vessel segmentation technique based on supervised classification using an ensemble classifier of boosted and bagged decision trees. We have used a nine-dimensional (9-D) feature vector which consists of the vessel map obtained from the orientation analysis of the gradient vector field, the morphological transformation, line strength measures, and the Gabor filter response which encodes information to successfully handle both normal and pathological retinas.

The important feature of a bagged ensemble is that the reliable estimates of the classification accuracy and feature importance are obtained during the training process without supplying test data. The ensemble classifier was constructed by using 200 weak learners

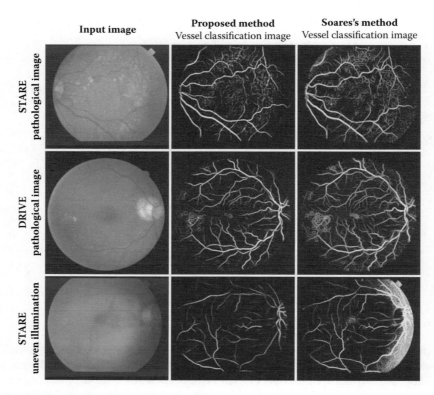

FIGURE 3.12
Comparison of segmentation results on pathological and uneven illumination images.

and is trained on 200,000 training samples randomly extracted from the training set of the DRIVE database and 75,000 samples from the STARE database. These parameters are chosen by empirically analyzing the out-of-bag classification for a given number of training samples and the decision trees. The out-of-bag classification error as a function of the number of decision trees was used to construct the ensemble, and the number of training samples used in ensemble training is illustrated in Figure 3.3. The number of training samples used is much less than in other classification-based methods proposed by Lupascu [46] and Soares [34] where 789,914 and 10^6 samples are used respectively.

Our algorithm renders better AUC accuracy, sensitivity, and specificity measures than other state of the art algorithms for both the DRIVE and STARE databases, being fractionally outperformed in terms of accuracy only by Ricci [36] and Lupascu [46] (for DRIVE only). This observation gains more importance by the fact that Lupascu's [46] technique used a 41-D feature vector as compared with a 9-D feature vector (4-D in the case of reduced feature set, Table 3.6) used by our algorithm and approximately four times more training samples than this work. The Ricci method has proved to be very dependent on the training set, as with cross-training the accuracy dropped from 0.9595 to 0.9266 whereas the drop in accuracy of this work is from 0.9480 to 0.9456; thus the technique appears to be more robust due to the training set used. This training set robustness allows our algorithm to be used on multiple data sets without retraining, which is very useful for large-scale screening programs. The algorithm achieves best accuracy in the case of the cross-trained classifier for DRIVE, and for STARE the cross-trained accuracy of Marin [47] is slightly better. However, as reported, this is due in part to the preprocessing performed for contrast, illumination, and background normalization. The proposed method does not include any preprocessing of retinal images before feature extraction with the goal of improving computational performance and avoiding the risk of thin vessel removal.

In addition, the simplicity of the method should also be highlighted. The method computes only nine features for pixel classification and only four features in the case of the reduced feature set, thus utilizing less computational time. The time required to train the classifier for the DRIVE database with 2×10^4 training samples and 200 decision trees is 100 s and the ensemble for STARE with 75,000 training samples and 200 decision trees takes 49 s. In comparison, the Gaussian Mixture Model classifier used by Soares [34] is trained in approximately 8 hours. The total time required to process a single image is approximately 1 m 40 s, running on a PC with an Intel Core2Duo CPU at 2.27 GHz and 4 GB of RAM. Since this method is experimentally implemented in MATLAB® 7.13, this performance might still be improved.

The performance metrics of most of the vessel segmentation algorithms in the literature are calculated on a small number of images of adults with particular morphological characteristics. The morphological characteristics of retinal images of premature infants and children are very different than those of the adult retina. Choroidal vessels are more visible alongside the retinal vessels in retinal images taken from premature infants [38]. A bright central reflex on the vessels and illumination artifacts contributes to challenges in image processing when retinal images from school children are considered [38]. The limited range of images in the DRIVE and STARE databases do not cater for a variable range of image-related characteristics such as interimage and intraimage variability in luminance, drift in contrast, and uneven background gray-level values. The resolution of images from the STARE and DRIVE data sets are limited to 0.4 and 0.3 megapixels respectively. While this lower resolution is acceptable for certain analyses such as fractal dimension or tortuosity, calculating the vessel diameter normally requires higher resolution images to achieve higher precision. Therefore, a new data set of retinal images acquired from multiethnic school children along with vessel segmentation ground truths has been made publicly available. The new data set is a subset of images from CHASE, which aims to study the cardiovascular risk factors in children of different ethnic origin. Images can be downloaded from the database website. This data set is intended to facilitate the development and comparison of vessel segmentation and vessel measurement algorithms.

The demonstrated performance, effectiveness, and robustness, along with its simplicity and speed in training as well as in classification, make this ensemble-based method for blood vessel segmentation a suitable tool to be integrated into a complete retinal image analysis system for clinical purposes and for large population studies in particular. In future we aim to incorporate the vessel width and tortousity measures into the algorithm and to develop an interactive vessel analysis software tool for ophthalmologists.

References

1. H. Leung, et al., Relationships between age, blood pressure, and retinal vessel diameters in an older population, *Investigative Ophthalmology and Visual Science*, 44: 2900–2904, 2003.
2. J. J. Kanski and B. Bowling, *Clinical Ophthalmology: A Systematic Approach*, 7th edn. London: Elsevier Health Sciences, 2011.
3. H. E. Jelinek and M. J. Cree, *Automated Image Detection of Retinal Pathology.* Boca Raton, FL: CRC Press Taylor & Francis Group, 2009.

4. G. Quellec, et al., A multiple-instance learning framework for diabetic retinopathy screening, *Medical Image Analysis*, 16: 1228–1240, 2012.

5. C. Heneghan, et al., Characterization of changes in blood vessel width and tortuosity in retinopathy of prematurity using image analysis, *Medical Image Analysis*, 6: 407–429, 2002.

6. M. Niemeijer, et al., Automated measurement of the arteriolar-to-venular width ratio in digital color fundus photographs, *IEEE Transactions on Medical Imaging*, 30: 1941–1950, 2011.

7. M. Foracchia, Extraction and quantitative description of vessel features in hypertensive retinopathy fundus images, in *Book Abstracts 2nd International Workshop on Computer Assisted Fundus Image Analysis*, E. Grisan, Ed., p. 6, 2001.

8. M. K. Ikram, et al., Retinal vessel diameters and risk of hypertension, *Hypertension*, 47: 189–194, 2006.

9. D. E. Becker, et al., Image processing algorithms for retinal montage synthesis, mapping, and real-time location determination, *IEEE Transactions on Biomedical Engineering*, 45: 105–118, 1998.

10. A. M. Broehan, et al., Real-time multimodal retinal image registration for a computer-assisted laser photocoagulation system, *IEEE Transactions on Biomedical Engineering*, 58: 2816–2824, 2011.

11. A. Can, et al., A feature-based, robust, hierarchical algorithm for registering pairs of images of the curved human retina, *IEEE Transactions on Pattern Analysis and Machine Intelligence*, 24: 347–364, 2002.

12. L. Shijian and L. Joo Hwee, Automatic optic disc detection from retinal images by a line operator, *IEEE Transactions on Biomedical Engineering*, 58: 88–94, 2011.

13. L. Huiqi and O. Chutatape, Automated feature extraction in color retinal images by a model based approach, *IEEE Transactions on Biomedical Engineering*, 51: 246–254, 2004.

14. C. Köse and C. İki'baş, A personal identification system using retinal vasculature in retinal fundus images, *Expert Systems with Applications*, 38: 13670–13681, 2011.

15. C. M. Wilson, et al., Computerized analysis of retinal vessel width and tortuosity in premature infants, *Investigative Ophthalmology & Visual Science*, 49: 3577–3585, 2008.

16. C. G. Owen, et al., Retinal arteriolar tortuosity and cardiovascular risk factors in a multi-ethnic population study of 10-year-old children; the child heart and health study in England (CHASE), *Arteriosclerosis, Thrombosis, and Vascular Biology*, 31: 1933–1938, 2011.

17. M. D. Abràmoff, et al., Retinal imaging and image analysis, *IEEE Reviews in Biomedical Engineering*, 3: 169–208, 2010.

18. M. M. Fraz, et al., Blood vessel segmentation methodologies in retinal images: A survey, *Computer Methods and Programs in Biomedicine*, 108: 407–433, 2012.

19. B. S. Y. Lam and Y. Hong, A novel vessel segmentation algorithm for pathological retina images based on the divergence of vector fields, *IEEE Transactions on Medical Imaging*, 27: 237–246, 2008.

20. F. Zana and J. C. Klein, Segmentation of vessel-like patterns using mathematical morphology and curvature evaluation, *IEEE Transactions on Image Processing*, 10: 1010–1019, 2001.

21. B. Zhang, et al., Retinal vessel extraction by matched filter with first-order derivative of Gaussian, *Computers in Biology and Medicine*, 40(4): 438–445, 2010.

22. J. Staal, et al., Ridge-based vessel segmentation in color images of the retina, *IEEE Transactions on Medical Imaging*, 23: 501–509, 2004.

23. A. D. Hoover, et al., Locating blood vessels in retinal images by piecewise threshold probing of a matched filter response, *IEEE Transactions on Medical Imaging*, 19: 203–210, 2000.

24. M. M. Fraz. CHASE_DB1, Available at: http://sec.kingston.ac.uk/retinal/CHASE_DB1, 2011.

25. M. M. Fraz, et al., An ensemble classification-based approach applied to retinal blood vessel segmentation, *IEEE Transactions on Biomedical Engineering*, 59: 2538–2548, 2012.

26. R. Polikar, Ensemble based systems in decision making, *IEEE Circuits and Systems Magazine*, 6: 21–45, 2006.

27. L. Breiman, Bagging predictors, *Machine Learning*, 24: 123–140, 1996.

28. R. Schapire, The boosting approach to machine learning: An overview, in *MSRI Workshop on Nonlinear Estimation and Classification*, 2002.

29. R. Polikar, Bootstrap-inspired techniques in computation intelligence, *IEEE Signal Processing Magazine*, 24: 59–72, 2007.

30. R. E. Schapire, The strength of weak learnability, in *30th Annual Symposium on Foundations of Computer Science*, pp. 28–33, 1989.

31. J. Friedman, et al., Additive logistic regression: A statistical view of boosting, *The Annals of Statistics*, 28: 337–374, 2000.

32. D. Onkaew, et al., Automatic extraction of retinal vessels based on gradient orientation analysis, in *Eighth International Joint Conference on Computer Science and Software Engineering (JCSSE)*, pp. 102–107, 2011.

33. J. R. Movellan, Tutorial on Gabor filters, Tutorial paper, Available at: http://mplab.ucsd.edu/tutorials/gabor.pdf, 2008.

34. J. V. B. Soares, et al., Retinal vessel segmentation using the 2-D gabor wavelet and supervised classification, *IEEE Transactions on Medical Imaging*, 25: 1214–1222, 2006.

35. R. Zwiggelaar, et al., Linear structures in mammographic images: Detection and classification, *IEEE Transactions on Medical Imaging*, 23: 1077–1086, 2004.

36. E. Ricci and R. Perfetti, Retinal blood vessel segmentation using line operators and support vector classification, *IEEE Transactions on Medical Imaging*, 26: 1357–1365, 2007.

37. C. G. Owen, et al., Retinal arteriolar tortuosity and cardiovascular risk factors in a multi-ethnic population study of 10-year-old children; the child heart and health study in England (CHASE), *Arteriosclerosis, Thrombosis, and Vascular Biology*, 31: 1933–1938, 2011.

38. C. G. Owen, et al., Measuring retinal vessel tortuosity in 10-year-old children: Validation of the computer-assisted image analysis of the retina (CAIAR) program, *Investigative Ophthalmology & Visual Science*, 50: 2004–2010, 2009.

39. J. Xiaoyi and D. Mojon, Adaptive local thresholding by verification-based multithreshold probing with application to vessel detection in retinal images, *IEEE Transactions on Pattern Analysis and Machine Intelligence*, 25: 131–137, 2003.

40. A. M. Mendonca and A. Campilho, Segmentation of retinal blood vessels by combining the detection of centerlines and morphological reconstruction, *IEEE Transactions on Medical Imaging*, 25: 1200–1213, 2006.

41. B. Al-Diri, et al., An active contour model for segmenting and measuring retinal vessels, *IEEE Transactions on Medical Imaging*, 28: 1488–1497, 2009.

42. B. S. Y. Lam, et al., General retinal vessel segmentation using regularization-based multiconcavity modeling, *IEEE Transactions on Medical Imaging*, 29: 1369–1381, 2010.

43. M. S. Miri and A. Mahloojifar, Retinal image analysis using curvelet transform and multistructure elements morphology by reconstruction, *IEEE Transactions on Biomedical Engineering*, 58: 1183–1192, 2011.

44. M. M. Fraz, et al., An approach to localize the retinal blood vessels using bit planes and centerline detection, *Computer Methods and Programs in Biomedicine*, 108: 600–616, 2012.

45. X. You, et al., Segmentation of retinal blood vessels using the radial projection and semi-supervised approach, *Pattern Recognition*, 44: 2314–2324, 2011.

46. C. A. Lupascu, et al., FABC: Retinal vessel segmentation using AdaBoost, *IEEE Transactions on Information Technology in Biomedicine*, 14: 1267–1274, 2010.

47. D. Marin, et al., A new supervised method for blood vessel segmentation in retinal images by using gray-level and moment invariants-based features, *IEEE Transactions on Medical Imaging*, 30: 146–158, 2011.

4

Computer Vision Algorithms Applied to Retinal Vessel Segmentation and Quantification of Vessel Caliber

Muhammad Moazam Fraz and Sarah A. Barman

CONTENTS

4.1 Introduction

With the development of digital imaging and computational efficiency, image-processing, analysis, and modeling techniques are increasingly used in all fields of medical sciences, particularly in ophthalmology. The blood vessel structure in retinal images is unique in the sense that it is the only part of the blood circulation system that can be directly observed noninvasively, and can be easily photographed and used in digital image analysis. Noticeable developments in image processing relevant to ophthalmology over the last decade include the progress made toward the development of automated diagnostic systems for ophthalmologic disorders (Bernardes et al. 2011). The quantification of the width and morphology of blood vessels in the retina has been a heavily researched area in recent years (Abràmoff et al. 2010). The accurate extraction of the retinal vascular tree forms the backbone of many automated computer-aided systems for screening and diagnosis of cardiovascular and ophthalmic diseases.

Retinal vessel segmentation and quantification of morphological attributes of retinal blood vessels, such as length, width, tortuosity, and branching pattern and angles, are utilized for diagnosis, screening, treatment, and evaluation of various cardiovascular (Leung et al. 2003) and ophthalmologic diseases (Kanski and Bowling 2011) such as hypertension, arteriosclerosis, choroidal neovascularization, and diabetes (Jelinek and Cree 2009). Automatic detection and analysis of the vasculature can assist in the implementation of screening programs for diabetic retinopathy (Quellec et al. 2012), evaluation of retinopathy of prematurity (Heneghan et al. 2002), foveal avascular region detection (Niemeijer et al. 2009a), arteriolar narrowing (Niemeijer et al. 2011), assessment of the relationship between vessel tortuosity and hypertensive retinopathy (Foracchia 2001), vessel diameter measurement in relation to diagnosis of hypertension (Ikram et al. 2006), and computer-assisted laser surgery (Becker et al. 1998; Broehan et al. 2011). Automatic generation of retinal maps and extraction of branch points have been used for temporal or multimodal image registration (Broehan et al. 2011), retinal image mosaic synthesis (Can et al. 2002), optic disc identification (Shijian and Joo Hwee 2011), and fovea localization (Huiqi and Chutatape 2004). Moreover, besides the other widely used methods, which include face, fingerprint, hand palm, ear, gait, signature, voice, and iris, the retinal vascular tree can be used for biometric identification (Köse and İki˙baş 2011). Manual segmentation of retinal blood vessels is a long and tedious task that requires training and skill. It is commonly accepted by the medical community that automatic quantification of retinal vessels is the first step in the development of a computer-assisted diagnostic system for ophthalmic disorders (Fraz et al. 2012b).

In this chapter, a detailed review, analysis, and categorization of retinal vessel segmentation and caliber measurement techniques are presented. The objective is to provide a detailed resource of the algorithms employed for vessel segmentation and width measurement as a ready reference. The key points are highlighted, the differences and performance measures are illustrated, and the advantages and disadvantages of various approaches are discussed. The current trends, the future directions, and the open problems in automated blood vessel segmentation are also discussed. A summary of the publicly available databases of retinal images is also provided as this has stimulated research and innovation in ophthalmology by providing a means of direct comparison between the algorithms of automated retinal image analysis.

This chapter begins by introducing retinal photography, challenges associated with retinal vessel segmentation, the public archives of retinal images, and quantitative measures of performance for vessel segmentation. A classification of the segmentation methods and brief description of the papers within each category are given in Section 4.3. Section 4.4 lays out the review of vessel caliber measurement techniques. The discussion is given in Section 4.5. Finally, the conclusion and future directions are presented in Section 4.6.

4.2 Retinal Image Processing

4.2.1 Retinal Imaging

Retinal photography requires the use of a complex optical system, called a fundus camera (Saine and Tyler 2002). It is a specialized, low-power microscope with an attached camera, capable of simultaneously illuminating and imaging the retina. It is designed to image the interior surface of the eye, which includes the retina, optic disc, macula, and posterior pole (Cassin and Solomon 1990). The fundus camera normally operates in three modes. In color photography the retina is examined in full color under the illumination of white light. In red-free photography, the imaging light is filtered to remove the red color and the vessels and other structures are improved in contrast. Fluorescent angiograms are acquired using the dye tracing method. A sodium fluorescein or indocyanine green is injected into the blood, and then the angiogram is obtained by photographing the fluorescence emitted after illumination of the retina with blue light at a wavelength of 490 nm.

4.2.2 Challenges in Retinal Vessel Segmentation

The retinal vasculature is composed of arteries and veins appearing as piecewise linear structures, with their tributaries visible within the retinal image, shown in Figure 4.1(a). The wide range of vessel widths ranges from 1 to 20 pixels, depending on both the width of the vessel and the image resolution. Other structures appearing in the retinal images include the retina boundary, the optic disc, and pathologies in the form of microaneurysms, cotton wool spots, bright and dark lesions, and exudates, as shown in Figure 4.1(d–g). These types of pathologies are particularly challenging for automatic vessel extraction

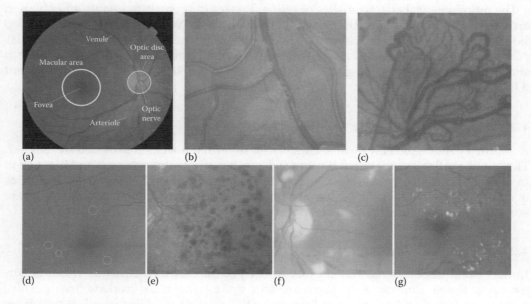

FIGURE 4.1
Structures in retina: (a) macula centered retinal image; (b) vessels with central reflex; (c) new vessel growth in retina; (d) microaneurysms; (e) dot and blot hemorrhages; (f) cotton wool spots; and (g) hard exudates.

because they may appear as a series of bright spots, sometimes with narrow, darker gaps in between, and may have similar attributes to vessels.

The vessel cross-sectional intensity profiles approximate a Gaussian shape or a mixture of Gaussians in the case where a central vessel reflex is present. The orientation and gray level of a vessel do not change abruptly; they are locally linear and gradually change in intensity along their lengths. The vessels can be expected to be connected and, in the retina, form a binary treelike structure. However, the shape, size, and local gray level of blood vessels can vary hugely and the central intensity of some vessels varies very little in comparison with the background gray level. Narrow vessels often have the lowest contrast.

Vessel crossing and branching can further complicate the profile model. As with the processing of most medical images, signal noise, drift in image intensity, and lack of image contrast pose significant challenges to the extraction of blood vessels. Retinal vessels also show evidence of a strong reflection along their centerline known as a central vessel reflex, as evident in Figure 4.1(b), which is more apparent in arterioles than venules, is stronger at images taken at longer wavelengths, and typically found in the retinal images of younger patients.

Images acquired in a controlled environment are high quality and hence facilitate retinal image processing. However, the quality of retinal images acquired during large population-based studies and screening programs is frequently reduced due to a number of factors. This includes the pressure of taking retinal scans of a large number of patients in a stipulated time, which in turn increases subjective errors in image acquisition by the human operator. Moreover, there are specular reflections from the cornea and lens and the light is scattered from ocular media turbidity, which causes large regional variations in the image intensity. This results in very dark and very bright regions within the same image with widely different contrast between the blood vessels and the background. This degradation of image quality may significantly encumber visual inspection and make automated retinal image processing more difficult.

The morphological characteristics of retinal images of premature infants and children are very different from those of the adult retina. Choroidal vessels are more visible alongside the retinal vessels in retinal images taken from premature infants (Wilson et al. 2008). A bright central reflex on the vessels (Figure 4.1(b)) and illumination artifacts contribute to challenges in image processing when retinal images from schoolchildren are considered (Owen et al. 2011).

4.2.3 Retinal Imaging Public Archives

A summary of the publicly available databases of retinal images is provided in Table 4.1. The public availability of retinal image databases has stimulated research and innovation in ophthalmology by providing a means of direct comparison between the algorithms of automated retinal image analysis. Most retinal vessel segmentation methodologies are evaluated on two databases (DRIVE and STARE).

4.2.4 Performance Measures

In the retinal vessel segmentation process, any pixel is classified either as vessel or surrounding tissue. Consequently, there are four events: two classifications (true positive and true negative) and two misclassifications (false positive and false negative), which are defined in Table 4.2.

The accuracy (Acc) is measured by the ratio of the total number of correctly classified pixels by the number of pixels in the image FOV. Sensitivity (SN) reflects the ability of an

TABLE 4.1

Retinal Image Databases in Public Domain

Database	Year	Retinal Images	FOV and Image Size	Measurement and Reference Standard
STARE (Hoover et al. 2000)	2000	20 nonmydriatic; 10 are normal and 10 are pathological.	45° 768 × 584	Vessel segmentation ground truths marked by two human observers.
DRIVE (Image Sciences Institute n.d.)	2004	40 nonmydriatic; divided into 20 test and 20 training images. In total 7 are pathological and the rest are normal.	35° 650 × 500	Ground truths marked by two human observers for vessel segmentation.
ARIA online (Farnell et al. 2008)	2006	92 images with AMD, 59 images with DR, 61 images in control group.	50° 768 × 576	Reference standard for blood vessel tracing, OD and fovea location by two image analysis experts.
ImageRet, DIARETDB0, and DIARETDB1 (Kauppi et al. 2007)	2008	DIARETDB0: 130 in which 20 are normal and 110 with DR. DIARETDB0: 89 out of which 5 are normal and 84 proliferative DR.	50° 1500 × 1152	Microaneurysms, hemorrhages, hard and soft exudates marked by four experts.
Messidor project (Messidor 2004)	2008	1200 images with different pathologies; 800 are mydriatic.	45° 1440 × 960, 2240 × 1488, 2304 × 1536	Reference standard contains the grading for diabetic retinopathy and the risk of macular edema.
REVIEW (Al-Diri et al. 2008)	2008	16 mydriatic images with 193 annotated vessel segments consisting of 5066 profile points.		Vessel width is manually marked by three observers. Reference standard is their average.
ROC microaneurysm data set (Niemeijer et al. 2009b)	2009	100: 50 training and 50 test images.	45° 768 × 576, 1058 × 1061, 1389 × 1383	Reference standard indicating the location of microaneurysms is provided with the training set.
VICAVR (Ortega Hortas and Penas Centeno n.d.)	2010	58 images.	768 × 584	Caliber of the vessels measured at different radii from the optic disc as well as the vessel type (artery/vein) labeled by three experts.
CHASE_DB1 (Fraz 2011)	2011	28 nonmydriatic retinal images of multiethnic children divided into sets of 20 test and 8 training. 32 annotated vessel segments consisting of 1605 profile points.	30° 1280 × 960.	Vessel segmentation ground truths marked by two human observers. Width is marked by two experts and reference standard is their average.

Note: DR, diabetic retinopathy; AMD, age-related macular degeneration; OD, optic disc.

algorithm to detect the vessel pixels. Specificity (SP) is the ability to detect nonvessel pixels. These metrics are defined in Table 4.3, which is based on the terms in Table 4.2.

In addition, the performance of the algorithm is also measured with the area under receiver operating characteristic (ROC) curve (AUC). The ROC curve is a plot of true-positive fractions (SN) versus false-positive fractions (1-SP) by varying the threshold on the probability map image.

TABLE 4.2

Vessel Classification

	Vessel Present	**Vessel Absent**
Vessel detected	True positive (TP)	False positive (FP)
Vessel not detected	False negative (FN)	True negative (TN)

TABLE 4.3

Performance Measures for Retinal Vessel Segmentation

Measure	Description
TPR	TP/vessel pixel count
FPR	FP/nonvessel pixel count
SN	TP/(TP + FN)
SP	TN/(TN + FP)
Acc	(TP + TN)/(TP + FP + TN + FN)

4.3 Retinal Vessel Segmentation Approaches

A common categorization of algorithms for segmentation of vessel-like structures in medical images is found in Kirbas and Quek (2004). A review of some of the methodologies presented in this chapter was previously published in a journal paper (Fraz et al. 2012b). In this chapter, in addition to a review of the vessel caliber measurement techniques, more vessel segmentation techniques are included in the survey, including a denser theoretical review and analysis of performance. The papers are categorized according to the image-processing technique employed. We have divided the retinal vessel segmentation algorithms into seven main categories: (1) pattern recognition techniques, (2) matched filtering, (3) vessel tracking/tracing, (4) mathematical morphology, (5) multiscale approaches, (6) model-based approaches, and (7) parallel/hardware-based approaches. Each segmentation method category is briefly described and the papers for each category are summarized. The performance measures used by the segmentation algorithms are tabulated at the end of each subsection. The reviewed papers are summarized in Table 4.4 on the basis of the image-processing technique used for segmentation. The fourth column illustrates the performance metrics used to evaluate the algorithm. The penultimate column indicates the capability of the algorithm in handling noisy images, pathological images, and images containing a central vessel reflex. "Nse," "Pth," and "Cvr" values in this column indicate that the algorithm is capable of handling the noisy, pathological, and central vessel reflex images, respectively.

4.3.1 Pattern Classification and Machine Learning

The algorithms based on pattern recognition deal with the automatic detection or classification of retinal blood vessel features and other nonvessel objects including background. Pattern recognition techniques for vessel segmentation are divided into two categories: supervised approaches and unsupervised approaches. Supervised methods exploit some prior labeling information to decide whether a pixel belongs to a vessel or not, while

TABLE 4.4

Categorization Retinal Vessel Segmentation Methods

Algorithm	Image-Processing Technique	Performance Metrics	N/P/C Images	Section
Akita and Kuga 1982	Artificial neural networks	Visual	No	Supervised classification methods 4.3.1.1
Nekovei and Ying 1995	Back propagation neural network	Visual	No	
Sinthanayothin et al. 1999	Principal component analysis and neural network	SN, SP	No	
Niemeijer et al. 2004	Gaussian derivative and k-NN classifier	Acc, AUC	No	
Staal et al. 2004	Image ridges and k-NN classifier	Acc, AUC	No	
Soares et al. 2006	Gabor filter and Gaussian mixture model (GMM) classifier	Acc, AUC	No	
Ricci and Perfetti 2007	Line operator and support vector Machine (SVM)	Acc, AUC	Nse/Cvr	
Xu and Luo 2010	Wavelets, Hessian matrix and SVM	SN, Acc	No	
Lupascu et al. 2010	Feature-based AdaBoost classifier	SN, Acc, AUC	No	
You et al. 2011	Radial projection and semisupervised classification using SVM	SN, SP, Acc	No	
Marin et al. 2011	Gray level and moment invariant-based features with neural network	SN, SP, Acc, AUC	Nse/Pth/Cvr	
Condurache and Mertins 2012	Hysteresis binary-classification paradigm	SN, SP, Acc	No	
Fraz et al. 2012c	Ensemble classifier of decision trees	SN, SP, Acc, AUC FDR, PPV	Nse/Pth/Cvr	
Tolias and Panas 1998	Fuzzy C-means clustering	Visual	No	Unsupervised classification methods 4.3.1.2
Ng et al. 2010	Maximum likelihood estimation of scale-space parameters	TPR, FPR	No	
Simó and de Ves 2001	Bayesian image analysis and statistical parameter estimation	Visual, TPR, FPR	No	
Kande et al. 2009	Spatially weighted fuzzy C-means clustering	AUC	Pth	
Salem et al. 2007	Radius-based Clustering ALgorithm (RACAL)	SN, SP	No	
Villalobos-Castaldi et al. 2010	Local entropy and co-occurrence matrix (GLCM)	SN, SP, Acc	No	
Chaudhuri et al. 1989	Two-dimensional Gaussian matched filter (MF)	Acc, AUC	No	Matched filtering 4.3.2
Hoover et al. 2000	MF and threshold probing	SN, SP, Acc	No	
Kochner et al. 1998	Steerable filters		No	
Gang et al. 2002	Amplitude-modified second-order Gaussian filter	Visual	No	
Xiaoyi and Mojon 2003	Verification-based multithreshold probing	Acc, AUC	No	
Al-Rawi et al. 2007	Improved Gaussian-matched filter	Acc, AUC	No	
Sukkaew et al. 2007	Statistically optimized Laplacian of Gaussian (LOG) skeletonization	SN, SP	Nse	

(continued)

TABLE 4.4   (Continued)

Categorization Retinal Vessel Segmentation Methods

Algorithm	Image-Processing Technique	Performance Metrics	N/P/C Images	Section
Yao and Chen 2009	Gaussian MF and pulse-coupled neural network	TPR, FPR	No	
Cinsdikici and Aydin 2009	Matched filter and ANT colony algorithm	SN, SP, Acc	No	
Lei et al. 2009	Modified matched filter with double-sided threshold	SN, SP, Acc	Pth	
Zhang et al. 2010	Gaussian-matched filter in combination with first-order derivative	Acc, AUC	Pth	
Amin and Yan 2010	Phase concurrency and log-Gabor filter	TPR, FPR	No	
Ramlugun et al. 2012	2-D Gabor filter followed by hysteresis thresholding	SN, SP, Acc	No	
Fathi and Naghsh-Nilchi 2013	Wavelet-based segmentation	SN, SP, Acc	No	
Zana and Klein 2001	Morphological processing and cross-curvature evaluation	TPR, Acc, AUC	Nse	Morphological processing 4.3.3
Ayala et al. 2005	Fuzzy mathematical morphology	TPR, FPR	No	
Mendonca and Campilho 2006	Difference of offset Gaussian filter and multiscale morphological reconstruction	Acc, AUC	No	
Yang et al. 2008	Mathematical morphology and fuzzy clustering	Visual	No	
Sun et al. 2010	Multiscale morphology, fuzzy filter, and watershed transformation	Visual	No	
Fraz et al. 2012a	Vessel centerline detection and morphological bit-plane slicing	TPR, FPR, SN, SP, Acc, PPV	No	
Miri and Mahloojifar 2011	Curvelet transform and multistructure elements morphology by reconstruction	TPR, FPR, Acc	Nse	
Liu and Sun 1993	Adaptive tracking	Visual	No	Vessel tracing/ tracking 4.3.4
Liang et al. 1994	Matched filter-based iterative tracking with manual intervention	Visual	No	
Chutatape et al. 1998	Gaussian and Kalman filters	Visual	No	
Quek and Kirbas 2001	Wave propagation and trace back	Visual	Nse	
Ali et al. 1999	Recursive tracking with directional templates	Visual	No	
Kelvin et al. 2007	Optimal contour tracking	Acc	Nse	
Delibasis et al. 2010	Model-based tracing	SN, SP, Acc	No	
Yin et al. 2012	Probabilistic line tracking	Segmentation matching factor	No	
Frangi et al. 1998	Eigen decomposition of Hessian and Frobenius norm	Visual	No	Multiscale approaches 4.3.5
Martinez-Perez et al. 1999	Scale-space analysis of maximum principal curvature	Visual	No	
Martinez-Perez et al. 2007	Maximum principal curvature, gradient magnitude, and region growing	TPR, FPR, Acc	No	

TABLE 4.4 (Continued)

Categorization Retinal Vessel Segmentation Methods

Algorithm	Image-Processing Technique	Performance Metrics	N/P/C Images	Section
Perez et al. 2007	ITK serial implementation	TPR, FPR, Acc	No	
Wink et al. 2004	Vector-valued multiscale representation	Visual	Nse	
Sofka and Stewart 2006	Likelihood ratio test with confidence and edge measures	Visual	Nse/Pth	
Anzalone et al. 2008	Scale-space analysis and parameter search	TPR, FPR, Acc	No	
Farnell et al. 2008	Multiscale line operator and region growing	AUC	No	
Vlachos and Dermatas 2009	Multiscale line tracking	SN, SP, Acc	Nse	
Li et al. 2012	Multiscale production of matched filters	SN, SP, Acc	Nse	
Moghimirad et al. 2012	Multiscale medialness function	SN, SP, Acc, AUC	Nse/Pth	
Vermeer et al. 2004	Laplacian profile model	SN, SP	C	Vessel profile models 4.3.6.1
Mahadevan et al. 2004	Vessel profile model	Visual	Nse/Pth	
Li et al. 2007	Multiresoution hermite model	SN, SP	Nse/Cvr	
Lam and Hong 2008	Divergence of vector fields	Acc, AUC	Nse/Pth	
Lam et al. 2010	Multiconcavity modeling	Acc, AUC	Nse/Pth	
Narasimha-Iyer et al. 2007	Dual-Gaussian profile model	Visual	Nse/Cvr	
Zhu 2010	Log-Gabor filters, phase concurrency, and Fourier domain	Visual	Nse	
Espona et al. 2007	Snakes in combination with blood vessel topological properties	SN, SP, Acc	No	Deformable models 4.3.6.2
Espona et al. 2008	Snakes in combination with morphological processing	SN, SP, Acc	No	
Al-Diri et al. 2009	Ribbon of twin active contour model	SN, SP	Cvr	
Sum and Cheung 2008	Chan–Vese contour model	Visual	Nse	
Zhang et al. 2009	Nonlinear projections, variational calculus	TPR, FPR, Acc	No	
Yuan et al. 2011	Local line integrals and variational optimization	AUC	Nse/Pth	
Alonso-Montes et al. 2005	CNN-based algorithm	Visual	No	Parallel hardware-based implementations 4.3.7
Alonso-Montes et al. 2008	Pixel-level snakes, pixel-parallel approach	Acc	No	
Renzo et al. 2007	CNN with virtual template expansion	Acc, AUC	No	
Costantini et al. 2010	CNN with virtual template expansion	Acc, AUC	No	
Palomera-Perez et al. 2010	ITK parallel implementation	TPR, FPR, Acc	No	

Notes: Performance metrics: Visual, visual comparison; SN, sensitivity; SP, specificity; Acc, accuracy; AUC, area under curve.

N/P/C images means noisy images/pathological images/central vessel reflex images. "Nse," "Pth," and "Cvr" values in this column indicate that the algorithm is capable of handling noisy, pathological, and central vessel reflex images, respectively.

unsupervised methods perform the vessel segmentation without any prior labeling knowledge.

4.3.1.1 Supervised Methods

In supervised methods, the rule for vessel extraction is learned by the algorithm on the basis of a training set of manually processed and segmented reference images often termed as the gold standard. This vascular structure in these ground truth or gold standard images is precisely marked by an ophthalmologist. However, as noted by Hoover et al. (2000) there is significant disagreement in the identification of vessels even among expert observers. In a supervised method, the classification criteria are determined by the ground truth data based on given features. Therefore, the prerequisite is the availability of the already classified ground truth data, which may not be available in real-life applications. As supervised methods are designed based on preclassified data, their performance is usually better than that of unsupervised ones and can produce very good results for healthy retinal images.

Artificial neural networks have been extensively investigated for segmenting retinal features such as the vasculature (Akita and Kuga 1982), making classifications based on statistical probabilities rather than objective reasoning. Nekovei and Ying (1995) describe an approach using a back-propagation network for the detection of blood vessels in angiography. The method applies the neural network directly to the angiogram pixels without prior feature detection. The feature vectors are formed by grayscale values from the subwindow centered on the pixel being classified. The use of principal component analysis (PCA) followed by neural networks is demonstrated by Sinthanayothin et al. (1999) for localization of anatomical structures in retinal images. Niemeijer et al. (2004) extract a feature vector for each pixel that consists of the green plane of the RGB image and the responses of a Gaussian matched filter and its first- and second-order derivatives at multiple scales and use the k-nearest neighbor (k-NN) (Duda et al. 2000) classifier for pixel classification. The methodology presented by Staal et al. (2004) is based on an extraction of image ridges, which are natural indicators of vessels and coincide approximately with vessel centerlines. The k-NN classifier with 27 features per pixel is used for vessel classification. The use of a two-dimensional (2-D) Gabor wavelet and supervised classification for retinal vessel segmentation has been demonstrated by Soares et al. (2006). Each pixel is represented by a feature vector composed of the pixel's intensity and 2-D Gabor wavelet transform responses taken at multiple scales. A Gaussian mixture model (GMM) (Duda et al. 2000) classifier is used to classify each pixel as either a vessel or nonvessel pixel. The algorithm takes into account the information local to each pixel through image filters, ignoring useful information from shapes and structures present in the image. It does not work very well on images with nonuniform illumination as it produces false detection in some images on the border of the optic disc, hemorrhages, and other types of pathologies that present strong contrast. The application of line operators as a feature vector and a support vector machine (SVM) (Duda et al. 2000) for pixel classification is proposed by Ricci and Perfetti (2007). Two orthogonal line detectors that are based on the evaluation of the average gray level along lines of fixed length passing through the target pixel at different orientations are applied to construct a feature vector for supervised classification using a SVM. The algorithm requires fewer features, feature extraction is computationally simpler, and fewer examples are needed for training. The line detector used is robust with respect to nonuniform illumination and contrast and its behavior in the presence of a central reflex is satisfactory. The combination of several image-processing techniques, which include adaptive image normalization, multiscale wavelet analysis, and line detectors, to produce a 12-D feature vector with SVM classification for vessel segmentation is proposed by Xu and Luo (2010). Lupascu et al. (2010) introduce another supervised method known as the feature-based AdaBoost classifier (FABC) (Duda et al. 2000) for vessel segmentation. The 41-D feature vector is a rich collection of measurements at different spatial scales including the output of various filters (Gaussian and derivatives of Gaussian filters, matched filters, and 2-D Gabor wavelet transform) and the likelihood of structures like edges and ridges (principal and mean curvatures, principal directions, and root mean square gradient). An AdaBoost classifier is trained on 789,914 samples of vessel and nonvessel pixels. The strength of the FABC lies in its capture of a rich collection of shape and structural information, in addition to local information at multiple spatial scales in the feature vector. FABC does not address issues related to the connection of broken vessel segments and some local ambiguities present due to the convergence of multiple and various bent vessels.

The combination of the radial projection and the semisupervised self-training method using a SVM is employed by You et al. (2011) for vessel segmentation. The vessel centerlines and the narrow and low-contrast blood vessels are located using radial projections. A modified steerable complex wavelet is employed for vessel enhancement. The line strength measures are applied to the vessel-enhanced image to generate the feature vector. The SVM classifier is used in a semisupervised self-training to extract the major structure of vessels. The segmented vasculature is obtained by the union of the two. The algorithm self-learns from human-labeled data and weakly labeled data, therefore yielding good results with a decrease in the detection of false vessels. The method is very good in detecting narrow and low-contrast vessels, but is prone to errors in case of pathologies. Marin et al. (2011) presented a neural network-based supervised methodology for the segmentation of retinal vessels. The methodology uses a 7-D feature vector composed of gray-level and moment invariant-based features. A multilayer feed-forward neural network is utilized for training and classification. The method proves to be effective and robust with different image conditions and on multiple image databases even if the neural network is trained on only one database. A binary classifier designing technique termed as hysteresis binary-classification paradigm (Condurache and Mertins 2012) has been proposed for vessel segmentation. This technique uses two classifiers: the pessimistic, which is designed to yield a zero false-positive rate (FPR) and a high false-negative rate; and the optimistic, which works with a practically zero false-negative rate and a high FPR. Then, based on the prior knowledge about vessel connectivity, the pessimist classification can be used to select true vessels from among the optimist classification.

The performance measures for evaluating the efficiency of supervised classification of retinal vessels are illustrated in Table 4.5, which shows the high performance of ensemble classification (Fraz et al. 2012c).

4.3.1.2 Unsupervised Methods

The approaches based on unsupervised classification attempt to find inherent patterns of blood vessels in retinal images that can then be used to determine that a particular pixel belongs to a vessel or not. The training data or hand-labeled ground truths do not contribute directly to the design of the algorithm in these approaches.

Tolias and Panas (1998) develop a fuzzy C-means (FCM) clustering algorithm that uses linguistic descriptions like *vessel* and *nonvessel* to track fundus vessels in retinal angiogram images. The fuzzy vessel-tracking process is based on finding the membership functions

TABLE 4.5

Performance Measures for Supervised Methods

Methodology	Database	Sensitivity	Specificity	Accuracy	Area under ROC
Human observer	DRIVE	0.7763	0.9723	0.9470	–
	STARE	0.8951	0.9384	0.9348	–
Sinthanayothin et al. 1999	Local data set	0.833	0.91	–	–
Niemeijer et al. 2004	DRIVE	0.7145	–	0.9416	0.9294
Staal et al. 2004	DRIVE	–	–	0.9442	0.952
	STARE	–	–	0.9516	0.9614
Soares et al. 2006	DRIVE	–	–	0.9466	0.9614
	STARE	–	–	0.9480	0.9671
Ricci and Perfetti 2007	DRIVE	–	–	0.9563	0.9558
	STARE	–	–	0.9584	0.9602
Lupascu et al. 2010	DRIVE	0.72	–	0.9597	0.9561
Xu and Luo 2010	DRIVE	0.7760	–	0.9328	–
You et al. 2011	DRIVE	0.7410	0.9751	0.9434	–
	STARE	0.7260	0.9756	0.9497	–
Marin et al. 2011	DRIVE	0.7067	0.9801	0.9452	0.9588
	STARE	0.6944	0.9819	0.9526	0.9769
Condurache and Mertins 2012	DRIVE	0.9094	0.9591	0.9516	0.9726
	STARE	0.8902	0.9673	0.9595	0.9791
Fraz et al. 2012c	DRIVE	0.7406	0.9807	0.9480	0.9747
	STARE	0.7548	0.9763	0.9534	0.9768

of the two linguistic values. First, the optic nerve and its bounding circle, which is a salient image region in fundus images, is detected and used as the starting point of the algorithm. Then, the FCM algorithm is applied to segment the points in the bounding circle as vessel and nonvessel. The striking features of the algorithm are that it does not utilize any edge information to locate the exact location of the vessels and this reduces the effects of noise in the tracking procedure. Also, the algorithm uses only fuzzy image intensity information and makes no assumptions for the shape model of the vessels. Moreover, no parametric tuning and initialization are needed. The algorithm resulted in good tracking of well-defined vessels in the image and missed only vessels of small diameter and low contrast. Salem et al. (2007) proposed a RAdius-based Clustering ALgorithm (RACAL), which uses a distance-based principle to map the distributions of the image pixels in combination with a partial supervision strategy. The performance of RACAL algorithms is compared with that of k-NN and they are found to be better in the detection of small vessels. An unsupervised fuzzy-based vessel segmentation approach, proposed by Kande et al. (2009), uses the intensity information from red and green channels of the same retinal image to correct nonuniform illumination, followed by matched filtering and a spatially weighted fuzzy C-means clustering.

Bayesian image analysis for the segmentation of arteries, veins, and the fovea in retinal angiograms is employed by Simó and de Ves (2001). The methodology is tested on various ocular fundus images and proved to be robust against added salt and pepper noise. Ng et al. (2010) proposed a generative model using a Gaussian-profiled valley for the detection of blood vessels along with a Gaussian model of noise. The covariance of a multiscale second-derivative Gaussian filter that outputs to the isotropic noise is calculated. The image and noise models are incorporated into a maximum likelihood estimator to estimate the width, contrast, and direction of the blood vessel at each point in the image and to detect the vessel centerline. The vessel is marked by combining the centerline and the estimated width parameter. The performance of this algorithm approximates with that of threshold probing (Hoover et al. 2000) and the RISA system (Martinez-Perez et al. 2002). The local entropy information in combination with the gray-level co-occurrence matrix (GLCM) is used by Villalobos-Castaldi et al. (2010) for vessel segmentation. First, a matched filter is used to enhance the vessels followed by the computation of the GLCM, from which a statistical feature is calculated, to act as a threshold value. Later, local entropy thresholding is employed to segment the vessel network.

Table 4.6 depicts the performance measures reported by various methodologies of retinal vessel segmentation based on unsupervised classification, with a high accuracy reported by Villalobos-Castaldi et al. (2010) using GLCM.

4.3.2 Matched Filtering

Matched filtering for the detection of the vasculature convolves a 2-D kernel with the retinal image. The kernel is designed to model a feature in the image at some unknown position and orientation, and the matched filter response (MFR) indicates the presence of the feature. The following three properties are exploited in order to design the matched filter kernel: vessels usually have a limited curvature and may be approximated by piecewise linear segments; the diameter of the vessels decrease as they move radially outward from the optic disc; and the cross-sectional pixel intensity profile of these line segments approximates a Gaussian curve. The convolution kernel may be quite large and needs to be applied at several rotations resulting in a computational overhead. In addition, the kernel responds optimally to vessels that have the same standard deviation of the underlying Gaussian function specified by the kernel. As a consequence, the kernel may not respond to those vessels that have a different profile. The retinal background variation and presence of pathologies in the retinal image also increase the number of false responses because the pathologies can exhibit the same local attributes as the vessels. An MFR method is found to be effective when used in conjunction with additional processing techniques.

Chaudhuri et al. (1989) proposed a 2-D linear kernel with a Gaussian profile for segmentation of the retinal vessels. The kernel is rotated in 15° increments to fit into vessels

TABLE 4.6

Performance Measures for Unsupervised Methods

Methodology	Database	Sensitivity	Specificity	Accuracy	Area under ROC
Ng et al. 2010	STARE	0.7000	0.9530	–	–
Kande et al. 2009	DRIVE	–	–	0.8911	0.9518
	STARE	–	–	0.8976	0.9298
Salem et al. 2007	STARE	0.8215	0.9750	–	–
Villalobos-Castaldi et al. 2010	DRIVE (without FOV)	0.9648	0.9480	0.9759	–

of different orientations. The highest response of the filter is selected for each pixel and is thresholded to provide a binary vessel image. Further postprocessing is then applied to prune and identify the vessel segments. Hoover et al. (2000) analyze the MFR image, formulated by Chaudhuri et al. (1989), in pieces and apply thresholding with iterative threshold probing based on local and region-based properties for each pixel as vessel or nonvessel. A reduction of false positives of as much as 15 times over the basic MFR and a true-positive rate (TPR) of up to 75% have been reported.

Steerable filters (Freeman and Adelson 1991), that is, a filter with arbitrary orientation, can be synthesized from the linear combination of basis filters. This class of filters is not applied in many directions. Rather, it is applied in only two basic directions and the response is calculated in other directions from a combination of the responses from these two directions. This approach has the advantage of faster computation for reasonable accuracy. Kochner et al. (1998) employed a steerable filter for vessel segmentation. The amplitude-modified second-order Gaussian filter (Gang et al. 2002) has also been utilized for vessel detection. It proves that the vessel width can be measured in a linear relationship with the spreading factor of the matched Gaussian filter when the magnitude coefficient of the Gaussian filter is suitably assigned. An adaptive local thresholding framework based on a verification-based multithreshold probing scheme (Xiaoyi and Mojon 2003) has also been investigated for vessel detection. This includes an application-dependent verification procedure that incorporates the domain-specific knowledge about blood vessels including curvilinear angle, width, contrast, and size. The methodology works very well for healthy retinal images but is prone to increased FPRs with pathological retinal images. An automated algorithm (Sukkaew et al. 2007) for detection of the blood vessels in low-quality and noisy retinal images of premature infants employs a statistically optimized Laplacian of Gaussian (LOG) edge detection filter, Otsu thresholding, medial axis transform skeletonization followed by pruning, and edge thinning for vessel segmentation. Al-Rawi et al. (2007) improved Chaudhuri et al.'s (1989) matched filter (MF) by using an exhaustive search optimization procedure on 20 retinal images of the DRIVE database to find the best parameters for matched filter size, the standard deviation, and threshold value. Yao and Chen (2009) use a 2-D Gaussian matched filter for retinal vessel enhancement and then a simplified pulse coupled neural network (Thomas and Jason 1998) is employed to segment the blood vessels by firing neighborhood neurons. Next, a fast 2-D Otsu algorithm is used to search the best segmentation results. Finally, the complete vessel tree is obtained via analysis of the regional connectivity.

A hybrid model of the matched filter and ANT colony algorithm (Marco and Thomas 2004) for retinal vessel segmentation is proposed by Cinsdikici and Aydin (2009). After some preprocessing, the image is passed through the matched filter and ANT algorithm in parallel. The results are then combined followed by length filtering to extract the complete vasculature. The algorithm is computationally fast enough but the accuracy decreases with pathological retinas.

The classical matched filter is generalized and extended (Zhang et al. 2010) with the first-order derivative of the Gaussian (MF-FDOG) to exploit the following property of blood vessels in the retina: the Gaussian-shaped cross-section is symmetric with respect to its peak position whereas the nonvessel edges, for example, the step edge for lesions, are asymmetric. The methodology uses a pair of filters, the zero-mean Gaussian filter (MF), and the first-order derivative of the Gaussian (FDOG) to detect the vessels. The methodology significantly reduces the false detections produced by the original MF and detects many fine vessels that are missed by the MF. A modified matched filter is also proposed by Lei et al. (2009); it uses a local vessel cross-section analysis using double-sided thresholding to reduce false responses to the pathologies. A high-speed detection of retinal blood vessels using phase congruency has been proposed by Amin and Yan (2010). Initially, phase congruency of the retinal image is generated, which is a soft classification of vessels that is invariant due to the change in image luminosity and contrast. A bank of log-Gabor filters are used for measuring phase congruency and a binary vessel tree is obtained by thresholding. The algorithm detects the vessels from images in the DRIVE and STARE databases in 10 sec. Ramlugun et al. (2012) segment the blood vessels using a 2-D Gabor filter on a histogram-equalized image followed by hysteresis thresholding. The method proposed by Fathi and Naghsh-Nilchi (2013) is based on complex continuous wavelet analysis where the line structures are distinguished from edge structures using the real and imaginary parts of the employed wavelet. The final vessel network is obtained by integrating the modulus values of the wavelet coefficients in the optimal scales and applying an adaptive thresholding method along with length filtering.

The comparison of selected performance measures for the methodologies based on matched filtering is illustrated in Table 4.7, where the highest accuracy is achieved by the improved matched filter method of Fathi and Naghsh-Nilchi (2013).

4.3.3 Morphological Processing

Morphological image processing (Serra 1983) is a collection of techniques for digital image processing based on mathematical morphology. Morphological operators apply structuring elements (SE) to images and typically use binary images but can be extended to gray-level images. The two main morphological operators are dilation and erosion. *Dilation* expands objects by a defined structuring element, filling holes, and connecting the disjoint regions. *Erosion* shrinks the objects by a structuring element. The other two operations are *closing*, which is a dilation followed by an erosion, and *opening*, that is, an erosion followed by a dilation. Two algorithms used in medical image segmentation and related to mathematical morphology are the *top hat* and *watershed* transformations. The enhancement effect of a top-hat transformation is due to the estimation of local background by a

TABLE 4.7

Performance Measures for the Methods Based on Matched Filtering

Methodology	Database	Sensitivity	Specificity	Accuracy	Area under ROC
Chaudhuri et al. 1989	DRIVE	–	–	0.8773	0.7878
Hoover et al. 2000	STARE	0.6751	0.9567	0.9267	–
Xiaoyi and Mojon 2003	DRIVE	–	–	0.9212	0.9114
	STARE	–	–	0.9337	0.8906
Yao and Chen 2009	STARE	0.8035	0.972	–	–
Al-Rawi et al. 2007	DRIVE	–	–	0.9535	0.9435
Zhang et al. 2010	DRIVE	0.7120	0.9724	0.9382	–
	STARE	0.7177	0.9753	0.9484	–
Cinsdikici and Aydin 2009	DRIVE	–	–	0.9293	0.9407
Lei et al. 2009	STARE	0.7286	0.9628	0.9416	–
Amin and Yan 2010	DRIVE	–	–	0.92	0.94
Ramlugun et al. 2012	DRIVE	0.6413	0.9767	0.9340	–
Fathi and Naghsh-Nilchi 2013	DRIVE	0.7768	0.9759	0.9581	–
	STARE	0.8061	0.9717	0.9591	–

morphology opening operation, which is subtracted from the original image resulting in enhanced vessels.

The basic morphology of the vasculature is known *a priori* to be comprised of connected linear segments. Morphological processing for identifying specific shapes has the advantage of speed and noise resistance. The main disadvantage of exclusively relying on morphological methods is that they do not exploit the known vessel cross-sectional shape. In addition, the use of an overly long structuring element may cause difficulty in fitting to highly tortuous vessels.

The combination of morphological filters for vessel enhancement and cross-curvature evaluation to identify linearly coherent structures is employed by Zana and Klein (1999, 2001). Ayala et al. (2005) define an average of fuzzy sets by making use of the average distance of Baddeley et al. (1995) and the mean of Vorob'ev (Stoyan and Stoyan 1994). The segmentation procedures presented by Zana and Klein (2001), Chaudhuri et al. (1989), and Heneghan et al. (2002) have been revisited and modified using these new averages. All these procedures produce grayscale images with enhanced blood vessels after low-level processing. The threshold will be applied to this vessel-enhanced image to generate a binary vessel tree. For the Zana and Klein (2001) method, the segmentation result is heavily dependent on the length of the linear structuring element. A fuzzy set of structuring elements with varied length is defined and then the final result is obtained with the aggregation of a proposed fuzzy set average. A decrease in the FPR is observed with this method.

A difference of offset Gaussian (DoOG) filter in combination with multiscale morphological reconstruction (Mendonca and Campilho 2006) is utilized for retinal vasculature extraction. The vessel centerlines are extracted by applying the DoOG filter and the vessels are enhanced by applying a modified top-hat operator with variable size circular structuring elements aimed at enhancement of vessels with different widths. The binary maps of the vessels are obtained at four scales by using morphological reconstruction with a double threshold operator. A final image with the segmented vessels is obtained by an iterative seeded region growing process of the centerline image with the set of four binary maps. An automatic hybrid method comprising of the combination of mathematical morphology and a fuzzy clustering algorithm is presented by Yang et al. (2008). The blood vessels are enhanced and the background is removed with a morphological top-hat operation, then the vessels are extracted by fuzzy clustering. Sun et al. (2010) combined morphological multiscale enhancement, fuzzy filtering, and watershed transformation for the extraction of the vascular tree in the angiogram. The fuzzy filter is shown to be insensitive to the added Gaussian noise in the angiograms. Fraz et al. (2012a, 2011) proposed a unique combination of vessel centerline detection and morphological bit plane slicing to extract the blood vessel tree from the retinal images. The centerlines are extracted by using the first-order derivative of a Gaussian filter in four orientations and then evaluation of derivative signs and average derivative values is performed. The shape and orientation map of blood vessels is obtained by applying a multidirectional morphological top-hat operator with a linear structuring element followed by bit plane slicing of the vessel-enhanced grayscale image. The centerlines are combined with these maps to obtain the segmented vessel tree. The combination of fast discrete curvelet transform (FDCT) and multistructure mathematical morphology (Miri and Mahloojifar 2011) is also employed for vessel detection.

Table 4.8 summarizes the results of various morphological image processing-based retinal vessel segmentation techniques evaluated on the DRIVE and STARE databases. A high accuracy is reported by Mendonca and Campilho (2006) when applied to the DRIVE data set.

TABLE 4.8

Performance Measures for Morphological Processing Methodologies

Methodology	Database	Sensitivity	Specificity	Accuracy	Area under ROC
Zana and Klein 2001	DRIVE	0.6971	–	0.9377	0.8984
Mendonca and Campilho 2006	DRIVE	0.7344	0.9764	0.9452	–
	STARE	0.6996	0.9730	0.9440	–
Fraz et al. 2012a	DRIVE	0.7152	0.9769	0.9430	–
	STARE	0.7311	0.9680	0.9442	–
Miri and Mahloojifar 2011	DRIVE	0.7352	0.9795	0.9458	–

4.3.4 Vessel Tracing/Tracking

Vessel-tracking algorithms segment a vessel between two points using local information and work at the level of a single vessel rather than the entire vasculature. The center of the longitudinal cross-section of a vessel is determined with various properties of the vessel including average width, gray-level intensity, and tortuosity measured during tracking. Tracking consists of following vessel centerlines guided by local information, usually trying to find the path that best matches a vessel profile model. The main advantage of vessel tracking methods is that they provide highly accurate vessel widths and can provide information about individual vessels that is usually unavailable using other methods. Noting that vessels are connected in the retina, these systems can follow a whole tree without wasting time examining the vast majority of the image that does not contain vessel. Vessel tracking can thus give information on vessel structure such as branching and connectivity. There are some complications relating to the technique that include the vessel-tracking algorithms being unable to detect vessels or vessel segments that have no seed-points and, in addition, missing any bifurcation points can result in undetected subtrees. Generally, the vessel-tracking algorithms are used in conjunction with matched filters of morphological operators. Some modifications and improvements are also suggested in the literature to deal with the above-mentioned problems. To deal with the problem of the central light reflex area, Xiaohong et al. (2001) supposed the vessel intensity profiles can be modeled as twin Gaussian functions.

Adaptive tracking (Liu and Sun 1993) is applied to detection of the vasculature in retinal angiograms, where the local vessel trajectories are estimated after giving an initial point within a vessel. Liang et al. (1994) developed an algorithm, involving the Gaussian matched filter, to find the course of the vessel centerline and measure the diameter and tortuosity of a single vessel segment, although only diameter measurements are reported. The algorithm needs manual intervention for start and end points and definition of the tracking direction. Chutatape et al. (1998) use a tracking strategy with Gaussian and Kalman filters for blood vessel detection in retinal images. The second-order Gaussian matched filter is employed to estimate the vessel centerline midpoint and then the tracking process is started from the circumference of the optic disc. The Kalman filter is employed to estimate the next vessel segment location using not only the parameters of the current segment but all previous vessel segments as well, similar to tracking a flying object in a radar system. The algorithm is sensitive to vessels with a central reflex. A wave propagation and traceback mechanism (Quek and Kirbas 2001) is proposed for the extraction of the vasculature from retinal angiography images. A vessel likelihood image is obtained by using a dual sigmoidal filter, which is used to compute a cost function in the form of refractive indexes, and then a digital wave is propagated through the image from the base of the vascular tree. This wave washes over the vasculature, ignoring local noise perturbations. The vasculature is obtained by tracing the wave along the local normal to the waveform. Wave propagation and traceback allows the extraction of not only the individual vessels, but the vascular connection morphology as well. The algorithm is evaluated on a set of six neurovascular angiogram images and it successfully detects 106 vessels out of 110. Ali et al. (1999) describe a real-time algorithm based on recursively tracking the vessels starting from initial seed-points, using directional templates. Each directional template is designed to give the maximum response for an edge oriented in a particular direction. Around each candidate vessel point, the templates are applied on either side of the point at varying distances. The edges are marked at points that yield the maximum response for the templates. The algorithm takes a step in the direction of maximum response and the procedure is repeated at the new point. This algorithm is very fast and prioritized versions have been used for real-time feature extraction and registration at frame rates of 30 frames/s. For dealing with the problem of real-time extraction of crossing and bifurcation of retinal vessels, Hong et al. (2001) describe an optimal algorithm to schedule the vascular tracing computations. A heuristic estimate of the optimal schedule is developed and used to guide the design of realizable scheduling algorithms. A semiautomated method for the segmentation of vascular images is proposed by Kelvin et al. (2007). The method incorporates the multiscale vesselness filtering (Frangi et al. 1998) into the conventional Livewire framework (Barrett and Mortensen 1997) to efficiently compute optimal medial axes. Sparse seed-points along the vessel boundary are determined and optimal contours connecting these points are found using Dijkstra's algorithm. The cost function incorporates Frangi's multiscale vesselness measure, vessel direction consistency, the edge evidence, and the spatial and radius smoothness constraints.

A probabilistic tracking method (Yin et al. 2012) is proposed to detect blood vessels in retinal images. During the tracking process, vessel edge points are detected iteratively using local gray-level statistics and vessel continuity properties. Local vessel sectional intensity profiles are estimated by a Gaussian-shaped curve. A Bayesian method with the maximum *a posteriori* (MAP) probability criterion is then used to identify local vessel structure and find out the edge points from these candidates. Different geometric shapes and noise levels are used for computer simulated images, whereas real retinal images from the REVIEW database are tested. Evaluation performance is performed using the segmentation matching factor (SMF) as a quality parameter.

4.3.5 Multiscale Approaches

The width of a vessel decreases as it travels radially outward from the optic disc and such a change in vessel caliber is a gradual one. Therefore, a vessel is defined as a contrasted pattern with a Gaussian-shaped cross-section profile, piecewise connected, and locally linear, with a gradually decreasing vessel width. Therefore, the idea behind scale-space representation for vascular extraction is to separate out information related to the blood vessel having varying widths at different scales.

Frangi et al. (1998) examined the multiscale second-order local structure of an image (Hessian) in the context of developing a vessel enhancement filter. A vesselness measure is obtained on the basis of the eigenvalue analysis of the Hessian, which finds out the principal directions in which the local second-order structure of the image can be decomposed.

This directly gives the direction of the smallest curvature along the vessel. Two gray-level invariant geometric ratios are defined on the basis of eigenvalues and the Frobenius norm matrix is computed. The final vesselness measure is defined using the geometric ratios, the eigenvalues, and the Frobenius norm matrix. Many of the multiscale algorithms are based on this vessel enhancement filter. Martinez-Perez et al. (1999) present a method based on scale-space analysis from which the width, size, and orientation of retinal blood vessels are obtained by using two main geometrical features based upon the first and the second derivative of the intensity (edges and the maximum principal curvature) along the scale space, which give information about the topology of the image. The algorithm is tested on both red-free and fluorescein retinal images and shows promising results. Based on the work of Martinez-Perez et al. (1999), a semiautomatic method to measure and quantify geometrical and topological properties of the retinal vascular tree is also described (Martinez-Perez et al. 2002). The procedure consists of a semiautomatic labeling of the skeleton trees followed by an automatic procedure for measurement of length, area, diameter, and branching angle of vessels. Several geometrical and topological indexes are extracted. The methods are validated by comparison with manual measurements and applied to a pilot study of ten normal and ten hypertensive subjects, and differences between groups in the morphological properties are investigated. An extension (Martinez-Perez et al. 2007) of Martinez-Perez et al.'s work (1999) is demonstrated by exploiting the observation that the intensity of an image is proportional to the amount of blood in the light path corresponding to the particular pixel during image capture. Therefore, a diameter-dependent equalization factor is applied to the multiscale information. The algorithm (Martinez-Perez et al. 1999) is further improved in Perez et al. (2007) by using the insight segmentation and registration toolkit (ITK) (Ibanez et al. 2003).

Wink et al. (2004) have developed a method for central axis extraction that finds a minimum cost path using the vector-valued multiscale representation of a feature. The methodology is tested on synthetic and real angiograms and shows its potential to cope with severe stenosis or imaging artifacts in the image. A likelihood ratio test (Sofka and Stewart 2006) has been used for vessel centerline extraction that combines matched-filter responses, confidence measures, and vessel boundary measures using a 6-D feature vector. This vesselness likelihood ratio is used by a vessel-tracing framework to produce the complete tree of vessel centerlines. Anzalone et al. (2008) proposed a modular supervised algorithm for vessel segmentation in red-free retinal images. The image background is normalized for uneven illumination conditions followed by vessel enhancement using scale-space theory. A supervised optimization procedure is used to determine the optimal scale factor and threshold for binarization of the segmented image followed by a cleaning operation for spur removal. The multiscale line operator (MSLO) (Farnell et al. 2008) is also investigated for segmentation of retinal vessels. A Gaussian pyramid of subsampled images is constructed by using a series of images at consecutively coarser length scales via Gaussian sampling with respect to the original retinal image. The line operator is applied to the images on each level of the pyramid separately. This algorithm is evaluated on the STARE and ARIA (http://cgi.csc.liv.ac.uk/~hanafi/in) databases and the reported AUC are 0.940 and 0.895, respectively. A multiscale line tracking for vasculature segmentation is presented by Vlachos and Dermatas (2009). After luminosity and contrast normalization, the seeds for line tracking are derived from a brightness selection rule from a normalized histogram. The line tracking is initialized at multiple scales to accommodate varying vessel widths. Several cross-sectional profile conditions are defined for termination conditions for line tracking. The multiscale confidence image map is derived after combining the results of multiscale line tracking. The methodology is very much dependent upon initial selection of seeds for line tracking. Li et al. (2012) use multiscale production of MFRs for vessel segmentation and width estimation. The scale production is used to enhance the edges and suppress noise so that some small weak vessels with low local contrast are detected with good width estimation. The medial lines of vessels are extracted by employing a weighted 2-D multiscale medial function (Moghimirad et al. 2012). The function response is multiplied with eigenvalues of the Hessian matrix. The noise reduction and reconstruction procedure are used to obtain vessel centerlines followed by radius estimation to construct the complete vascular tree.

The performance measures including TPR, FPR, sensitivity, specificity, accuracy, and AUC for the methods based on multiscale approaches are illustrated in Table 4.9, showing the scale-space approach to achieve the highest accuracy when applied to a range of retinal images from the DRIVE and STARE data sets (Martinez-Perez et al. 1999, 2007).

4.3.6 Model-Based Approaches

These approaches apply the explicit vessel models to extract the retinal vessels. We classify the model-based approaches into two categories: (1) vessel profile models and (2) deformable models.

4.3.6.1 Vessel Profile Models

The vessel cross-sectional intensity profiles approximate a Gaussian shape or a mixture of Gaussians in the case where a central vessel reflex is present. Other profiles such as the second-order derivative Gaussian, the cubic spline, or hermite polynomial profile can be readily substituted. The more complex scenario is to include the nonvessel features like bright or dark lesions and the background characteristics in the vessel detection model to increase the segmentation accuracy in difficult imaging conditions. The flat background has also been assumed in some profile models for the vessel section. Vessel crossing and branching can further complicate the profile model.

TABLE 4.9

Performance Measures for Multiscale Approaches

Methodology	Database	Sensitivity	Specificity	Accuracy	Area under ROC
Martinez-Perez et al. 1999	DRIVE	0.6389	–	0.9181	–
Martinez-Perez et al. 2007	DRIVE	0.7246	0.9655	0.9344	–
	STARE	0.7506	0.9569	0.9410	–
Perez et al. 2007	DRIVE	0.660	0.9612	0.9220	–
	STARE	0.779	0.9409	0.9240	–
Anzalone et al. 2008	DRIVE	–	–	0.9419	–
Farnell et al. 2008	STARE	–	–	–	0.940
	ARIA	–	–	–	0.895
Vlachos and Dermatas 2009	DRIVE	0.747	0.955	0.929	–
Li et al. 2012	DRIVE	0.7154	0.9716	0.9343	–
	STARE	0.7191	0.9687	0.9407	–
Moghimirad et al. 2012	DRIVE	0.7852	0.9935	0.9659	0.9580
	STARE	0.7177	0.9753	0.9484	0.9678

Vermeer et al. (2004) modeled the vessel profile as Laplacian to incorporate the central vessel reflex. Mahadevan et al. (2004) present a set of algorithms for a robust and modular framework for vessel detection in noisy images. The authors presented the estimation of the log likelihood of vessel parameters in a noisy environment using three models: Huber's censored likelihood ratio test (Huber 1965), the ranked ordered test (Field and Smith 1994) for log likelihood, and the robust model selection (Ronchetti 1985) based on nonlinear least-squares fitting. The framework is adaptable to incorporate a variety of vessel profile models including Gaussian, derivatives of Gaussian and dual Gaussian, and various noise models like Gaussian noise and Poisson noise. The framework is tested on a synthetic phantom as well as sequences of clinical images and the results are compared with those of the matched filter (Chaudhuri et al. 1989) and the direct exploratory vessel tracing algorithm (Ali et al. 1999) and report an improvement of 43.7% and 145.7%, respectively. An extension (Narasimha-Iyer et al. 2008) of this vessel detection framework is also proposed by the authors with the inclusion of a generalized dual-Gaussian cross-sectional profile for improved detection of vessels containing a central vessel reflex.

A multiresolution hermite model is proposed for vascular segmentation by Li et al. (2007), which employs a 2-D hermite function intensity model in a quad-tree structure over a range of spatial resolutions. The vessel modeling and estimation technique is based on a hermite polynomial instead of a Gaussian mixture (Narasimha-Iyer et al. 2007; Xiaohong et al. 2001) to incorporate the central light reflex. A block-based multiresolution approach is used in combination with an expectation-maximization (EM) optimization scheme to fit the local model parameters. The local models of vessel segments and bifurcations are linked using a stochastic Bayesian approach to infer the global vascular structure. Lam and Hong (2008) proposed a novel vessel segmentation algorithm for pathological retinal images based on the divergence of vector fields. In this method, the centerlines are detected using the normalized gradient vector field, and then the blood vessel-like objects are detected using the gradient vector field of a pixel. All the pathological retinal images in the STARE database are used to evaluate the proposed method and an average accuracy of 0.9474 and an AUC of 0.9392 are reported. The algorithm presented by Lam et al. (2010) is based on regularization-based multiconcavity modeling and is able to handle both normal and pathological retinas with bright and dark lesions simultaneously. Three different concavity measures are proposed to detect blood vessels and each of these measures is designed to address the negative impact produced by the lesions for identifying the normal vessels. The features obtained from these concavity measures are combined according to their statistical and geometrical properties and later a lifting technique is used for optimizing the regularized solution toward the ideal vessel shape. The dual-Gaussian model initially used by Xiaohong et al. (2001) is extended to estimate the cross-sectional intensity profile of retinal vessels in dual-wavelength images recorded at 560 and 600 nm (Narasimha-Iyer et al. 2007). A universal representation of vessel cross-sectional profiles that includes modeling of normal vessels as well as for branch points and crossovers, in the Fourier domain, utilizing phase congruency is proposed by Zhu (2010).

4.3.6.2 Deformable Models

Active contour models, informally known as *snakes* (Kass et al. 1988), are the curves defined within an image domain that can move under the influence of internal forces within the curve itself and external forces derived from the image data. The internal and external forces are defined so that the snake will conform to an object boundary or other desired features within an image. The *internal (smoothing) forces* produce *tension* and *stiffness* that constrain the behavior of the snake and the *external* forces may be specified by a supervising process or a human user. Some of the advantages of snakes over classical feature attraction techniques are that they are autonomous and self-adapting in their search for a minimal energy state. They can also be easily manipulated using external image forces. They can be used to track dynamic objects in temporal as well as spatial dimensions. The main limitation of the models is that they usually only incorporate edge information, ignoring other image characteristics, possibly combined with some prior expectation of shape. Due to this, they often overlook minute features in the process of minimizing the energy over the entire path of their contours. They are required to be initialized close to the feature of interest if they are to avoid being trapped by other local minima. Their accuracy is governed by the convergence criteria used in the energy minimization technique; higher accuracies require tighter convergence criteria and hence, longer computation times. Snakes are often used in applications like object tracking, shape recognition, segmentation, edge detection, and stereo matching. A number of authors have investigated the use of active contour models in retinal vascular segmentation.

Espona et al. (2007) use the classical snake in combination with blood vessel topological properties to extract the vasculature from a retinal image. The algorithm is further improved (Espona et al. 2008) by introducing morphological operations for vessel crease extraction and the fine-tuning of snake energy-minimizing parameters. Al-Diri and Hunter (2005) introduce ribbon of twin (ROT), a parametric active contour model in which two twins of contours (one inside and one outside the vessel) represent a ribbon along a vessel. The two outside contours are connected by pull forces to the inside contours, while the inside contours are connected by push forces with each other. The model converges when the maximum distance between both contours inside the twin are less than a certain threshold. The edges of the vessel are captured from both sides by inside and outside contours. The distance between the inside contours gives the measure of vessel width. The model exhibits robust behavior on retinal images with noise and those that have closely parallel vessels, blurred vessel edges, central vessel reflex, and very fine vessels. The ROT model is utilized to extract vessel segments and width measures (Al-Diri et al. 2009). Initially, the tramline filter is used to locate an initial set of potential vessel segment centerline pixels, which are used for initializing the ROT active contour model. Later, the junction resolution algorithm extends the discrete segments and resolves various crossings, junctions, and joinings. The algorithm accurately locates the vessel edges under challenging conditions, including noisy blurred edges, very closely located parallel vessels, light reflex phenomena, and very fine vessels. The junction resolution algorithm is evaluated on the first five images of DRIVE for detection of bifurcations and crossovers and resulted in precision rates of 89%, 95%, and 90%, respectively. The width measurement is reported on the REVIEW database (Al-Diri et al. 2008). Yuan et al. (2011) analyze the vesselness measures proposed by Krissian et al. (1998), Li et al. (2003), and Frangi et al. (1998) and propose a new method based on local line integrals and variational optimization that produces accurate vesselness measures and vessel direction estimations that are less subject to local intensity abnormalities. The methodology performed well on synthetic images as well as on DRIVE and STARE.

The geometric models for active contours are based on the theory of curve evolution geometric flows. These models are usually implemented using the level-set based numerical algorithm. The level set method (LSM) is a numerical technique for tracking interfaces and shapes. The advantage of the level set method is that numerical computations involving curves and surfaces can be performed on a fixed Cartesian grid without having to parameterize these objects. Sum and Cheung (2008) proposed a modification in the Chan–Vese model (Chan and Vese 2001) by incorporating the local image contrast into a level-set-based active contour to handle nonuniform illumination. The approach is evaluated with experiments involving both synthetic images and clinical angiograms. A methodology based on nonlinear projections is proposed by Zhang et al. (2009). The segmented vessel tree is obtained by an adaptive thresholding method based on the variational image binarization algorithm (Tong et al. 2005).

The performance of model-based approaches for retinal vessel segmentation is summarized in Table 4.10, where the highest accuracy is reported for Lam et al. (2010), an algorithm based on the divergence of vector fields, on the DRIVE and STARE data sets.

4.3.7 Parallel Hardware-Based Implementations

The high computational cost of retinal vessel segmentation algorithms and requirements for real-time performance are addressed by parallel hardware-based implementation of algorithms. One attractive paradigm for parallel real-time image processing is represented by cellular neural networks (CNN) (Chua and Yang 1988; Roska and Chua 1993), which can be implemented on very-large-scale integration (VLSI) chips. The Insight segmentation and registration ToolKit (ITK) (Ibanez et al. 2003) is also used for parallel implementation for vessel segmentation algorithms in high-resolution images. The toolkit provides leading-edge segmentation and registration algorithms in two, three, and more dimensions and is implemented in C++, and it is wrapped for Tcl, Python, and Java. Alonso-Montes et al. (2005) presented a hardware-based algorithm where the segmentation is obtained through CNN-based histogram equalization and modification, local adaptive thresholding, and morphological opening. Pixel-level snakes (PLS) (Vilariño and Rekeczky 2005), a topographic iterative active contour technique, are used to extract the vascular tree using the initial contour of vessels and their external potential image. The algorithm is simulated in

TABLE 4.10

Performance Measures for the Model-Based Methodologies

Methodology	Database	Sensitivity	Specificity	Accuracy	Area under ROC
Vermeer et al. 2004	GDx (local database)	0.924	0.921	–	–
	STARE	–	–	0.9287	0.9187
Li et al. 2007	DRIVE	0.780	0.978	–	–
	STARE	0.752	0.980	–	–
Lam and Hong 2008	STARE	–	–	0.9474	0.9392
Lam et al. 2010	DRIVE	–	–	0.9472	0.9614
	STARE	–	–	0.9567	0.9739
Espona et al. 2007	DRIVE	0.6634	0.9682	0.9316	–
Espona et al. 2008	DRIVE	0.7436	0.9615	0.9352	–
Al-Diri et al. 2009	DRIVE	0.7282	0.9551	–	–
	STARE	0.7521	0.9681	–	–
Zhang et al. 2009	DRIVE		0.9772	0.9610	–
	STARE	0.7373	0.9736	0.9087	–
Yuan et al. 2011	DRIVE	–	–	–	0.9641
	STARE	–	–	–	0.9715

the MATCNN (Rekeczky 1997) environment using 3×3 linear CNN templates and implemented on a CNN chip-set architecture based on the CNN universal machine (CNNUM) (Roska and Chua 1993) paradigm.

A pixel-parallel approach for fast retinal vessel extraction is presented (Alonso-Montes et al. 2008), which in fact redefines the original proposal (Alonso-Montes et al. 2005) in terms of local dynamic convolutions and morphological operations together with arithmetic and logical operations to be implemented and tested in a fine-grain single-instruction multiple data (SIMD) parallel processor array (Dudek and Carey 2006). The exterior of vessels is found by parallel active contour, the PLS (Vilarino and Rekeczky 2004). The above-mentioned methods rely on several design parameters: the scaling factors of local mean and variance, the neighborhood size, and the structuring element for morphological operations. Since no guidelines are available for their settings, they must be empirically tuned. Moreover, nonlinear CNN templates are required for local estimation of the variance in the image. To overcome these issues, Renzo et al. (Costantini et al. 2010; Renzo et al. 2007) exploited the geometrical properties of blood vessels by calculating the line strength measures (Ricci and Perfetti 2007; Zwiggelaar et al. 2004) for the blood vessels in the green plane of the colored retinal image. The line strength image could be realized with simple CNN templates in a multistep operation with virtual template expansion. The proposed CNN algorithm requires only linear space-invariant 3×3 templates, so it could be implemented using one of the existing CNN chips. For example, the ACE16K chip is a 128×128 array with 7-bit accuracy, 8 analog grayscale memories per cell, and 32 stored templates (Linan et al. 2002). The algorithm gives better AUC and accuracy values for the same neighborhood size as compared with Alonso-Montes et al.'s algorithm (2008).

A parallel implementation (Palomera-Perez et al. 2010) of a multiscale vessel segmentation algorithm based on ITK (Perez et al. 2007) is capable of achieving accuracy comparable to its serial counterpart while processing eight to ten times faster, which is advantageous for handling for higher-resolution images and larger data sets. Table 4.11 illustrates the performance metrics for the algorithms based on parallel hardware implementations.

4.4 Retinal Vessel Width Measurement Algorithms

Many different techniques have been used to estimate vessel diameters, all of which are predicated upon the idea of measuring a vessel perpendicular to its local longitudinal orientation. Each method defines a cross-section and defines the vessel boundaries on

TABLE 4.11

Performance Measures for Parallel Hardware Implementation-Based Methods

Methodology	Database	Sensitivity	Specificity	Accuracy	Area under ROC
Renzo et al. 2007	DRIVE	–	–	0.9348	0.9261
Alonso-Montes et al. 2008	DRIVE	–	–	0.9185	0.9011
Palomera-Perez et al. 2010	DRIVE	0.64	0.967	0.9250	–
	STARE	0.769	0.9449	0.926	–

the cross-section between which the width is measured. Brinchmann-Hansen and Heier (1986) introduced a technique to measure blood vessel width from an intensity profile orthogonal to a retinal vessel. Their approach is called full width half maximum (FWHM), which identifies the minimum and maximum intensity levels on either side of the initial estimated midpoint of the profile. The half maximum is determined for both left and right sides of the profile by taking the mean of the minimum and maximum points on the left and repeating the process on the right. The FWHM estimate of the profile width is then the distance between the half maximums. Gregson et al. (1995) proposed an alternative approach to measure the width of an intensity profile. This model consists of a rectangular profile of a fixed height that is fitted to the profile data. The height of the rectangle profile is calculated by subtracting the minimum intensity level from the maximum intensity level. The width of the rectangular profile is then adjusted until the area under the rectangular profile is equal to the area under the profile data.

Heneghan et al. (2002) present the characterization of changes in blood vessel width and tortuosity in retinopathy of prematurity using image analysis. The method locates the blood vessel structure as a binary image by using morphological operations and a second derivative operator. The width at a particular point in the binary image is defined as the largest line segment passing through that point that can be contained within the foreground of the binary image, at all possible rotations. For this purpose, the line segment is extended from both sides of that point until a black (nonvessel) pixel is encountered. The distance between last two white (vessel) pixels encountered is taken as the width for that rotation. The smallest distance over all rotations is taken as the vessel width. Gang et al. (2002) have proposed the use of amplitude-modified second-order Gaussian filters to measure vessel width. It proves that the vessel width can be measured in a linear relationship with the spreading factor of the matched Gaussian filter when the magnitude coefficient of the Gaussian filter is suitably assigned. In the method proposed by Lowell et al. (2004), the diameter measurements are made by fitting a 2-D model, which resembles an idealized cross-sectional profile running along the length of a vessel segment in a small region of interest (ROI). The model is fitted on an intensity image produced by extracting the green channel from an original color digital image. Delibasis et al. (2010) presented a model-based tracing algorithm for vessel segmentation and diameter estimation. The algorithm utilizes a parametric model of a vessel composed of a "stripe" that exploits geometric properties for parameter definitions. A measure of match (MoM) is defined that quantifies the similarity between the model and the vessel profile in the given image. The seed-points for vessel tracking are indentified by splitting the binary output in nonoverlapping square blocks and picking a random nonzero pixel as a seed. The algorithm finds optimal model parameters at each seed-point that include strip orientation, strip width, and the MoM. There is a linear dependency between vessel diameter and model width parameter. Al-Diri et al. (2009) proposed an algorithm for segmentation and measurement of retinal blood vessels by growing a "ribbon of twins" active contour model, the extraction of segment profiles (ESP) algorithm, which uses two pairs of contours to capture each vessel edge. Most recently, an algorithm was proposed by Xu et al. (2011) to measure the width of retinal vessels in fundus photographs using a graph-based approach. A vessel centerline image is derived from the vesselness map and the bifurcation points and crossing points are excluded to obtain vessel segments. The two borders of the vessel segments are then processed simultaneously by transforming the first derivative of the vessel pixel intensities into a two-slice 3-D surface segmentation problem, which is further converted into the problem of computing a minimum closed set in a node-weighted graph.

4.5 Discussion

The performance of algorithms based on supervised classification is better in general than that of their counterparts. Almost all the supervised methods report an AUC of approximately 0.95 and among them Soares et al. (2006) reported the highest. However, these methods do require ground truth for training, which is often not available in case of screening programs and large population-based studies. Matched filtering has been extensively used for automated retinal vessel segmentation. Many improvements and modifications are proposed since the introduction of the Gaussian-matched filter by Chaudhuri et al. (1989). The parametric optimization of the matched filter using exhaustive search (Al-Rawi et al. 2007) and ant optimization (Cinsdikici and Aydin 2009) resulted in an improvement of segmentation accuracy from 0.8773 to 0.9535. The concept of steerable filters (Kochner et al. 1998) helps in the reduction of processing time. Matched filtering alone cannot handle vessel segmentation in pathological retinal images; therefore it is often employed in a multiscale manner and in combination with other image-processing techniques (Cinsdikici and Aydin 2009; Sofka and Stewart 2006). The problem of the central vessel reflex is solved by employing a mixture of the Gaussian model (Narasimha-Iyer et al. 2007; 2008) and ribbon of twin active contour (Al-Diri et al. 2009). The confidence measures and edge measures defined by Sofka and Stewart (2006) deal with the problem of overlapping of the nonvessel structures like the retinal boundary and the optic disc in vasculature extraction. The use of multiconcavity modeling (Lam et al. 2010) and the divergence of vector fields (Lam and Hong 2008) is quite successful in dealing with pathologies in the form of cotton wool spots, bright and dark lesions, and exudates. The supervised methods that have used moment invariant-based features with a neural network (Marin et al. 2011) and a decision tree-based ensemble classifier (Fraz et al. 2012c) are observed to be training set robust. The classifier is trained on the DRIVE database and the application to the STARE database yields high accuracy. The combination of radial projections with steerable wavelets and semisupervised classification (You et al. 2011) resulted in very good performance in the detection of narrow and low-contrast vessels, thus producing the highest sensitivity. A new view of vesselness measure based on local line integrals and variational optimization (Yuan et al. 2011) has been proposed with a discussion on the limitations of Hessian-based vessel enhancement methods. The Gabor wavelets are very useful in retinal image analysis. Besides vessel segmentation (Soares et al. 2006; Osareh and Shadgar 2009) and optic disc detection (Rangayyan et al. 2010), the Gabor wavelet transform has also been utilized for the robust fractal analysis of the retinal vasculature (Azemin et al. 2011).

The performance metrics based on contingency tables (Table 4.2) have been widely used for performance evaluation of binary classification. The metrics from this family include TPR (sensitivity), FPR (1-specificity), accuracy, positive predictive value, false discovery rate, and AUC. These metrics are based on measurement of success or failure rate in the detected pixels, obtained by means of pixel-to-pixel comparison between the automated segmentation and a manually labeled reference image. A new function for the evaluation of global quality in retinal vessel segmentation is proposed (Gegundez-Arias et al. 2012). It is based on the characterization of vascular structures as connected segments with measurable area and length and its design is meant to be sensitive to anatomical vascularity features. Therefore, this function gives a high degree of match with human quality perception and can be used to enhance evaluation in retinal vessel segmentation.

4.6 Conclusion and Future Directions

The segmentation of the blood vessels in the retina has been a heavily researched area in recent years. The accurate extraction of the retinal vascular tree forms the backbone of many automated computer-aided systems for screening and diagnosis of cardiovascular and ophthalmic diseases. Even though many promising techniques and algorithms have been developed, there is still room for improvement in blood vessel segmentation methodologies. Few of the reviewed algorithms serve for pathological and noisy retinal images (Lam and Hong 2008; Lam et al. 2010; Mahadevan et al. 2004; Sum and Cheung 2008; Zhu 2010) and there are even less that are suitable for analysis of images where vessels contain a central reflex (Al-Diri et al. 2009; Marin et al. 2011; Ricci and Perfetti 2007), as illustrated in Table 4.4. Most of the techniques available in the literature are evaluated on a limited range of data sets, which include 20 images each from the DRIVE and STARE databases. The performance measures presented in most of the papers are calculated on a small number of images of particular morphological characteristics. The limited range of images in the DRIVE and STARE databases do not cater for the image-related characteristics such as interimage and intraimage variability in luminance, drift in contrast, and uneven background gray-level values. The development of techniques that work for images acquired from different imaging equipment, under different environmental conditions, is also an open area for research in vessel segmentation algorithms.

One of the real-life practical applications of automatic blood vessel segmentation in health care is diabetic screening programs. The development of research software applications that integrate various computer-assisted retinal image analysis algorithms such as vessel extraction, registration, landmark tracing for pathologies, vessel caliber measurement, and branching and crossover detection is a new research direction. These kinds of applications can facilitate progress in studying the correlations of ocular fundus anatomy with retinal diseases.

To improve screening programs involving the evaluation of large image data sets, collaboration between experts and health-care centers is needed. In this direction, System for the Integration of Retinal Images Understanding Services (Sirius) (Ortega et al. 2010) is a web-based system for retinal image analysis that provides a collaborative framework for experts. Sirius consists of a web-based client user interface, a web application server for service delivery, and the service module for image-processing tasks. The system allows the sharing of images and processed results between remote computers and provides automated methods to diminish interexpert variability in the analysis of the images. A service module for the analysis of retinal microcirculation using a semiautomatic methodology for the computation of the arteriovenous ratio (AVR) is included in the framework. The service module could be further extended to include vessel width and tortuosity measures and detection of other pathologies in retinal images. Retinopathy Online Challenge (ROC) (Niemeijer et al. 2009b), a multiyear online competition for various aspects of diabetic retinopathy detection, is also an excellent collaborative effort for improving the computer-aided detection and diagnosis of diabetic retinopathy. The Retinal Image Vessel Extraction and Registration System (RIVERS) project (Stewart and Roysam; Tsai et al. 2008) can also be considered as an initiative in this direction. Vascular Assessment and Measurement Platform for Images of the REtina (VAMPIRE) (Perez-Rovira et al. 2011a) is a software application for semiautomatic quantification of retinal vessel properties. The system aims to provide efficient and reliable detection of retinal landmarks (optic disc, retinal zones, main vasculature) and quantify key parameters used frequently in investigative studies, including vessel width, vessel branching coefficients, and tortuosity measures. The creation of ground truths for vessel segmentation is a crucial task that entails training and skill. Live-Vessel (Kelvin et al. 2007) is a semi-automatic and interactive medical image segmentation software tool for locating vessels and vascular trees in 2-D color medical images.

Vessel extraction is often the first stage of processing before pathology detection algorithms are applied. There are thousands of images acquired from various types of fundus camera. In addition, most of the published algorithms are evaluated on the limited image data sets of DRIVE and STARE. The resolutions of images from the STARE and DRIVE data sets are limited to 0.4 and 0.3 megapixels, respectively. While this lower resolution is acceptable for certain analyses like fractal dimension or tortuosity, calculating the vessel diameter normally requires higher-resolution images to achieve higher precision. Mosher et al. (2006) have compared central retinal artery equivalents (CRAE) and central retinal vein equivalents (CRVE) of vessels measured from images of 6.3 megapixel resolution captured with a digital camera and digitized images taken with a film camera. Some artifacts like the nerve fiber are more visible in the higher-resolution images and may result in more false positives. The classification of retinal blood vessels into arterioles and venules is essential in clinical diagnosis for vessel caliber measurement and to calculate the CRAE/CRVE/AVR. Therefore, in order to expand the utility of vessel segmentation algorithms for health care, there is a need to create larger data sets with available ground truths that include the labeling of vessels and other anatomical structures and classification of arterioles and venules. Besides DRIVE and STARE, the other publicly available retinal image databases include CHASE_DB1 (Fraz 2011) for vessel segmentation and width measurement in child retinal images; REVIEW (Al-Diri et al. 2008) for vessel width measures; Messidor (2004), ImageRet (Kauppi et al. 2007), and ARIA Online (Damian Farnell 2006) for diabetic retinopathy; ROC microaneurysm set (Niemeijer et al. 2009b) for microaneurysm detection; and the VICAVR database (Ortega Hortas and Penas Centeno n.d.) for the computation of AVR.

Most segmentation methodologies are evaluated on the retinal images of adults. The morphological characteristics of retinal images of premature infants, babies, and children are very different from those of the adult retina. Choroidal vessels are more visible alongside the retinal vessels in retinal images taken from premature infants (Wilson et al. 2008). A bright central reflex on the vessels and illumination artifacts contribute to challenges in image processing when retinal images from schoolchildren are considered (Owen et al. 2009).

Advances in ophthalmic imaging systems (Bernardes et al. 2011) make it possible to gather high volumes of patient images for screening. Processing of these images in computer-aided diagnostic systems requires fast segmentation algorithms robust enough to process the images acquired from various image capture systems and imaging conditions. The algorithms exploiting parallel and hardware-based implementations (Alonso-Montes et al. 2005; Palomera-Perez et al. 2010; Renzo et al. 2007) offer a solution providing high computation speed that is required in real-time applications.

Three-dimensional optical coherence tomography (3-D OCT) imaging is used to obtain detailed images from within the retina and therefore improves visualization and mapping of the retinal microstructure. The availability of ultrawide field retinal images provided by Optos technologies (Optos, n.d.) and 3-D OCT triggers the need to develop faster, more accurate 3-D segmentation techniques, particularly focusing on retinal images taken from an ultrawide field of view, with pathologies and backgrounds of uneven intensity and illumination distribution. Perez-Rovira et al. (2011b) present improvement in this direction.

There are a relatively small number of anatomical structures visible in the retinal image obtained with a fundus camera if compared with other human organs, for example, the brain, heart, and lungs. Moreover, the expected morphology, size, and color variation across a population is expected to be high. Tobin et al. (2007) present a report on estimating retinal anatomic structure using a single retinal image, which can be the first step in the construction of a statistical retinal atlas using data from a large number of subjects.

Accuracy and robustness of the segmentation process is essential to achieve a more precise and efficient computer-aided diagnostic system. It is not expected that vessel segmentation systems will replace experts in diagnosis; rather they will reduce the workload of the experts in processing the sheer volume of medical images. This chapter provides a survey of current retinal blood vessel segmentation and caliber methods. We have covered both early and recent literature focusing on retinal vessel segmentation algorithms and techniques. Our aim was to introduce the current segmentation techniques, give the reader a framework for the existing research, and introduce the array of retinal vessel segmentation algorithms found in the literature. The current trends, the future directions, and the open problems in automated blood vessel segmentation are also discussed.

References

Abràmoff, M.D., M.K. Garvin and M. Sonka. 2010. Retinal imaging and image analysis. *IEEE Reviews in Biomedical Engineering*, 3: 169–208.

Akita, K. and H. Kuga. 1982. A computer method of understanding ocular fundus images. *Pattern Recognition*, 15(6): 431–443.

Al-Diri, B. and A. Hunter. 2005. A ribbon of twins for extracting vessel boundaries. In *The 3rd European Medical and Biological Engineering Conference*. Prague, Czech Republic.

Al-Diri, B., A. Hunter and D. Steel. 2009. An active contour model for segmenting and measuring retinal vessels. *IEEE Transactions on Medical Imaging*, 28(9): 1488–1497.

Al-Diri, B., A. Hunter, D. Steel, M. Habib, T. Hudaib and S. Berry. 2008. Review: A reference data set for retinal vessel profiles. In *30th Annual International Conference of the IEEE Engineering in Medicine and Biology Society*, pp. 2262–2265.

Ali, C., S. Hong, J.N. Turner, H.L. Tanenbaum and B. Roysam. 1999. Rapid automated tracing and feature extraction from retinal fundus images using direct exploratory algorithms. *IEEE Transactions on Information Technology in Biomedicine*, 3(2): 125–138.

Alonso-Montes, C., D.L. Vilarino and M.G. Penedo. 2005. CNN-based automatic retinal vascular tree extraction. In *9th International Workshop on Cellular Neural Networks and Their Applications*, pp. 61–64.

Alonso-Montes, C., D.L. Vilario, P. Dudek and M.G. Penedo. 2008. Fast retinal vessel tree extraction: A pixel parallel approach. *International Journal of Circuit Theory and Applications*, 36(5–6): 641–651.

Al-Rawi, M., M. Qutaishat and M. Arrar. 2007. An improved matched filter for blood vessel detection of digital retinal images. *Computers in Biology and Medicine*, 37(2): 262–267.

Amin, M.A. and H. Yan. 2010. High speed detection of retinal blood vessels in fundus image using phase congruency. *Soft Computing*, 15(6): 1217–1230.

Anzalone, A., F. Bizzarri, M. Parodi and M. Storace. 2008. A modular supervised algorithm for vessel segmentation in red-free retinal images. *Computers in Biology and Medicine*, 38(8): 913–922.

Ayala, G., T. Leon and V. Zapater. 2005. Different averages of a fuzzy set with an application to vessel segmentation. *IEEE Transactions on Fuzzy Systems*, 13(3): 384–393.

Azemin, M.Z.C., D.K. Kumar, T.Y. Wong, R. Kawasaki, P. Mitchell and J.J. Wang. 2011. Robust methodology for fractal analysis of the retinal vasculature. *IEEE Transactions on Medical Imaging*, 30(2): 243–250.

Baddeley, A.J., I.S. Molchanov, A.J. Baddeley and I.S. Molchanov. 1995. Averaging of random sets based on their distance functions. *Journal of Mathematical Imaging and Vision*, 8: 79–92.

Barrett, W.A. and E.N. Mortensen. 1997. Interactive live-wire boundary extraction. *Medical Image Analysis*, 1(4): 331–341.

Becker, D.E., A. Can, J.N. Turner, H.L. Tanenbaum and B. Roysam. 1998. Image processing algorithms for retinal montage synthesis, mapping, and real-time location determination. *IEEE Transactions on Biomedical Engineering*, 45(1): 105–118.

Bernardes, R., P. Serranho and C. Lobo. 2011. Digital ocular fundus imaging: A review. *Ophthalmologica*, 226(4): 161–181.

Brinchmann-Hansen, O. and H. Heier. 1986. The apparent and true width of the blood column in retinal vessels. *Acta Ophthalmologica*, 64(179): 29–32.

Broehan, A.M., T. Rudolph, C.A. Amstutz and J.H. Kowal. 2011. Real-time multimodal retinal image registration for a computer-assisted laser photocoagulation system. *IEEE Transactions on Biomedical Engineering*, 58(10): 2816–2824.

Can, A., C.V. Stewart, B. Roysam and H.L. Tanenbaum. 2002. A feature-based, robust, hierarchical algorithm for registering pairs of images of the curved human retina. *IEEE Transactions on Pattern Analysis and Machine Intelligence*, 24(3): 347–364.

Cassin, B., S.A.B. Solomon and M.L. Rubin. 1990. *Dictionary of Eye Terminology*, 2nd ed. Triad: Gainesville, FL.

Chan, T.F. and L.A. Vese. 2001. Active contours without edges. *IEEE Transactions on Image Processing*, 10(2): 266–277.

Chaudhuri, S., S. Chatterjee, N. Katz, M. Nelson and M. Goldbaum. 1989. Detection of blood vessels in retinal images using two-dimensional matched filters. *IEEE Transactions on Medical Imaging*, 8(3): 263–269.

Chua, L.O. and L. Yang. 1988. Cellular neural networks: Theory. *IEEE Transactions on Circuits and Systems*, 35(10): 1257–1272.

Chutatape, O., Z. Liu and S.M. Krishnan. 1998. Retinal blood vessel detection and tracking by matched Gaussian and Kalman filters. In *Proceedings of the 20th Annual International Conference of the IEEE Engineering in Medicine and Biology Society*, vol. 6, pp. 3144–3149.

Cinsdikici, M.G. and D. Aydin. 2009. Detection of blood vessels in ophthalmoscope images using MF/ant (matched filter/ant colony) algorithm. *Computer Methods and Programs in Biomedicine*, 96(2): 85–95.

Condurache, A.P. and A. Mertins. 2012. Segmentation of retinal vessels with a hysteresis binary-classification paradigm. *Computerized Medical Imaging and Graphics*, 36(4): 325–335.

Costantini, G., D. Casali and M. Todisco. 2010. A hardware-implementable system for retinal vessel segmentation. In *Proceedings of the 14th WSEAS International Conference on Computers: Part of the 14th WSEAS CSCC Multiconference – Vol. II*, pp. 568–573. WSEAS; Stevens Point, Wisconsin, USA: World Scientific and Engineering Academy and Society.

Delibasis, K.K., A.I. Kechriniotis, C. Tsonos and N. Assimakis. 2010. Automatic model-based tracing algorithm for vessel segmentation and diameter estimation. *Computer Methods and Programs in Biomedicine*, 100(2): 108–122.

Duda, R.O., P.E. Hart and D.G. Stork. 2000. *Pattern Classification*. 2nd ed. Wiley-Interscience: Hoboken, NJ.

Dudek, P. and S.J. Carey. 2006. General-purpose 128 × 128 SIMD processor array with integrated image sensor. *Electronics Letters*, 42(12): 678–679.

Espona, L., M.J. Carreira, M. Ortega and M.G. Penedo. 2007. A snake for retinal vessel segmentation. Paper presented at the *Proceedings of the 3rd Iberian Conference on Pattern Recognition and Image Analysis*, Part II, Girona, Spain.

Espona, L., M.J. Carreira, M.G. Penedo and M. Ortega. 2008. Retinal vessel tree segmentation using a deformable contour model. In *19th International Conference on Pattern Recognition*, pp. 1–4.

Farnell, D.J.J., F.N. Hatfield, P. Knox, M. Reakes, S. Spencer, D. Parry and S.P. Harding. 2008. Enhancement of blood vessels in digital fundus photographs via the application of multiscale line operators. *Journal of the Franklin Institute*, 345(7): 748–765.

Fathi, A. and A.R. Naghsh-Nilchi. 2013. Automatic wavelet-based retinal blood vessels segmentation and vessel diameter estimation. *Biomedical Signal Processing and Control*, 8(1): 71–80.

Field, C. and B. Smith. 1994. Robust estimation: A weighted maximum-likelihood approach. *International Statistical Review*, 62(3): 405–424.

Foracchia, M. 2001. Extraction and quantitative description of vessel features in hypertensive retinopathy fundus images. In Grisan, E. (ed.), *Book Abstracts 2nd International Workshop on Computer Assisted Fundus Image Analysis*, p. 6.

Frangi, A.F., W.J. Niessen, K.L. Vincken, M.A. Viergever, W. William, C. Alan and D. Scott. 1998. Multiscale vessel enhancement filtering. In *Medical Image Computing and Computer-Assisted Intervention Miccai™98*, p. 130. Springer: Berlin/Heidelberg.

Fraz, M.M. 2011. Child Health and Heart Study in England. Chase_db1. Kingston University: London. http://sec.kingston.ac.uk/retinal/CHASE_DB1.

Fraz, M.M., S.A. Barman, P. Remagnino, A. Hoppe, A. Basit, B. Uyyanonvara, A.R. Rudnicka and C.G. Owen. 2012a. An approach to localize the retinal blood vessels using bit planes and centerline detection. *Computer Methods and Programs in Biomedicine*, 108(2): 600–606.

Fraz, M.M., S.A. Barman, P. Remagnino, A. Hoppe, A. Basit, B. Uyyanonvara, A.R. Rudnicka and C.G. Owen. 2012b. Blood vessel segmentation methodologies in retinal images—A survey. *Computer Methods and Programs in Biomedicine*, 108(1): 407–433.

Fraz, M.M., P. Remagnino, A. Hoppe, B. Uyyanonvara, A.R. Rudnicka, C.G. Owen and S.A. Barman. 2012c. An ensemble classification based approach applied to retinal blood vessel segmentation. *IEEE Transactions on Biomedical Engineering*, 59(9): 2538–2548.

Fraz, M.M., P. Remagnino, A. Hoppe, B. Uyyanonvara, C. Owen, A. Rudnicka and S. Barman. 2011. Retinal vessel extraction using first-order derivative of Gaussian and morphological processing. In Bebis, G., Boyle, R., Parvin, B., Koracin, D., Wang, S., Kyungnam, K., Benes, B., et al. (eds), *Advances in Visual Computing*. Springer: Berlin, pp. 410–420.

Freeman, W.T. and E.H. Adelson. 1991. The design and use of steerable filters. *IEEE Transactions on Pattern Analysis and Machine Intelligence*, 13: 891–906.

Gang, L., O. Chutatape and S.M. Krishnan. 2002. Detection and measurement of retinal vessels in fundus images using amplitude modified second-order Gaussian filter. *IEEE Transactions on Biomedical Engineering*, 49(2): 168–172.

Gegundez-Arias, M.E., A. Aquino, J.M. Bravo and D. Marin. 2012. A function for quality evaluation of retinal vessel segmentations. *IEEE Transactions on Medical Imaging*, 31(2): 231–239.

Gregson, P.H., Z. Shen, R.C. Scott and V. Kozousek. 1995. Automated grading of venous beading. *Computers and Biomedical Research*, 28(4): 291–304.

Heneghan, C., J. Flynn, M. O'Keefe and M. Cahill. 2002. Characterization of changes in blood vessel width and tortuosity in retinopathy of prematurity using image analysis. *Medical Image Analysis*, 6(4): 407–429.

Hong, S., B. Roysam, C.V. Stewart, J.N. Turner and H.L. Tanenbaum. 2001. Optimal scheduling of tracing computations for real-time vascular landmark extraction from retinal fundus images. *IEEE Transactions on Information Technology in Biomedicine*, 5(1): 77–91.

Hoover, A.D., V. Kouznetsova and M. Goldbaum. 2000. Locating blood vessels in retinal images by piecewise threshold probing of a matched filter response. *IEEE Transactions on Medical Imaging*, 19(3): 203–210.

Huber, P.J. 1965. A robust version of the probability ratio test. *The Annals of Mathematical Statistics*, 36(6): 1753–1758.

Huiqi, L. and O. Chutatape. 2004. Automated feature extraction in color retinal images by a model based approach. *IEEE Transactions on Biomedical Engineering*, 51(2): 246–254.

Ibanez, L., W. Schroeder, L. Ng and J. Cates. 2003. The ITK software guide. Kitware. http://www.itk.org/ItkSoftwareGuide.pdf.

Ikram, M.K., J.C.M. Witteman, J.R. Vingerling, M.M.B. Breteler, A. Hofman and P.T.V.M. De Jong. 2006. Retinal vessel diameters and risk of hypertension. *Hypertension*, 47(2): 189–194.

Image Sciences Institute. n.d. Drive: Digital retinal images for vessel extraction. http://www.isi.uu.nl/Research/Databases/DRIVE/.

Jelinek H.E. and M.J. Cree. 2009. *Automated Image Detection of Retinal Pathology.* CRC Press: Boca Raton, FL.

Kanski, J.J. and B. Bowling. 2011. *Clinical Ophthalmology: A Systematic Approach.* 7th ed. London: Elsevier Health Sciences.

Kande, G.B., P.V. Subbaiah and T.S. Savithri. 2009. Unsupervised fuzzy based vessel segmentation in pathological digital fundus images. *Journal of Medical Systems,* 34(5): 849–858.

Kass, M., A. Witkin and D. Terzopoulos. 1988. Snakes: Active contour models. *International Journal of Computer Vision,* 1(4): 321–331.

Kauppi, T., V. Kalesnykiene, J.-K. Kamarainen, L. Lensu, I. Sorri, A. Raninen, R. Voutilainen, J. Pietilä, H. Kälviäinen and H. Uusitalo. 2007. *Diaretdb1* diabetic retinopathy database and evaluation protocol. In *Medical Image Understanding and Analysis (MIUA2007),* pp. 61–65. Aberystwyth.

Kelvin, P., H. Ghassan and A. Rafeef. 2007. Live-vessel: Extending livewire for simultaneous extraction of optimal medial and boundary paths in vascular images. Paper presented at the *Proceedings of the 10th International Conference on Medical Image Computing and Computer-Assisted Intervention,* Brisbane, Australia.

Kirbas, C. and F. Quek. 2004. A review of vessel extraction techniques and algorithms. *ACM Computing Surveys,* 36(2): 81–121.

Kochner, B., D. Schuhmann, M. Michaelis, G. Mann and K.-H. Englmeier. 1998. Course tracking and contour extraction of retinal vessels from color fundus photographs: Most efficient use of steerable filters for model-based image analysis. In *Medical Imaging 1998: Image Processing,* pp. 755–761. San Diego, CA: SPIE.

Köse, C. and C. İki̇'baş. 2011. A personal identification system using retinal vasculature in retinal fundus images. *Expert Systems with Applications,* 38(11): 13670–13681.

Krissian, K., G. Maladain, R. Vaillant, Y. Trousset and N. Ayache. 1998. Model-based multiscale detection of 3D vessels. In *Proceedings of the IEEE Computer Society Conference on Computer Vision and Pattern Recognition,* pp. 722–727.

Lam, B.S.Y. and Y. Hong. 2008. A novel vessel segmentation algorithm for pathological retina images based on the divergence of vector fields. *IEEE Transactions on Medical Imaging,* 27(2): 237–246.

Lam, B.S.Y., G. Yongsheng and A.W.C. Liew. 2010. General retinal vessel segmentation using regularization-based multiconcavity modeling. *IEEE Transactions on Medical Imaging,* 29(7): 1369–1381.

Lei, Z., L. Qin, J. You and D. Zhang. 2009. A modified matched filter with double-sided thresholding for screening proliferative diabetic retinopathy. *IEEE Transactions on Information Technology in Biomedicine,* 13(4): 528–534.

Leung, H., J.J. Wang, E. Rochtchina, A.G. Tan, T.Y. Wong, R. Klein, L.D. Hubbard and P. Mitchell. 2003. Relationships between age, blood pressure, and retinal vessel diameters in an older population. *Investigative Ophthalmology & Visual Science,* 44(7): 2900–2904.

Li, Q., S. Sone and K. Doi. 2003. Selective enhancement filters for nodules, vessels, and airway walls in two- and three-dimensional CT scans. *Medical Physics,* 30(8): 2040–2051.

Li, Q., J. You and D. Zhang. 2012. Vessel segmentation and width estimation in retinal images using multiscale production of matched filter responses. *Expert Systems with Applications,* 39(9): 7600–7610.

Li, W., A. Bhalerao and R. Wilson. 2007. Analysis of retinal vasculature using a multiresolution hermite model. *IEEE Transactions on Medical Imaging,* 26(2): 137–152.

Liang, Z., M.S. Rzeszotarski, L.J. Singerman and J.M. Chokreff. 1994. The detection and quantification of retinopathy using digital angiograms. *IEEE Transactions on Medical Imaging,* 13(4): 619–626.

Linan, G., A. Rodriguez-Vazquez, S. Espejo and R. Dominguez-Castro. 2002. ACE16k: A 128 × 128 focal plane analog processor with digital i/o. In *Proceedings of the 2002 7th IEEE International Workshop on Cellular Neural Networks and Their Applications,* pp. 132–139.

Liu, I. and Y. Sun. 1993. Recursive tracking of vascular networks in angiograms based on the detection-deletion scheme. *IEEE Transactions on Medical Imaging,* 12(2): 334–341.

Lowell, J., A. Hunter, D. Steel, A. Basu, R. Ryder and R.L. Kennedy. 2004. Measurement of retinal vessel widths from fundus images based on 2-D modeling. *IEEE Transactions on Medical Imaging,* 23(10): 1196–1204.

Lupascu, C.A., D. Tegolo and E. Trucco. 2010. FABC: Retinal vessel segmentation using adaboost. *IEEE Transactions on Information Technology in Biomedicine*, 14(5): 1267–1274.

Mahadevan, V., H. Narasimha-Iyer, B. Roysam and H.L. Tanenbaum. 2004. Robust model-based vasculature detection in noisy biomedical images. *IEEE Transactions on Information Technology in Biomedicine*, 8(3): 360–376.

Marco, D. and S. Thomas. 2004. *Ant Colony Optimization*. Bradford Company: Scituate, MA.

Marin, D., A. Aquino, M.E. Gegundez-Arias and J.M. Bravo. 2011. A new supervised method for blood vessel segmentation in retinal images by using gray-level and moment invariants-based features. *IEEE Transactions on Medical Imaging*, 30(1): 146–158.

Martinez-Perez, M.E., A.D. Hughes, A.V. Stanton, S.A. Thorn, N. Chapman, A.A. Bharath and K.H. Parker. 2002. Retinal vascular tree morphology: A semi-automatic quantification. *IEEE Transactions on Biomedical Engineering*, 49(8): 912–917.

Martinez-Perez, M.E., A.D. Hughes, A.V. Stanton, S.A. Thom, A.A. Bharath and K.H. Parker. 1999. Retinal blood vessel segmentation by means of scale-space analysis and region growing. In *Proceedings of the Second International Conference on Medical Image Computing and Computer-Assisted Intervention*, pp. 90–97. London, UK: Springer-Verlag.

Martinez-Perez, M.E., A.D. Hughes, S.A. Thom, A.A. Bharath and K.H. Parker. 2007. Segmentation of blood vessels from red-free and fluorescein retinal images. *Medical Image Analysis*, 11(1): 47–61.

Mendonca, A.M. and A. Campilho. 2006. Segmentation of retinal blood vessels by combining the detection of centerlines and morphological reconstruction. *IEEE Transactions on Medical Imaging*, 25(9): 1200–1213.

Messidor. 2004. Messidor: Methods to evaluate segmentation and indexing techniques in the field of to retinal ophthalmology. http://messidor.crihan.fr/download-en.php.

Miri, M.S. and A. Mahloojifar. 2011. Retinal image analysis using curvelet transform and multistructure elements morphology by reconstruction. *IEEE Transactions on Biomedical Engineering*, 58(5): 1183–1192.

Moghimirad, E., S. Hamid Rezatofighi and H. Soltanian-Zadeh. 2012. Retinal vessel segmentation using a multi-scale medialness function. *Computers in Biology and Medicine*, 42(1): 50–60.

Mosher, A., B.E.K. Klein, R. Klein, M.D. Knudtson and N.J. Ferrier. 2006. Comparison of retinal vessel measurements in digital vs film images. *American Journal of Ophthalmology*, 142(5): 875–878.

Narasimha-Iyer, H., J.M. Beach, B. Khoobehi and B. Roysam. 2007. Automatic identification of retinal arteries and veins from dual-wavelength images using structural and functional features. *IEEE Transactions on Biomedical Engineering*, 54(8): 1427–1435.

Narasimha-Iyer, H., V. Mahadevan, J.M. Beach and B. Roysam. 2008. Improved detection of the central reflex in retinal vessels using a generalized dual-gaussian model and robust hypothesis testing. *IEEE Transactions on Information Technology in Biomedicine*, 12(3): 406–410.

Nekovei, R. and S. Ying. 1995. Back-propagation network and its configuration for blood vessel detection in angiograms. *IEEE Transactions on Neural Networks*, 6(1): 64–72.

Ng, J., S.T. Clay, S.A. Barman, A.R. Fielder, M.J. Moseley, K.H. Parker and C. Paterson. 2010. Maximum likelihood estimation of vessel parameters from scale space analysis. *Image and Vision Computing*, 28(1): 55–63.

Niemeijer, M., M.D. Abràmoff and B. Van Ginneken. 2009a. Fast detection of the optic disc and fovea in color fundus photographs. *Medical Image Analysis*, 13(6): 859–870.

Niemeijer, M., B. Van Ginneken, M.J. Cree, A. Mizutani, G. Quellec, C.I. Sanchez, B. Zhang, et al. 2009b. Retinopathy online challenge: Automatic detection of microaneurysms in digital color fundus photographs. *IEEE Transactions on Medical Imaging*, 29(1): 185–195.

Niemeijer, M., J.J. Staal, B. van Ginneken, M. Loog and M.D. Abràmoff. 2004. Comparative study of retinal vessel segmentation methods on a new publicly available database. In Fitzpatrick, J.M. and Sonka, M. (eds), *SPIE Medical Imaging*. SPIE, vol. 5370, pp. 648–656.

Niemeijer, M., X. Xiayu, A.V. Dumitrescu, P. Gupta, B. Van Ginneken, J.C. Folk and M.D. Abramoff. 2011. Automated measurement of the arteriolar-to-venular width ratio in digital color fundus photographs. *IEEE Transactions on Medical Imaging*, 30(11): 1941–1950.

Optos. n.d. Optomap image library. http://www.optos.com/en-us/Professionals/Image-library/ (accessed July 2012).

Ortega, M., N. Barreira, J. Novo, M.G. Penedo, A. Pose-Reino and F. Gómez-Ulla. 2010. Sirius: A web-based system for retinal image analysis. *International Journal of Medical Informatics*, 79(10): 722–732.

Ortega Hortas, M. and M. Penas Centeno. n.d. VICAVR database. http://www.varpa.es/vicavr.html.

Osareh, A. and B. Shadgar. 2009. Automatic blood vessel segmentation in color images of retina. *Iranian Journal of Science and Technology Transaction B-Engineering*, 33(B2): 191–206.

Owen, C.G., A.R. Rudnicka, R. Mullen, S.A. Barman, D. Monekosso, P.H. Whincup, J. Ng and C. Paterson. 2009. Measuring retinal vessel tortuosity in 10-year-old children: Validation of the computer-assisted image analysis of the retina (CAIAR) program. *Investigative Ophthalmology & Visual Science*, 50(5): 2004–2010.

Owen, C.G., A.R. Rudnicka, C.M. Nightingale, R. Mullen, S.A. Barman, N. Sattar, D.G. Cook and P.H. Whincup. 2011. Retinal arteriolar tortuosity and cardiovascular risk factors in a multi-ethnic population study of 10-year-old children; the child heart and health study in England (CHASE). *Arteriosclerosis, Thrombosis, and Vascular Biology*, 31(8):1933–1938.

Palomera-Perez, M.A., M.E. Martinez-Perez, H. Benitez-Perez and J.L. Ortega-Arjona. 2010. Parallel multiscale feature extraction and region growing: Application in retinal blood vessel detection. *IEEE Transactions on Information Technology in Biomedicine*, 14(2): 500–506.

Perez-Rovira, A., T. Macgillivray, E. Trucco, K.S. Chin, K. Zutis, C. Lupascu, D. Tegolo, et al. 2011a. Vampire: Vessel assessment and measurement platform for images of the retina. In *2011 Annual International Conference of the IEEE Engineering in Medicine and Biology Society, EMBC*, pp. 3391–3394.

Perez-Rovira, A., K. Zutis, J.P. Hubschman and E. Trucco. 2011b. Improving vessel segmentation in ultra-wide field-of-view retinal fluorescein angiograms. In *2011 Annual International Conference of the IEEE Engineering in Medicine and Biology Society, EMBC*, pp. 2614–2617.

Perez, M.E.M., A.D. Hughes, S.A. Thorn and K.H. Parker. 2007. Improvement of a retinal blood vessel segmentation method using the insight segmentation and registration toolkit (ITK). In *29th Annual International Conference of the IEEE Engineering in Medicine and Biology Society*, pp. 892–895.

Quek, F.K.H. and C. Kirbas. 2001. Vessel extraction in medical images by wave-propagation and traceback. *IEEE Transactions on Medical Imaging*, 20(2): 117–131.

Quellec, G., M. Lamard, M.D. Abràmoff, E. Decencière, B. Lay, A. Erginay, B. Cochener and G. Cazuguel. 2012. A multiple-instance learning framework for diabetic retinopathy screening. *Medical Image Analysis*, 16(6): 1228–1240.

Ramlugun, G.S., V.K. Nagarajan and C. Chakraborty. 2012. Small retinal vessels extraction towards proliferative diabetic retinopathy screening. *Expert Systems with Applications*, 39(1): 1141–1146.

Rangayyan, R., X. Zhu, F. Ayres and A. Ells. 2010. Detection of the optic nerve head in fundus images of the retina with Gabor filters and phase portrait analysis. *Journal of Digital Imaging*, 23(4): 438–453.

Rekeczky, C. 1997. MATCNN: Analogic simulation toolbox for Matlab. Analogic and Neural Computing Laboratory, Computer and Automation Institute.

Renzo, P., R. Elisa, C. Daniele and C. Giovanni. 2007. Cellular neural networks with virtual template expansion for retinal vessel segmentation. *IEEE Transactions on Circuits and Systems II: Express Briefs*, 54(2): 141–145.

Ricci, E. and R. Perfetti. 2007. Retinal blood vessel segmentation using line operators and support vector classification. *IEEE Transactions on Medical Imaging*, 26(10): 1357–1365.

Ronchetti, E. 1985. Robust model selection in regression. *Statistics & Probability Letters*, 3(1): 21–23.

Roska, T. and L.O. Chua. 1993. The CNN universal machine: An analogic array computer. *IEEE Transactions on Circuits and Systems II: Analog and Digital Signal Processing*, 40(3): 163–173.

Saine, P.J. and M.E. Tyler. 2002. *Ophthalmic Photography: Retinal Photography, Angiography, and Electronic Imaging*. 2nd ed. Boston: Butterworth-Heinemann.

Salem, S., N. Salem and A. Nandi. 2007. Segmentation of retinal blood vessels using a novel clustering algorithm (RACAL) with a partial supervision strategy. *Medical and Biological Engineering and Computing*, 45(3): 261–273.

Serra, J. 1983. *Image Analysis and Mathematical Morphology*. Orlando, FL: Academic Press.

Shijian, L. and L. Joo Hwee. 2011. Automatic optic disc detection from retinal images by a line operator. *IEEE Transactions on Biomedical Engineering*, 58(1): 88–94.

Simó, A. and E. De Ves. 2001. Segmentation of macular fluorescein angiographies. A statistical approach. *Pattern Recognition*, 34(4): 795–809.

Sinthanayothin, C., J.F. Boyce, H.L. Cook and T.H. Williamson. 1999. Automated localisation of the optic disc, fovea, and retinal blood vessels from digital colour fundus images. *British Journal of Ophthalmology*, 83(8): 902–910.

Soares, J.V.B., J.J.G. Leandro, R.M. Cesar, H.F. Jelinek and M.J. Cree. 2006. Retinal vessel segmentation using the 2-D Gabor wavelet and supervised classification. *IEEE Transactions on Medical Imaging*, 25(9): 1214–1222.

Sofka, M. and C.V. Stewart. 2006. Retinal vessel centerline extraction using multiscale matched filters, confidence and edge measures. *IEEE Transactions on Medical Imaging*, 25(12): 1531–1546.

Staal, J., M.D. Abràmoff, M. Niemeijer, M.A. Viergever and B. Van Ginneken. 2004. Ridge-based vessel segmentation in color images of the retina. *IEEE Transactions on Medical Imaging*, 23(4): 501–509.

Stewart, C.V. and B. Roysam. Rivers: Retinal image vessel extraction and registration system. Rensselaer Computer Science, Troy, NY. http://cgi-vision.cs.rpi.edu/cgi/RIVERS/.

Stoyan, D. and H. Stoyan. 1994. *Fractals, Random Shapes and Point Fields: Methods of Geometrical Statistics*. New York: John Wiley.

Sukkaew, L., B. Uyyanonvara, S. Barman, A. Fielder and K. Cocker. 2007. Automatic extraction of the structure of the retinal blood vessel network of premature infants. *Journal of the Medical Association of Thailand*, 90(9): 1780–1792.

Sum, K.W. and P.Y.S. Cheung. 2008. Vessel extraction under non-uniform illumination: A level set approach. *IEEE Transactions on Biomedical Engineering*, 55(1): 358–360.

Sun, K., Z. Chen, S. Jiang and Y. Wang. 2010. Morphological multiscale enhancement, fuzzy filter and watershed for vascular tree extraction in angiogram. *Journal of Medical Systems*, 35(5): 811–824.

Thomas, L. and M.K. Jason. 1998. *Image Processing Using Pulse-Coupled Neural Networks*. New York: Springer-Verlag.

Tobin, K.W., E. Chaum, V.P. Govindasamy and T.P. Karnowski. 2007. Detection of anatomic structures in human retinal imagery. *IEEE Transactions on Medical Imaging*, 26(12): 1729–1739.

Tolias, Y.A. and S.M. Panas. 1998. A fuzzy vessel tracking algorithm for retinal images based on fuzzy clustering. *IEEE Transactions on Medical Imaging*, 17(2): 263–273.

Tong, C.S., Y. Zhang and N. Zheng. 2005. Variational image binarization and its multi-scale realizations. *Journal of Mathematical Imaging and Vision*, 23(2): 185–198.

Tsai, C.L., B. Madore, M.J. Leotta, M. Sofka, G. Yang, A. Majerovics, H.L. Tanenbaum, C.V. Stewart and B. Roysam. 2008. Automated retinal image analysis over the internet. *IEEE Transactions on Information Technology in Biomedicine*, 12(4): 480–487.

Vermeer, K.A., F.M. Vos, H.G. Lemij and A.M. Vossepoel. 2004. A model based method for retinal blood vessel detection. *Computers in Biology and Medicine*, 34(3): 209–219.

Vilarino, D.L. and C. Rekeczky. 2004. Implementation of a pixel-level snake algorithm on a CNNUM-based chip set architecture. *IEEE Transactions on Circuits and Systems I: Regular Papers*, 51(5): 885–891.

Vilariño, D.L. and C. Rekeczky. 2005. Pixel-level snakes on the CNNUM: Algorithm design, on-chip implementation and applications. *International Journal of Circuit Theory and Applications*, 33(1): 17–51.

Villalobos-Castaldi, F., E. Felipe-Riverón and L. Sánchez-Fernández. 2010. A fast, efficient and automated method to extract vessels from fundus images. *Journal of Visualization*, 13(3): 263–270.

Vlachos, M. and E. Dermatas. 2009. Multi-scale retinal vessel segmentation using line tracking. *Computerized Medical Imaging and Graphics*, 34(3): 213–227.

Wilson, C.M., K.D. Cocker, M.J. Moseley, C. Paterson, S.T. Clay, W.E. Schulenburg, M.D. Mills, et al. 2008. Computerized analysis of retinal vessel width and tortuosity in premature infants. *Investigative Ophthalmology & Visual Science*, 49(8): 3577–3585.

Wink, O., W.J. Niessen and M.A. Viergever. 2004. Multiscale vessel tracking. *IEEE Transactions on Medical Imaging*, 23(1): 130–133.

Xiaohong, G., A. Bharath, A. Stanton, A. Hughes, N. Chapman and S. Thom. 2001. A method of vessel tracking for vessel diameter measurement on retinal images. In *International Conference on Image Processing*, pp. 881–884. Thessaloniki, Greece.

Xiaoyi, J. and D. Mojon. 2003. Adaptive local thresholding by verification-based multithreshold probing with application to vessel detection in retinal images. *IEEE Transactions on Pattern Analysis and Machine Intelligence*, 25(1): 131–137.

Xu, L. and S. Luo. 2010. A novel method for blood vessel detection from retinal images. *BioMedical Engineering OnLine*, 9(1): 14.

Xu, X., M. Niemeijer, Q. Song, M. Sonka, M.K. Garvin, J.M. Reinhardt and M.D. Abràmoff. 2011. Vessel boundary delineation on fundus images using graph-based approach. *IEEE Transactions on Medical Imaging*, 30(6): 1184–1191.

Yang, Y., S. Huang and N. Rao. 2008. An automatic hybrid method for retinal blood vessel extraction. *International Journal of Applied Mathematics and Computer Science*, 18(3): 399–407.

Yao, C. and H.-J. Chen. 2009. Automated retinal blood vessels segmentation based on simplified PCNN and fast 2D-Otsu algorithm. *Journal of Central South University of Technology*, 16(4): 640–646.

Yin, Y., M. Adel and S. Bourennane. 2012. Retinal vessel segmentation using a probabilistic tracking method. *Pattern Recognition*, 45(4): 1235–1244.

You, X., Q. Peng, Y. Yuan, Y.-M. Cheung and J. Lei. 2011. Segmentation of retinal blood vessels using the radial projection and semi-supervised approach. *Pattern Recognition*, 44(10–11): 2314–2324.

Yuan, Y., L. Yishan and A.C.S. Chung. 2011. VE-LLI-VO: Vessel enhancement using local line integrals and variational optimization. *IEEE Transactions on Image Processing*, 20(7): 1912–1924.

Zana, F. and J.C. Klein. 1999. A multimodal registration algorithm of eye fundus images using vessels detection and Hough transform. *IEEE Transactions on Medical Imaging*, 18(5): 419–428.

Zana, F. and J.C. Klein. 2001. Segmentation of vessel-like patterns using mathematical morphology and curvature evaluation. *IEEE Transactions on Image Processing*, 10(7): 1010–1019.

Zhang, B., L. Zhang, L. Zhang and F. Karray. 2010. Retinal vessel extraction by matched filter with first-order derivative of Gaussian. *Computers in Biology and Medicine*, 40(4): 438–445.

Zhang, Y., W. Hsu and M. Lee. 2009. Detection of retinal blood vessels based on nonlinear projections. *Journal of Signal Processing Systems*, 55(1): 103–112.

Zhu, T. 2010. Fourier cross-sectional profile for vessel detection on retinal images. *Computerized Medical Imaging and Graphics*, 34(3): 203–212.

Zwiggelaar, R., S.M. Astley, C.R.M. Boggis and C.J. Taylor. 2004. Linear structures in mammographic images: Detection and classification. *IEEE Transactions on Medical Imaging*, 23(9): 1077–1086.

5

Segmentation of the Vascular Network of the Retina

Ana Maria Mendonça, Behdad Dashtbozorg, and Aurélio Campilho

CONTENTS

5.1 Introduction

The retina is a unique region where the vascular condition can be observed *in vivo*. It is a window to the systemic vasculature, as the retinal blood vessels are exposed to the same stresses and pathologies as the whole vascular system. The retinal vasculature status can be evaluated with high-resolution eye fundus color images, and variations in the retinal microcirculation can be used as an indicator of a lesion in the cerebral microvasculature. The features measured on these images can characterize retinal arteriolar narrowing, which is a marker of hypertension, or diabetic retinopathy (DR).

Fundus photography is a well-established technique for retinal imaging and is widely used for screening and the large-scale detection of DR, glaucoma, and age-related macular degeneration, which are the leading causes of blindness in the developed world. From an analysis of retinal images, we are able to derive quantitative and objective indicators that reflect the retinal morphology and condition. During the last three decades, the image analysis research community has made many contributions, including: (a) the detection and segmentation of images of structures, such as the retinal vessels, the optic disc, and the fovea; and (b) the segmentation of retinal abnormalities, such as hemorrhages, micro-aneurysms, neovascularization, and drusen, among others.

In this chapter, we focus on the segmentation of the blood vessels in high-resolution retinal images. First, recent methods (from the last two to three years) for the analysis of retinal images are outlined based on a survey of papers on segmentation methodologies and their clinical applications. In the following sections, we detail our methodology for blood vessel retinal segmentation, with a special emphasis on the segmentation of high-resolution fundus images and its validation on the arteriovenous ratio (AVR) calculation.

The report presented herein is an extended version of a previous work by the authors, which applied to low-resolution retinal images [1]. The high-resolution fundus images, although presenting a more detailed representation of the vessels, particularly important in the thin vessels, also raise new challenges, as the presence of a central reflex is especially visible in the larger vessels. In this situation, the conventional approach usually gives rise to the separation of a blood vessel into two segments, which is an obstacle to obtaining reliable quantitative measures of the blood vessel. With the new approach described herein, we are able to overcome this oversegmentation problem. To validate our approach, we measured the AVR and compared our results with expert measurements.

5.2 Recent Research on Retinal Image Analysis

The medical imaging community is making great efforts to develop automatic methods to characterize retinal lesions, many of them requiring the characterization of the retinal vasculature. There are several approaches to the segmentation of the retinal blood vessels, with the main challenge being to accurately and automatically delineate the vessels in order to detect pathological changes. The authors of papers on blood vessel segmentation methods have proposed different image analysis approaches in order to improve the sensitivity and specificity of their methods. Efforts are being made to automate the process and to make the results independent or adaptive to images acquired under different conditions and by different apparatus. Several different labeled retinal data sets are publicly available to the research community to validate and compare its approaches. Segmentation is only the first step in the pathological categorization of the retinal status and the subsequent clinical diagnosis. To provide a global overview of the different issues involved in retinal image analysis, we briefly survey the recent research developments for vessel segmentation in retinal images, organizing the articles from an image analysis and a clinical application point of view, together with addressing the evaluation and validation efforts made so far. This brief survey on the recent methods, which have been published in the last 2–3 years, is organized as follows: (a) retinal data sets used for evaluation; (b) review and survey articles; (c) retinal blood vessel segmentation methodologies; and (d) clinical applications.

5.2.1 Retinal Data Sets Used for Evaluation

The archives of the fundus images that are commonly used to evaluate retinal vessel segmentation algorithms are detailed as follows.

The digital retinal image for vessel extraction (DRIVE) database [2] contains 40 color images of 565 × 584 pixels in size that were captured in digital form using a Canon CR5 nonmydriatic three-charge-coupled device (3CCD) camera at 45° field of view (FOV) as part of a screening program in the Netherlands. Two sets of manually segmented binary images showing the blood vessels were made available by the authors.

The image data in the structured analysis of the retina (STARE) archive are 700 × 605 red-green-blue (RGB) images [3,4]. The images were captured by a TopCon TRV-50 fundus camera at 35° FOV. The automated retinal image analyzer (ARIA) database contains images with a resolution of 768 × 576 pixels. In the ARIA database, the fundus images are in color and they were taken using a Zeiss FF450 + fundus camera with a 50° field width. The color fundus images contained in the STARE and ARIA archives are classified as normal and abnormal, according to the information provided with the archives.

To test the vessel caliber measurements, several authors use the retinal vessel image set for estimation of widths (REVIEW) database [5,6]. This database contains images that are of a higher resolution than the DRIVE images, ranging in size from 1360 × 1024 to 3584 × 2438 pixels. It consists of four image sets (high-resolution image set [HRIS], vascular disease image set [VDIS], central light reflex image set [CLRIS], and kick point image set [KPIS]), which include 16 images with 5066 locations of vessel segments that have been manually marked by three observers.

The Iowa normative set for processing images of the retina (INSPIRE-AVR) archive contains 40 high-resolution color images of 2392 × 2048 pixels. This data set can be used as a reference for measuring the AVR [7,8], which has been labeled by two experts.

The methods for evaluating segmentation and indexing techniques dedicated to retinal ophthalmology (MESSIDOR) archive [9] contains 1200 eye fundus color images. The images have 1440 × 960, 2240 × 1488, or 2304 × 1536 pixels. This archive can be used for testing the segmentation and indexing methods in eye fundus images with pathologies.

The data set CHASE_DB1 contains 28 retinal images of both eyes of 14 children [41]. The images were recorded with a handheld Nidek fundus camera NM-200-M, and were captured at 30° FOV with a resolution of 1280 × 960 pixels. Two independent observers labeled the blood vessels in the 28 images.

5.2.2 Review and Survey Articles

Recently, Fraz et al. [10] surveyed the methodologies for the image segmentation of retinal blood vessels. Their paper contains 135 references and examines different methodologies, categorizing them according to the image-processing methodology. In particular, the authors surveyed 69 papers from peer-reviewed publications. Pattern classification approaches were the most frequent, followed by matched-filtering methods. This review paper also provides good coverage on the different performance measure results, together with information on the database where the evaluation was performed.

With 187 papers referenced, Abràmoff et al. [11] reviewed the current status of retinal imaging methodologies (focusing on eye fundus imaging and optical coherence tomography), in image analysis methods and their clinical applications. Regarding the eye fundus image analysis methods, this paper is particularly focused on reviewing the main tasks that are frequently used in this field: the location of the segmentation of the retinal structures (the retinal vessels, optic disc, and fovea) and the segmentation of abnormalities (in the blood vessels, pigment epithelium, and choroid). Additionally, the paper reviews methods for the construction of fundus-imaging-based retinal atlases and the analysis of the optic nerve head morphology from fundus photographs.

The review by Bernardes et al. [12] mentions 165 papers, and gives an overview of the image segmentation techniques of the three main retinal structures (the retinal vessels, optic disc, and fovea). Their review also surveys some of the detection methods used for signs of disease onset and progression.

The aforementioned recent surveys provide good coverage of the main contributions in the field. In this chapter, we focus on the retinal vessel image analysis approaches for segmentation, classification, and measurement/evaluation that have been proposed in the last 2–3 years.

5.2.3 Retinal Blood Vessel Segmentation Methodologies

Generally, the strategies for the segmentation of blood vessels can be grouped as pixel processing-based methods (which include the kernel-based and classifier-based approaches) and tracking methods. The retinal blood vessel segmentation is an earlier phase that is required for artery–vein classification and blood vessel caliber measurement.

5.2.3.1 Pixel Processing-Based Methods

The pixel processing-based approaches often start by an enhancement phase giving more emphasis to vessel-like structures, followed by further processing steps for accurate vessel delineation. Matched filtering is an example of these pixel-based methods, which continues to be one of the most popular approaches. It basically consists of filtering the eye fundus image with a kernel function adapted to the intensity profile of the blood vessels independently of the local contrast changes and trying to cover the existing range of scales and orientations. An example of this is the paper by Li et al. [13] who proposed a multiscale extraction approach, including the product of the filtered responses in three scales in the image enhancement step. After matched filtering, the vessels are detected using a double-thresholding technique. Finally, postprocessing steps are introduced to (1) remove the false positives introduced by bright lesions and (2) link the broken vessels. This method was tested using the publicly available databases DRIVE and STARE. The authors compared their approach with other methods employing multiscale filters [14–15].

Ramlugun et al. [16] proposed an enhanced step based on an adaptive histogram equalization method followed by a two-dimensional (2-D) Gabor matched filter and a double thresholding for blood vessel detection. The performance was evaluated using the DRIVE database, and the authors concluded that the introduction of the histogram equalization step gave a better performance.

In the paper by Ramlugun et al. [17], matched filters were applied to equalized images. The filtered image was thresholded using a hysteresis method. The selection of parameters was studied in order to improve the segmentation of the small vessels. Twenty images of the DRIVE data set were used in the evaluation.

Bankhead et al. [18] presented an unsupervised classification method for both detection and measurement of the retinal blood vessels. The method uses wavelets for vessel segmentation by thresholding the wavelet coefficients, followed by a spline fitting to determine the vessel orientations, and find the zero crossings of the second derivative of the vessel profile. The segmentation was tested using the DRIVE database and the authors used the REVIEW data set for the caliber measurements.

Zhu [19] proposed a representation for vessel cross-sectional profiles that is useful for defining a new scheme of vessel detection based on symmetry and asymmetry in the Fourier domain. The approach was tested using the STARE and ARIA data sets [3]. The achieved results were comparable to the results of a modified Gaussian matched-filtering method.

Moghimirad et al. [20] proposed a multiscale approach for retinal vessel segmentation, based on their computation of the medial axis followed by a vessel centerline extraction, vessel reconstruction, and noise reduction. The method was evaluated using the STARE and DRIVE databases. Ng et al. [21] used a multiscale approach for estimating the vessel location and its parameters by fitting a vessel model to the output of the second derivative filters. The method was evaluated using the STARE database.

Saleh and Eswaran [22] applied a series of morphological and nonmorphological image-processing operations for enhancing, background removal, and vessel detection. The method was evaluated using the DRIVE data set.

Fraz et al. [23] presented a supervised scheme for the segmentation of the retinal blood vessels by using an ensemble classifier of bagged decision trees. The measured features were based on the line strength information of the blood vessels and the filter responses of a mixture of Gaussians and Gabor filters. The authors evaluated the system using the CHASE_DB1 data set.

5.2.3.2 Tracking Methods

In the vessel-tracking methods, the seed points are selected at the vessel edges or on the vessel centerline, and from this starting point the blood vessel is followed, taking into consideration the location, direction, and profile vessel information. Vlachos and Dermatas [24] proposed a multiscale line tracking approach for vessel segmentation. The procedure starts from a set of seeds and iteratively tracks the next pixel based on cross-sectional profile information. It terminates when this measure becomes invalid. Additional postprocessing steps are included for removing noisy lines and erroneous areas with invalid orientations. The authors evaluated their approach using the DRIVE database. Yin et al. [25] introduced a tracking method using a probabilistic maximum *a posteriori* (MAP) formulation to select the vessel configuration from three different cases: normal, bifurcation, and crossing. Adel et al. [26] had already proposed an initial version of this MAP approach. The tracker evolves based on the selected configuration and on other parameters measured in the previous iteration (such as the vessel edge points, center pixel, direction, and vessel diameter). This approach was evaluated using the REVIEW data set.

Table 5.1 provides an overview of the achieved results. In Table 5.1, we compare several methods using the following performance measures: (1) accuracy, as the ratio of the total number of correctly detected pixels to the total number of pixels; (2) the fraction of pixels correctly detected as vessel pixels (true-positive ratio [TPR] or the sensitivity); and (3) the fraction of pixels erroneously detected as vessel pixels (false-positive ratio [FPR]). The specificity (Sp) of the method is $Sp = 1 - FPR$.

5.2.3.3 Retinal Vessel Classification

Vázquez et al. [27] compared different feature sets and classification strategies, and they also tested the influence of the distance to the optic disc on their measurements. The achieved accuracy for classifying blood vessels as either an artery or a vein was 86.34%, in their database. Saez et al. [28], who are researchers from the same group, proposed a

TABLE 5.1

Comparison of Retinal Segmentation Performances Using One of the
Observers as a Reference

Paper	Database	Accuracy	Sensitivity (TPR)	Specificity (1-FPR)
Second observer	DRIVE	0.9473	0.7760	0.9725
Vlachos and Dermatas [25]	DRIVE	0.929	0.747	0.955
Mohmimirad et al. [21]	DRIVE		0.7852	0.9935
Bankhead et al. [19]	DRIVE	0.9371	0.7027	0.9717
Saleh and Eswaran [23]	DRIVE	0.9653	0.8431	0.9717
Ramlugun et al. [18]	DRIVE	0.9341	0.6413	0.9767
Second observer	STARE	0.9354	0.8949	0.9939
Mohmimirad et al. [21]	STARE	0.9756	0.8133	0.9909
Ng et al. [22]	STARE	–	0.70	0.953
Yin et al. [26]	REVIEW		0.925	0.9999

method for classifying retinal blood vessels as veins or arteries. After vessel segmentation, a set of pixel-based and profile-based feature vectors are measured and used as inputs to a k-means clustering approach. The methodology was evaluated in a local image database, manually labeled by three observers. In their method, the probability of an incorrect classification was 21.81% for arteries and 12.1% for veins.

Niemeijer et al. [8] followed a supervised approach, using as training a set of centerline pixels previously labeled and characterized by a set of 27 color and intensity features at four scales. The system attained an area under the receiver operating characteristic (ROC) curve of 0.84 for the artery–vein classification of the blood vessels in the 40 images of the INSPIRE-AVR data set.

5.2.3.4 Caliber Measurement

In their paper, Bankhead et al. [18] made vessel caliber measurements from the vessel edges found by the zero crossing of the second derivative of the vessel profile.

Active contours are used for fully automated vessel segmentation by the extraction of segment profiles algorithm [29]. Xu et al. [30] proposed a graph-based algorithm that starts by generating a vesselness map. The vessel orientations are identified by a principal component analysis of several adjacent centerline pixels. The vessel profiles used to generate a graph are derived along the estimated centerlines. A graph search is applied in order to determine the vessel edges by minimizing a cost function. This approach was evaluated using the REVIEW data set.

Zhu [31] proposed a phase congruency approach to define the representation of vessel cross-sectional profiles in the Fourier domain. The retinal blood vessel segmentation results were shown for the STARE and ARIA data sets. The performance of their approach for width measurement was also discussed for the ARIA data set. Table 5.2 gives an overview of the performance of the caliber measurements of several methods.

5.2.4 Clinical Applications

The AVR is a well-established, predictive value of hypertension, cerebral atrophy, stroke, and other cardiovascular events in adults. Retinal vessel segmentation and caliber

TABLE 5.2

Retinal Caliber Measurement Performances

Paper	Database	Mean	Standard Deviation	%[a]
Bankhead et al. [18]	REVIEW	4.66	0.32	99.3
Al-Diri et al. [29]	REVIEW	7.1		99.3
Xu et al. [30]	REVIEW	6.8	2.2	97.9

[a] Weighted percentage of vessel locations at which a meaningful measure of the vessel diameter was returned by the algorithm.

measurement can play an important role in the detection of these pathological conditions and other rare or irregular diseases such as hemorrhages and neovascularization. The segmentation of anatomical structures of the retina can also be an important step for the location and characterization of pathological conditions, such as vascular or optic disc abnormalities. The review paper by Faust et al. [32] gives several examples of this for hypertensive retinopathy characterization based on vessel tortuosity and focal vessel narrowing, or for hemorrhage detection in DR, or for grading DR in computer-aided diagnosis systems. Agurto et al. [33] proposed a multiscale amplitude-modulation frequency-modulation methodology for discriminating between normal and pathological retinal images, including neovascularization and hemorrhages. Akram and Khan [34] used blood vessel segmentation together with optic disc detection for lesion detection and segmentation and for the early detection of DR.

5.3 Retinal Blood Vessel Segmentation

This section describes a method that has been developed for the automated segmentation of the vascular structure in color images of the eye fundus. Mendonça and Campilho [1] previously published the original method and some of the results for low-resolution images. An extension of the proposed approach for segmenting high-resolution images will be presented in the following section.

Using the functional block diagram shown in Figure 5.1, the method can be schematically described. The three main processing phases can be identified as: (1) preprocessing: for background normalization and thin vessel enhancement; (2) vessel centerline detection: for defining a set of connected segments in the central part of the vessels; and (3) vessel segmentation: for finally labeling the pixels belonging to the vessels. These phases are further subdivided into several steps, as follows:

Preprocessing: (a) Background normalization is achieved by subtracting an estimate of the background generated by averaging with a large kernel; previously, the selected monochromatic component was submitted to a noise removal operation, followed by an image border extension for minimizing undesired border effects. (b) Thin vessel enhancement is achieved by processing with a set of line detection filters, corresponding to the four main orientations; for each pixel, the highest filter response is kept and added to the normalized image.

Vessel centerline detection: (a) Vessel centerline candidates are selected using directional information provided by a set of four directional difference of offset Gaussian (DoOG)

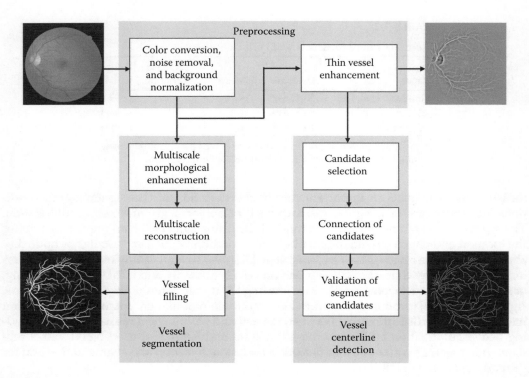

FIGURE 5.1
Retinal vessel segmentation functional diagram.

filters. (b) The candidate points that were obtained in the previous step are connected by a region-growing process guided by local image statistics. (c) The centerline segment candidates are validated based on the characteristics of the line segments; this operation is applied to each of the four directions and finally combined, resulting in a map of the detected vessel centerlines.

Vessel segmentation: (a) Multiscale morphological vessel enhancement is achieved by using a modified top-hat transform with variable-size structuring elements aimed at enhancing vessels with different widths. (b) Multiscale morphological vessel reconstruction is achieved by using a binary morphological reconstruction method, for generating binary maps of the vessels at four scales. (c) Vessel filling by a region-growing process is achieved by using as initial seeds the pixels within the centerlines; the growing process is successively applied to the four scales and in each growing region step, the seed image is the result of the previous aggregation.

Each of these phases is detailed and illustrated in the following subsections.

5.3.1.1 Preprocessing

Most of the image segmentation methodologies use the green channel as the natural basis for vessel segmentation because it normally presents the highest contrast between the blood vessels and the retinal background. Nevertheless, Mendonça and Campilho [1] have shown that other monochromatic components, extracted from different color space representations, can also be useful for this purpose. Independent of the component derived from the original color fundus images, in the work of Mendonça and Campilho the segmentation is always performed on a monochromatic image where the vessels show intensities higher than the background.

The background of retinal images is often characterized by a gradual intensity variation occurring from the periphery toward the central macular area; other retinal regions, such as the optic disc, also have distinctive intensity values. The blood vessels stand out from the background, but a more thorough analysis of local vessel intensities can reveal significant variations (normally dependent from neighboring conditions) that can negatively interfere in the complete vessel segmentation process. In order to decrease this influence, the monochromatic representation of the original color image is normalized by subtracting an estimate of the background, which is the result of averaging with an image size-dependent kernel. Before this background normalization step, the selected monochromatic component is filtered with a small-dimension Gaussian kernel for noise removal, and an image of the FOV border is extended following an approach similar to the one described by Soares et al. [14], aimed at minimizing some of the border effects that can occur as a consequence of the averaging operation required by the background estimation step. These two preprocessing operations were not included in the original version of the method described by Mendonça and Campilho [1].

To improve the discrimination between thin vessels and the background noise, the normalized image is processed with a set of line detection filters [35], and for each pixel, the highest filter response is kept and added to the normalized image. This preprocessed image is used as the input for the vessel centerline detection phase.

Figure 5.2 shows the results of the preprocessing phase for three original color images, two (top and middle) from the DRIVE database [2] and one (bottom) from the STARE database [3]. The monochromatic component for the top row image is the luminance, while the green component is depicted in the middle row; for the bottom row image, the a* component is displayed.

5.3.1.2 Detection of Vessel Centerlines

Vessel centerlines are herein defined as connected sets of pixels that correspond to the intensity maxima computed from the intensity profiles of the vessel cross sections. The first operation aimed at extracting the vessel centerline pixels is the application of a set of directional differential filters that are sensitive to the main vessel orientations. The underlying idea is that when a first-order derivative filter is applied orthogonally to the main orientation of the vessel, derivative values with opposite signs are obtained on the two vessel hillsides, which simply means that there will be positive values on one side of the vessel cross section and negative values on the other side. Since retinal vessels can occur in any direction, the selection of a set of four directional filters whose responses can be combined to cover the whole range of possible orientations is required. The particular kernels used are first-order derivative filters, known as the DoOG filters [36], with prevailing responses to horizontal (0°), vertical (90°), and diagonal (45°, 135°) directions. Each of the four directional images resulting from the DoOG filters is searched for specific combinations of signs on the expected direction of the vessel cross section; the search is performed on one pixel wide lines with an orientation corresponding to the vessel cross-profile, which means that the scanning direction is distinct for each of the four images under analysis. As real vessels do not have the ideal Gaussian profile, we empirically assessed the four combinations of the filter responses detailed by Mendonça and Campilho [1].

From each image containing the selected set of candidate points in one specific direction, an initial collection of the centerline segments is generated by a region-growing

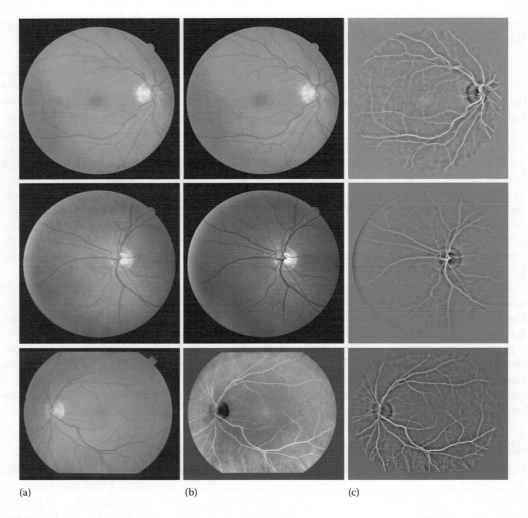

FIGURE 5.2
Preprocessed retinal images. (a) Original color image; (b) selected monochromatic component; and (c) background normalized image.

process, which starts with a set of seed points verifying restricted value conditions, and is afterward extended by aggregating other neighboring pixels with lower filter responses. Both the seed and the aggregation thresholds are defined based on statistics derived from a histogram of the image containing the set of candidate points; the values of the seeds are above a limit depending on the mean and the percentage α of the standard deviation of this distribution, while the aggregation threshold is the histogram mode.

The identification of the connected sets of points with a high probability of belonging to the vessel centerlines is preceded by a cleaning of the smallest segments, while keeping those with more than a specified number of points (*min_npoints*). To increase the discrimination between valid centerline segments and fragments associated with noise, each pixel of an image resulting from the region-growing process is multiplied by the corresponding pixel value in the background normalized image. This operation is particularly important for pixels associated with thin vessels, where the values of the directional gradients are similar to those in some background structures, but whose original intensities are usually higher.

For the final validation, each candidate segment is characterized by two features: the segment intensity, evaluated by the geometric mean of the average and maximum intensity values of its points, and the segment length, measured by the number of points. These two features are then compared with image-dependent reference values. As the validation process is applied independently to segments of the four directional sets, the reference values for the two features, intensity and length, are calculated from each of these sets. Global references for the two features are also obtained from a fifth set that gathers selected segments taken from the four directional sets; in this newly formed set, the segments keep all of their individual characteristics except their direction. The final reference value for a specific direction is the maximum between the calculated directional and global reference values.

Following an independent evaluation of the four directional sets of segments, those segments that are classified as belonging to the vessel centerlines are joined together into a binary image, which is the final result of the process for vessel centerline detection.

The intermediary and final results of the vessel centerline detection phase for the original fundus image of the top row in Figure 5.2 are depicted in Figure 5.3. The preprocessed image is shown in Figure 5.3a, while the other three images in the same row exemplify the detection of horizontal vessel centerline segments. Figure 5.3b presents the result of the differential operator, where negative values of the derivative correspond to the darkest points, while high intensities are associated with positive derivative signs. The initial set of candidates and the final validated segments are depicted in Figure 5.3c and d, respectively.

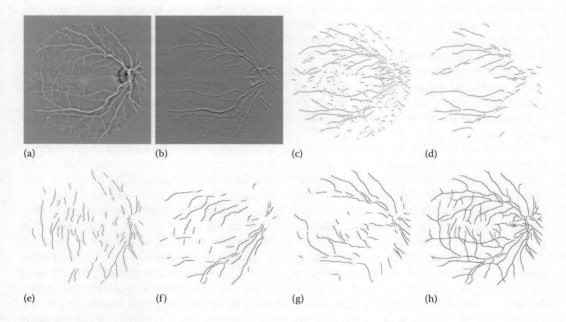

(a) (b) (c) (d)

(e) (f) (g) (h)

FIGURE 5.3
Vessel centerlines detection. (a) Preprocessed image; (b) result of DoOG filter (horizontal); (c) horizontal candidate segments; (d) horizontal centerline segments; (e) vertical segments; (f) diagonal segments (45°); (g) diagonal segments (135°); and (h) vessel centerlines.

The vessel centerlines for the other three directions are presented in Figure 5.3e–g, and the final combination is shown in Figure 5.3h.

5.3.1.3 Vessel Segmentation

Vessel filling is achieved by an iterative procedure that starts from the detected centerlines and, in each step, uses the output image from the previous iteration as seed for a simple region-growing algorithm, whose aggregation phase is limited by a binary mask representing vessel segments in a limited width range.

As in the previous step, a multiscale approach is followed, where a set of modified top-hat operators [37] using circular structuring elements of increasing radii is used for generating several enhanced representations of the vascular network, each one emphasizing vessels in a limited width range, from smaller to larger vessels. Image masks containing binary reconstructions of the main vessel segments within a specific size range are derived from the enhanced representations by morphological reconstruction. The option of using such a multiscale approach, instead of using a single-scale operator, is justified by the expected dependence of the operator response from the vessel width. The range of the radius of the structuring elements varies from 1 to 8 pixels, covering the overall range of vessel widths for the two image data sets used in this work. For images with a different resolution, the set of structuring elements radii should be adapted accordingly.

The four enhanced images resulting from the previous processing sequence are used for reconstructing potential vessel segments. For this task, a binary morphological reconstruction method, called the double threshold operator, is selected. This operator consists in thresholding each image for two ranges of gray values, one being included in the other; the image obtained with the narrow threshold range (marker image) is used as a seed for the reconstruction using the wide-range thresholded image (mask image) [38]. Based on the distinct emphasis placed on different widths by each specific top-hat transform, the correct selection of the marker and the mask images allows the generation of four binary images, each one containing a partial reconstruction of the vascular tree of the retina. For each vessel-enhanced image, the marker and the mask images are derived using threshold values directly calculated from the intensity histogram of the non-null pixels; each one of these thresholds is defined as the highest intensity value such that the number of pixels with intensities above this limit is greater or equal to a predefined percentage.

Figure 5.4 illustrates the generation of the four images containing partial reconstructions of the retinal vasculature. The series of enhanced images with increasing structuring elements is presented in the first column (Figure 5.4a); the corresponding marker, mask, and reconstructed images can be observed in the other three columns (Figure 5.4b–d).

A final image with the segmented vessels is obtained by iteratively combining the centerline image with the set of images that resulted from the vessel segments reconstruction phase. In the first iteration, the vessel centerline pixels are used as seeds for a region-growing algorithm, which breed these points by aggregating the pixels in the reconstructed image derived from the top-hat operator with the smallest structuring element size. The aggregation of the points is, as usual, conditioned by the connectivity restriction. In each of the subsequent three iterations, the reconstructed images corresponding to the vessels with increasing widths are, in turn, used for extending the output of the previous region-growing step.

The final vessel segmentation is obtained after a cleaning operation that is aimed at removing all the pixels that are completely surrounded by vessel points, but are not labeled

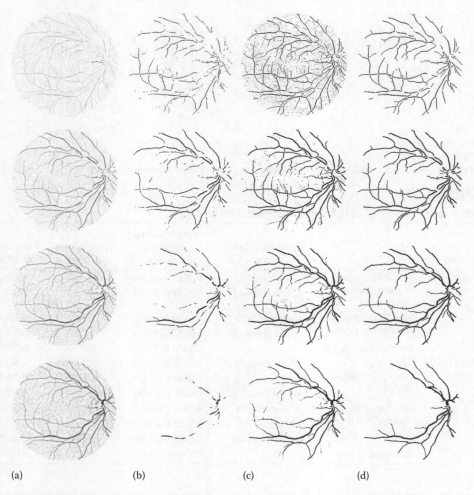

(a) (b) (c) (d)

FIGURE 5.4
Vessel segments reconstruction. (a) Images with the vessels enhanced with morphological top-hat operators using structuring elements of increasing sizes (from top to bottom); (b) marker images; (c) mask images; and (d) reconstructed images.

as part of a vessel. This is done by considering that each pixel with at least six neighbors that are classified as vessel points must also belong to a vessel.

The vessel-filling process is demonstrated in Figure 5.5, where the results of the four iterations are shown. The process starts with the vessel centerlines image, which is combined with the reconstructed image, shown on the top right of Figure 5.4, to produce the image in Figure 5.5a; in each of the following steps, the previous image is the basis for aggregating the neighboring pixels from one reconstructed image until the final image is generated, as presented in Figure 5.5d.

Table 5.3 shows the performance measures of the current implementation of the vessel segmentation algorithm for the images of the DRIVE and STARE databases. The values previously published by Mendonça and Campilho [1] and those achieved by an observer are also included in Table 5.3. The set of parameters for each database was kept unchanged, being identical to the set reported for the original method [1].

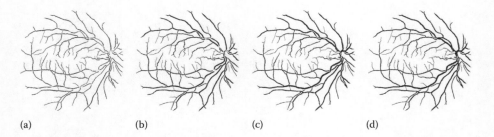

    (a)   (b)   (c)   (d)

FIGURE 5.5

Vessel filling. (a–c) Results of consecutive iterations; and (d) result of vessel segmentation.

TABLE 5.3

Performance Measures of the Vessel Segmentation Method

Database		Monochromatic Image	Average Accuracy (Standard Deviation)	Sensitivity (TPR)	Specificity (1-FPR)
DRIVE	Mendonça and Campilho this work	Gray intensity	0.9466 (0.0060)	0.7467	0.9762
		Green channel	0.9458 (0.0058)	0.7497	0.9749
	Mendonça and Campilho [1]	Gray intensity	0.9463 (0.0065)	0.7315	0.9781
		Green channel	0.9542 (0.0062)	0.7344	0.9764
	Second observer [2]		0.9473 (0.0048)	0.7761	0.9725
STARE (with FOV)	Mendonça and Campilho this work	a* component	0.9487 (0.0120)	0.7194	0.9759
		Gray intensity	0.9438 (0.0146)	0.6953	0.9731
		Green channel	0.9455 (0.0138)	0.7183	0.9725
	Mendonça and Campilho [1]	a* component	0.9479 (0.0123)	0.7123	0.9758
		Gray intensity	0.9421 (0.0151)	0.6764	0.9734
		Green channel	0.9440 (0.0142)	0.6996	0.9730
	Second observer		0.9354 (0.0171)	0.8949	0.939

5.4 Segmentation of Retinal Vessels in High-Resolution Images

Most of the algorithms that have been proposed in the literature for retinal vessel segmentation are not scale independent, because they frequently rely on features extracted at particular image scales or they are supported by kernel-based operations, such as image filtering or template matching. Although the method described in the previous section also presents this limitation, the adjustments required for dealing with high-resolution images were quite straightforward.

The changes introduced in the original algorithm are detailed in Section 5.4.1, whereas a modified solution using a low-resolution image for the intermediary stage of centerlines detection is described in Section 5.4.2. These two extensions of the original algorithm were evaluated on the 40 images of the INSPIRE-AVR data set [7].

5.4.1 Single-Resolution Method

The method described in Section 5.3 was extended to work with high-resolution images mainly by rescaling the dimension of the filters that are applied in both the preprocessing and the vessel-filling phases using a factor derived from the actual image resolution for the data set under analysis, establishing as reference the filter sizes that were defined in the original algorithm for the DRIVE and STARE databases. The values for the method parameters should be set for each database because they mainly depend on some characteristics of the images, namely, the contrast and the noise level, as well as the final application of the vessel segmentation result.

5.4.1.1 Preprocessing

The sequence of operations for image preprocessing was kept unchanged, except where the size of the two averaging filters used in this phase was concerned. The selected noise removal filter has a 15×15 Gaussian kernel (standard deviation = 3), while for the background estimation the original average filter of size 31×31 was replaced by a 91×91 Gaussian with a standard deviation value of 12 to avoid an excessive attenuation near vessel bifurcations and crossings. The result of this phase of the algorithm for an original image of the INSPIRE-AVR data set is presented in Figure 5.6.

5.4.1.2 Vessel Centerline Detection

No changes were required in the procedure initially delineated for the detection of vessel centerlines. The original DoOG kernels are still adequate for the calculation of image derivatives because the criterion used for selecting candidate points, based on the localization of a combination of derivative signs, proved to be insensitive to large variations in vessel widths. However, as the vessel central reflex is much accentuated in high-resolution images, the centerline segments detected in large caliber vessels are sometimes formed by pairs of ridgelines that run along vessel walls. This is not a problem for the proposed method, as the main role of this initial set of segments is to act as a guideline for the subsequent phase of vessel filling. The overall results of the vessel centerline detection for the green and a* components of the fundus photograph of Figure 5.6 are depicted in Figure 5.7a, whereas a more detailed view near the optic disc can be observed in Figure 5.7b.

5.4.1.3 Vessel Segmentation

In the last step of the method, the retinal vessels are segmented as described in Section 5.3. Due to the increase in the image resolution, the structuring elements of the top-hat transforms that were used for vessel enhancement were resized using a scale factor similar to

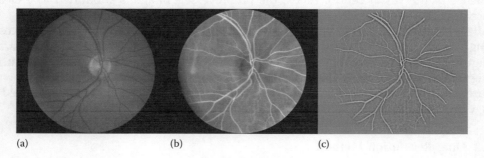

(a) (b) (c)

FIGURE 5.6
Preprocessing result. (a) Original image; (b) a* component; and (c) preprocessed image.

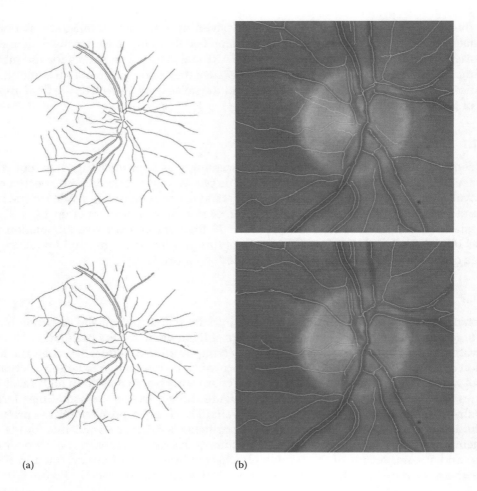

(a)   (b)

FIGURE 5.7
Results of vessel centerline detection using as input the green channel (top row) and the a* component (bottom row). (a) Detected centerlines; and (b) a detailed view of the result with the centerlines detected around the optic disc overlapped on the original image.

the one used for adapting the filters in the preprocessing phase. In order to reduce the influence of the vessel central reflex, the preprocessed image is submitted to a closing operator with a small square structuring element before enhancement.

After achieving the partial vessel reconstructed images, the four iterations of the vessel-filling procedure are applied for generating the segmented retinal vasculature, as illustrated in Figure 5.8. Figure 5.9 compares two segmented vascular structures for the original image of Figure 5.6, which were obtained after the final cleaning operation; the result shown in Figure 5.9a uses the green component as input, whereas the a* component produced the image presented in Figure 5.9b.

5.4.2 Dual-Resolution Method

An image containing the vessel centerlines is a fundamental intermediary result that essentially prevents the inclusion of noisy pixels, which result from the morphological

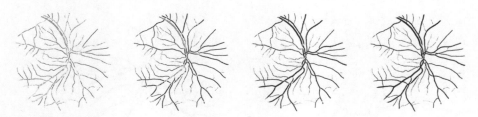

FIGURE 5.8
Results of the four iterations of the vessel-filling procedure (from left to right).

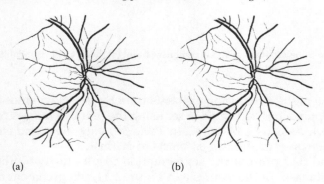

(a)   (b)

FIGURE 5.9
Final segmented vascular structures using as input: (a) the green component; and (b) the a* component.

enhancement process. As previously mentioned, centerline points are the seeds for the first iteration of the vessel-filling phase, and a vessel that does not contain at least one seed will not be included in the final segmentation. Although centerline detection is critical for the inclusion/exclusion of a particular vessel, it does not have great influence on the final vessel borders that are determined by the morphological enhancement and reconstruction steps.

As the vessel centerline detection phase is the most time consuming part of the algorithm, taking around one-half of the processing time, we have decided to evaluate the influence of using the low-resolution version of the original image in this intermediary phase. Thus, the size of the preprocessed image is reduced by a factor of four in each dimension before centerline detection, and the image containing the detected points is augmented by an identical factor before being used for vessel filling. All the other processing steps are performed on the full-resolution image.

The dual-resolution method is exemplified in Figure 5.10, which displays the centerlines detected using the low-resolution image (a) and the corresponding segmented retinal vasculature (b).

5.4.3 Comparison of Single-Resolution and Dual-Resolution Methods

The methods described in the previous two sections were compared using the 40 images of the INSPIRE-AVR database [7]. The dimension of the images is 2392×2048, with 8 bits per pixel. For this data set, both the green channel (RGB) and a* component (L*a*b*) were assessed as inputs for the vessel segmentation process.

A multiplicative factor equal to three was chosen for enlarging the size of the filters used in the preprocessing and vessel segmentation phases. The same factor was applied to

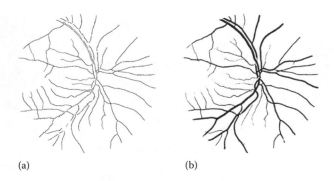

(a)   (b)

FIGURE 5.10
Result of the dual-resolution method. (a) Vessel centerlines; and (b) final vessel segmentation.

determine the size of the structuring elements used for vessel enhancement. The parameters of the two approaches, which were set using the first five images of the data set, are shown in Table 5.4. As can be observed in Table 5.4, only the parameters related to the centerlines detection step (α and *min_npoints*) are distinct.

Figures 5.11 and 5.12 present the segmentation results for two other images of the INSPIRE-AVR database. In the example in Figure 5.11, the green channel was used as the input, while Figure 5.12 displays the results for the a* component. Each figure shows the original fundus photograph and the vessel centerline and vessel segmented images generated by the proposed approaches. As can be observed, although some alterations can be found in the centerlines, the changes at the segmentation level are mostly related to the detection of thin vessels or background noise. In general, the segmentation of the major vessels is not affected by the use of a low-resolution image for centerline detection.

In order to obtain a quantitative assessment of the differences between the two vessel segmentations, the accuracy of the dual-resolution result was calculated using as ground truth the corresponding vascular structure generated by the single-resolution method. The average values of accuracy for the 40 images of the data set are shown in Table 5.5. The values represented in Table 5.5 demonstrate that no significant modification has been introduced when the dual-resolution solution is chosen, as, on average, less than 0.5% of the pixels have different labels in the two segmentation results.

TABLE 5.4

Parameter Settings

Parameter		Single-Resolution Method	Dual-Resolution Approach
α		−2.0	−0.75
min_npoints		40	10
Histogram% (marker image)/ histogram% (mask image)	$R_1 = 3; R_2 = 6$	5/8	5/8
	$R_3 = 9; R_4 = 12$	5/10	5/10
	$R_5 = 15; R_6 = 18$	2/11	2/11
	$R_7 = 21; R_8 = 24$	1/11	1/11

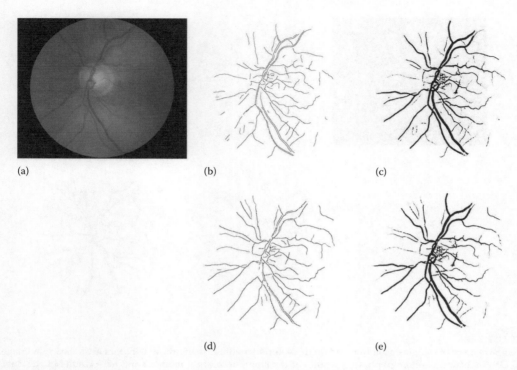

FIGURE 5.11
Comparison of the single-resolution and dual-resolution methods using the green channel as the input image. (a) Original fundus photograph; (b,c) results of the single-resolution method; and (d,e) results of the dual-resolution method.

5.5 Application for Arteriovenous Ratio Calculation

One important application for an accurate segmentation of the retinal vasculature is the possibility of quantifying alterations in the ratio between the widths of the arteries and veins, as it is now accepted that these changes are associated with an increase in the risk for stroke, cerebral atrophy, and myocardial infarction, among others [8].

In this section, the vessel segmentation results that were achieved with the two methods described in the preceding section will be validated through their use in calculating the AVR in the 40 images of the INSPIRE-AVR data set. For AVR determination, we have defined a procedure similar to the procedure described by Niemeijer et al. [8] that automates the protocol established by Knudtson et al. [39]. Starting from the segmentation of the retinal vasculature, the following sequence of steps is required: (1) region of interest (ROI) determination; (2) artery and vein identification; (3) vessel diameter estimation; and (4) AVR calculation.

The region to measure vessel calibers (ROI) is a standard area 0.5–1.0 disc diameter from the optic disc margin [39]. After locating the optic disc center using an automatic methodology based on the entropy of vascular directions [40], the ROI is positioned centered on this point just by considering a disc diameter of 360 pixels, as assumed by Niemeijer et al. [8]. The ROI determined for the first image of the INSPIRE-AVR data set

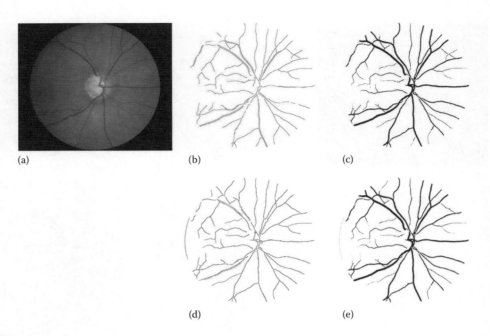

FIGURE 5.12
Comparison of the single-resolution and dual-resolution methods using the a* component as the input image.
(a) Original fundus photograph; (b,c) results of the single-resolution method; and (d,e) results of the dual-
resolution method.

TABLE 5.5

Average Value of Accuracy of the Dual-
Resolution Segmentation for INSPIRE-AVR
Database Using as Ground Truth the
Single-Resolution Result

Monochromatic Image	Average Accuracy (Standard Deviation)
a* component	0.9962 (0.0025)
Green channel	0.9958 (0.0016)

is shown in Figure 5.13 delimited by the two outer circles, whereas the optic disc margin
is represented by the innermost circle. The identification of arteries and veins within
the ROI is accomplished by a comparison with a manual classification performed by an
expert.

The retinal vasculature is then used for vessel diameter estimation. First, a distance
transform using a Euclidean metric is applied to the segmented binary image containing
the vessels, with the aim of assigning to each vessel point its distance to the background, d.
Then, the image is thinned in order to get a new centerline for the vessels passing through
the ROI. The vessel diameter, vd, for each centerline point is estimated by $vd = 2d - 1$.

A procedure similar to the one described by Niemeijer et al. [8] is applied for the AVR
measurement. The ROI is equidistantly sampled to provide six regions for performing
distinct AVR calculations. For each region, the six largest arteries and the six largest
veins are identified and the AVR value is computed based on the algorithm described by

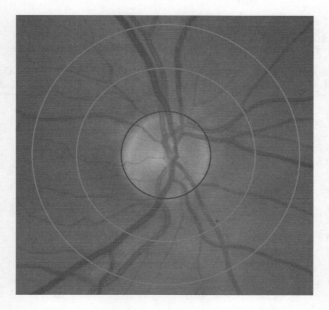

FIGURE 5.13
Original image with the ROI for AVR calculation (delimited by the two outer circles) and the optic disc margin (represented by the innermost circle).

Niemeijer et al. [8]. The final AVR estimate for the complete image is the average of the six regional values.

Table 5.6 summarizes the AVR values for the 40 images of the INSPIRE-AVR data set calculated using data obtained from both single-resolution and dual-resolution algorithms. Table 5.6 also includes two other AVR measures that were computed by two ophthalmologists using the semiautomated computer program, IVAN, developed at the University of Wisconsin [8]. The estimates for Observer 1 are used as reference for calculating the errors for the results of the two proposed methods and for Observer 2 results.

The analysis of the individual AVR and error values, as well as the global measures included in the last four rows of Table 5.6, allows the conclusion that vessel calibers directly estimated from the segmented vessels are useful for AVR computation; it confirms that no significant differences are introduced by the use of the low-resolution image for centerline detection; and it demonstrates that both methods are successful solutions for retinal blood vessel segmentation in high-resolution fundus photographs.

5.6 Conclusion

Most of the applications for analyzing the human retina demand the segmentation of the blood vessels. Although this is a hard task for specialists to perform, its use is also quite challenging in image analysis methodologies, thereby justifying vessel segmentation as an active field of research for more than two decades, with a great diversity of novel solutions being proposed every year. This fact was also confirmed by the brief review of proposals that was recently published.

TABLE 5.6

AVR Values for Each Image of the INSPIRE-AVR Data Set

Image Number	Reference AVR	Single-Resolution AVR	Single-Resolution Error	Dual-Resolution AVR	Dual-Resolution Error	Observer 2 AVR	Observer 2 Error
1	0.70	0.71	0.01	0.71	0.01	0.71	0.01
2	0.63	0.80	0.17	0.79	0.16	0.68	0.05
3	0.70	0.63	0.07	0.63	0.07	0.65	0.05
4	0.65	0.70	0.05	0.69	0.04	0.64	0.01
5	0.78	0.77	0.01	0.76	0.02	0.75	0.03
6	0.65	0.67	0.02	0.67	0.02	0.65	0.00
7	0.67	0.64	0.03	0.63	0.04	0.65	0.02
8	0.64	0.70	0.06	0.69	0.05	0.71	0.07
9	0.69	0.61	0.08	0.61	0.08	0.76	0.07
10	0.56	0.63	0.07	0.63	0.07	0.85	0.29
11	0.64	0.72	0.08	0.72	0.08	0.74	0.10
12	0.76	0.69	0.07	0.69	0.07	0.75	0.01
13	0.57	0.60	0.03	0.60	0.03	0.62	0.05
14	0.62	0.63	0.01	0.63	0.01	0.58	0.04
15	0.64	0.67	0.03	0.67	0.03	0.61	0.03
16	0.68	0.68	0.00	0.68	0.00	0.68	0.00
17	0.52	0.56	0.04	0.57	0.05	0.45	0.07
18	0.62	0.56	0.06	0.56	0.06	0.63	0.01
19	0.67	0.82	0.15	0.82	0.15	0.63	0.04
20	0.71	0.65	0.06	0.65	0.06	0.62	0.09
21	0.57	0.59	0.02	0.57	0.00	0.58	0.01
22	0.72	0.86	0.14	0.85	0.13	0.76	0.04
23	0.66	0.68	0.02	0.68	0.02	0.69	0.03
24	0.65	0.68	0.03	0.68	0.03	0.64	0.01
25	0.56	0.56	0.00	0.55	0.01	0.49	0.07
26	0.73	0.75	0.02	0.75	0.02	0.61	0.12
27	0.64	0.65	0.01	0.65	0.01	0.63	0.01
28	0.63	0.73	0.10	0.72	0.09	0.68	0.05
29	0.72	0.68	0.04	0.68	0.04	0.70	0.02
30	0.59	0.61	0.02	0.61	0.02	0.61	0.02
31	0.75	0.84	0.09	0.83	0.08	0.75	0.00
32	0.53	0.62	0.09	0.62	0.09	0.61	0.08
33	0.61	0.62	0.01	0.62	0.01	0.59	0.02
34	0.65	0.66	0.01	0.66	0.01	0.61	0.04
35	0.74	0.70	0.04	0.70	0.04	0.64	0.10
36	0.69	0.65	0.04	0.65	0.04	0.62	0.07
37	0.82	0.79	0.03	0.80	0.02	0.79	0.03
38	0.93	0.76	0.17	0.76	0.17	0.76	0.17
39	0.61	0.64	0.03	0.64	0.03	0.64	0.03
40	0.74	0.68	0.06	0.68	0.06	0.62	0.12
Mean	0.67	0.68	0.05	0.68	0.05	0.66	0.05
Standard deviation	0.08	0.07	0.04	0.07	0.04	0.08	0.05
Minimum	0.52	0.56	0.00	0.55	0.00	0.45	0.00
Maximum	0.93	0.86	0.17	0.85	0.17	0.85	0.29

In this chapter, we have presented an improved version of our method for segmenting the vascular structure of the retina that is able to deal with an increased image resolution by adjusting the size of the kernel of the filters that are required for preprocessing and vessel enhancement. We have also proved that vessel centerlines detected in lower-resolution images did not affect the final segmentation results. Vessel calibers directly calculated from the segmented vasculature were used for estimating the AVR in 40 images of the INSPIRE database and produced values comparable to those obtained by two ophthalmologists.

References

1. A. Mendonça, A. Campilho, Segmentation of retinal blood vessels by combining the detection of centerlines and morphological reconstruction, *IEEE Transactions on Medical Imaging*, 25(9): 1200–1213, 2006.
2. Image Sciences Institute. DRIVE database. DRIVE: Digital retinal images for vessel extraction. Available at: http://www.isi.uu.nl/Research/Databases/DRIVE/.
3. STARE database: Structured analysis of the retina. Available at: http://www.ces.clemson.edu/~ahoover/stare/.
4. A. Hoover, V. Kouznetsova, M. Goldbaum, Locating blood vessels in retinal images by piecewise threshold probing of matched filter response, *IEEE Transactions on Medical Imaging*, 19(3): 203–210, 2000.
5. B. Al-Diri, A. Hunter, D. Steel, M. Habib, T. Hudaib, S. Berry, REVIEW: A data set for retinal vessel profiles, In: *Proceedings of the 30th Annual International Conference of the IEEE Engineering in Medicine and Biology Society*, pp. 2262–2265, 2008.
6. University of Lincoln. 2010. Retinal image computing and understanding. REVIEW database. Available at: http://reviewdb.lincoln.ac.uk/.
7. University of Iowa Carver College of Medicine. INSPIRE-AVR database. Available at: http://webeye.ophth.uiowa.edu/component/k2/item/270.
8. M. Niemeijer, X. Xu, A. Dumitrescu, P. Gupta, B. van Ginneken, J. Folk, M. Abràmoff, Automated measurement of the arteriolar-to-venular width ratio in digital color fundus photographs, *IEEE Transactions on Medical Imaging*, 30(11): 1941–1950, 2011.
9. MESSIDOR Techno-Vision Project. 2008. MESSIDOR database. Available at: http://messidor.crihan.fr/index-en.php.
10. M. Fraz, P. Remagnino, A. Hoppe, B. Uyyanonvara, A. Rudnicka, C. Owen, S. Barman, Blood vessel segmentation methodologies in retinal images: A survey, *Computer Methods and Programs in Biomedicine*, 108: 407–433, 2012.
11. M. Abràmoff, M. Garvin, M. Sonka, Retinal imaging and image analysis, *IEEE Reviews in Biomedical Engineering*, 3: 169–208, 2010.
12. R. Bernardes, P. Serranho, C. Lobo, Digital ocular fundus imaging: A review, *Ophthalmologica*, 226(4): 161–181, 2011.
13. Q. Li, J. You, D. Zhang, Vessel segmentation and width estimation in retinal images using multiscale production of matched filter responses, *Expert Systems Applied*, 39(9): 7600–7610, 2012.
14. J. Soares, J. Leandro, R. Cesar Jr., H. Jelinek, M. Cree, Retinal vessel segmentation using the 2-Gabor wavelet and supervised classification, *IEEE Transactions on Medical Imaging*, 25(9): 1214–1222, 2006.
15. M. Martinez-Perez, A. Hughes, S. Thom, A. Bharath, K. Parker, Segmentation of blood vessels from red-free and fluorescein retinal images, *Medical Image Analysis*, 11: 47–61, 2007.
16. G. Ramlugun, V. Nagarajan, C. Chakraborty, Small retinal vessels extraction towards proliferative diabetic retinopathy screening, *Expert Systems Applied*, 39: 1141–1146, 2012.

17. G. Ramlugun, V. Nagarajan, C. Chakraborty, Small retinal vessels extraction towards proliferative diabetic retinopathy screening, *Expert Systems Applied*, 39(1): 1141–1146, 2012.
18. P. Bankhead, C. Scholfield, J. McGeown, T. Curtis, Fast retinal vessel detection and measurement using wavelets and edge location refinement, *PLoS ONE*, 7(3): e32435, 2012.
19. T. Zhu, Fourier cross-sectional profile for vessel detection on retinal images, *Computerized Medical Imaging and Graphics*, 34(3): 203–212, 2010.
20. E. Moghimirad, S. Rezatofighi, H. Soltanian-Zadeh, Retinal vessel segmentation using a multiscale medialness function, *Computers in Biology and Medicine*, 42(1): 50–60, 2012.
21. J. Ng, S. Clay, S. Barman, A. Fielder, M. Moseley, K. Parker, C. Paterson, Maximum likelihood estimation of vessel parameters from scale space analysis, *Image and Vision Computing*, 28: 56–63, 2010.
22. M. Saleh, C. Eswaran, An efficient algorithm for retinal blood vessel segmentation using h-maxima transform and multilevel thresholding, *Computer Methods in Biomechanics and Biomedical Engineering*, 15(5): 517–525, 2012.
23. M.M. Fraz, P. Remagnino, A. Hoppe, B. Uyyanonvara, A.R. Rudnicka, C.G. Owen, S.A. Barman, Ensemble classification system applied for retinal vessel segmentation on child images containing various vessel profiles, *Image Analysis and Recognition*, 7325: 380–390, 2012.
24. M. Vlachos, E. Dermatas, Multi-scale retinal vessel segmentation using line tracking, *Computerized Medical Imaging and Graphics*, 34(3): 213–227, 2010.
25. Y. Yin, M. Adel, S. Bourennane, Retinal vessel segmentation using a probabilistic tracking method, *Pattern Recognition*, 45(4): 1235–1244, 2012.
26. M. Adel, A. Moussaoui, M. Rasigni, S. Bourennane, L. Hamami, Statistical-based tracking technique for linear structures detection: Application to vessel segmentation in medical images, *IEEE Signal Processing Letters*, 7: 555–558, 2010.
27. S. Vázquez, N. Barreira, M. Penedo, M. Ortega, A. Reino, Improvements in retinal vessel clustering techniques: Towards the automatic computation of the arterio venous ratio, *Computing*, 90(3–4): 197–217, 2010.
28. M. Saez, S. González-Vázquez, M. González-Penedo, M. Barceló, M. Pena-Seijo, G. Coll de Tuero, A. Pose-Reino, Development of an automated system to classify retinal vessels into arteries and veins, *Computer Methods and Programs in Biomedicine*, 108(1): 367–376, 2012.
29. B. Al-Diri, A. Hunter, D. Steel, An active contour model for segmenting and measuring retinal vessels, *IEEE Transactions on Medical Imaging*, 28: 1488–1497, 2009.
30. X. Xu, M. Niemeijer, Q. Song, M. Sonka, M. Garvin, J. Reinhardt, M. Abràmoff, Vessel boundary delineation on fundus images using graph-based approach, *IEEE Transactions on Medical Imaging*, 30(6): 1184–1191, 2011.
31. T. Zhu, Fourier cross-sectional profile for vessel detection on retinal images, *Computerized Medical Imaging and Graphics*, 34(3): 203–212, 2010.
32. O. Faust, R. Acharya, E. Ng, K. Ng, J. Suri, Algorithms for the automated detection of diabetic retinopathy using digital fundus images: A review, *Journal of Medical Systems*, 36: 145–157, 2012.
33. C. Agurto, V. Murray, E. Barriga, S. Murillo, M. Pattichis, H. Davis, S. Russell, M. Abràmoff, P. Soliz, Multiscale AM-FM methods for diabetic retinopathy lesion detection, *IEEE Transactions on Medical Imaging*, 29(2): 502–512, 2010.
34. U. Akram, S. Khan, Automated detection of dark and bright lesions in retinal images for early detection of diabetic retinopathy, *Journal of Medical Systems*, 36(5): 3151–3162, 2012.
35. W.K. Pratt, *Digital Image Processing*, 3rd edn., New York: Wiley, 2001.
36. T.S. Yoo, G.D. Stetten, B. Lorensen, Basic image processing and linear operators, In: T.S. Yoo (ed.), *Insight into Images*, pp. 19–45. Wellesey, MA: A K Peters, Ltd., 2004.
37. P. Salembier, Comparison of some morphological segmentation algorithms based on contrast enhancement: Application to automatic defect detection, In: L. Torres, E. Masgrau, M.A. Lagunas (eds), *Signal Processing V: Theories and Applications*, pp. 833–836. Amsterdam: Elsevier, 1990.
38. P. Soille, *Morphological Image Analysis: Principles and Applications*, 2nd edn., pp. 199–201. Berlin: Springer-Verlag, 2003.

39. M. Knudtson, K. Lee, L. Hubbard, T. Wong, R. Klein, B. Klein, Revised formulas for summarizing retinal vessel diameters, *Current Eye Research*, 27(3): 143–149, 2003.

40. A. Mendonça, F. Cardoso, A. Sousa, A. Campilho, Automatic localization of the optic disc in retinal images based on the entropy of vascular directions, *Image Analysis and Recognition*, 7325: 424–431, 2012.

41. Kingston University Research. CHASE_DB1 database. Available at: http://sec.kingston.ac.uk/retinal.

6

Automatic Analysis of the Microaneurysm Turnover in a Web-Based Framework for Retinal Analysis

Noelia Barreira, Manuel G. Penedo, Sonia González,
Lucía Ramos, Brais Cancela, and Ana González

CONTENTS

Diabetic retinopathy is a well-known disease related to diabetes that can cause blindness in its later stages. Each stage of this disease is characterized by a different kind of retinal lesion. Microaneurysms are small red dots that appear in the first stages of diabetic retinopathy. For this reason, the detection of these structures from retinal images is a key issue for early diagnosis. Moreover, several studies have shown that microaneurysm turnover, that is, the formation rate of this kind of lesion, is a sign of worsening of the patient's condition. In this chapter, we propose an automatic procedure for the identification of microaneurysms from retinal images as well as a methodology for lesion registration in order to compute the rate of microaneurysm turnover. We also include an automatic procedure for evaluating the significance of the microaneurysms related to their position with respect to the fovea, which is responsible for sharp central vision. Moreover, we describe the integration of these algorithms in a web-based framework for retinal analysis.

6.1 Introduction

Diabetic retinopathy is a complication of diabetes mellitus (DM) that can cause vision loss and blindness. This pathology is present in most patients with Type 1 diabetes and 77% of patients with Type 2 diabetes. The World Health Organization (WHO) estimates that after 15 years of diabetes, approximately 2% of people become blind and about 10% develop severe visual impairment. In 2008, diabetes affected 347 million people around the world and its global prevalence is rising due to the effects of diet and lifestyle [1]. As a consequence, the number of patients affected by visual impairment will increase over time, as will the associated health care costs.

Diabetic retinopathy is mainly characterized by four kinds of retinal lesions (Figure 6.1). Microaneurysms are small circular red dots of blood caused by capillary breakage. When the break affects a vein or an artery, the lesion is larger and irregular so it is known as a microhemorrhage. Hard exudates are bright dots or groups of dots around the capillaries that are produced when vessels leak lipids into the retina. Finally, cotton wool or soft exudates are whitish areas caused by nerve fiber layer infarctions apparent in automatic analysis of the microaneurysm turnover in a web-based framework of the retina. The presence of these lesions in the retina establishes four stages in the development of the disease:

- *Mild nonproliferative diabetic retinopathy*: Microaneurysms and microhemorrhages appear in the eye fundus.

- *Moderate nonproliferative diabetic retinopathy*: This is characterized by the presence of soft exudates.

- *Severe nonproliferative diabetic retinopathy*: Retinal vessels become blocked, so the retina secretes a substance that stimulates the growth of new capillaries. Microaneurysms and microhemorrhages become severe and cover the whole of the retina.

- *Proliferative diabetic retinopathy*: New capillaries grow in the retina. Their walls are very thin and so the risk of hemorrhages increases. If the hemorrhages are located at the fovea, they can cause blindness.

Treatments are more effective in the early stages of the disease, but in these stages patients do not suffer significant changes in their vision and so in most cases the retinopathy is not

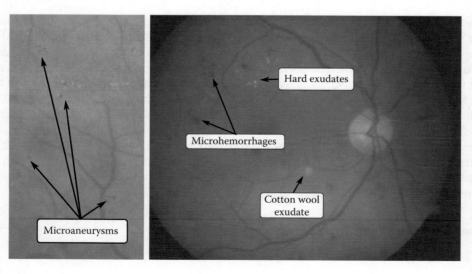

FIGURE 6.1
Typical retinal lesions of diabetic retinopathy.

diagnosed. Even though vision loss can be partially corrected by argon laser photocoagulation in the later stages, the retinopathy cannot be reversed. For this reason, early diagnosis and treatment are critical issues. The Diabetic Retinopathy Study [2] and the Early Treatment Diabetic Retinopathy Study [3] have shown that early treatment can reduce visual loss by up to 90%, as well as reducing cases of blindness from 50% to 5%. In this sense, one of the main directives of the WHO is screening programs for the early diagnosis and monitoring of diabetic retinopathy. To this end, retinographs are widely used in hospitals and primary health care centers.

Since diabetic retinopathy presents several progressive lesions in the retina, these lesions can be used to monitor the disease. Microaneurysms are the first sign of diabetic retinopathy. The amount of microaneurysms is variable and it is related to the seriousness of the retinopathy. In this sense, the microaneurysm formation rate or turnover is a well-known parameter in the study of the progress of the disease [4,5].

However, screening is not straightforward because identifying and matching retinal lesions over time and across different retinal images is a difficult, subjective, and time-consuming task, and the diabetic population is constantly growing. Therefore, numerous efforts have been made to develop automatic tools for diabetic retinopathy screening purposes.

In this chapter, we describe the stages of the development of a methodology for screening for the first stages of diabetic retinopathy and the analysis of microaneurysm turnover. Microaneurysms are detected from the retinal image by means of template matching and a set of specialized filters in an unsupervised manner. A registration technique aligns retinal images from the same patient in order to compute the turnover variable and analyze the disease progression. Finally, automatic detection of the fovea allows quantification of the significance of the lesions. We also describe the integration of this methodology in a web-based framework for retinal analysis. This task includes the development of a suitable interface for presenting the results as well as the efficient integration of image-processing techniques into the framework.

This chapter is organized as follows. Section 6.2 reviews the works presented in the literature in this field. Section 6.3 presents a methodology for microaneurysm detection and turnover analysis around the fovea. Section 6.4 describes a web framework for computer-aided diagnosis as well as a web interface for diabetic retinopathy screening. Finally, Section 6.5 presents the conclusions of this chapter.

6.2 State of the Art

Diabetic retinopathy is a well-known complication of diabetes. Thus, in the literature we can find several works that deal with the automatic detection and monitoring of various signs of this pathology. Some of these works have also led to the development of computer-aided diagnosis systems for detecting and grading diabetic retinopathy.

In 1997, Cree et al. [6] proposed one of the first tools for detecting microaneurysms and computing their turnover from angiographies. Their methodology was based on removing the vessel tree by means of morphological operators and detecting the candidate microaneurysms using a matched filter. These candidates were the input of a classifier that decided the final output. They achieved a sensitivity of 0.82 with 5.7 false positives per image. Frame et al. [7] compared several classification methods for detecting microaneurysms from angiographies. However, even though microaneurysms can be clearly detected in this kind of image, this imaging technique requires the injection of a contrast agent into the blood vessels. The use of noninvasive techniques, such as retinographies, is preferred nowadays.

In 2005, Niemeijer et al. published one of the most frequently cited works in this field [8]. First, they isolated the candidate points by removing other retinal structures. Then, they computed a set of features from the candidate points. These features were based on analysis of the shape, size, and color of typical microaneurysms. Finally, they used the *k*-nearest neighbor classifier to identify the lesions, achieving a sensitivity of 100% at a specificity of 87% on a data set with 100 images.

In 2007, Walter et al. [9] proposed a similar approach. First, they performed a contrast and shade normalization in the color fundus image. They then detected the candidate lesions using the diameter closing operator and, finally, several features computed from the candidate lesions were the input of a classifier. They obtained a sensitivity of 88.47% on a data set of 94 images.

In 2009, the Retinopathy Online Challenge was organized in order to compare several tools for microaneurysm detection on a data set of 100 images with an available gold standard [10]. Five research groups presented their algorithms [11–14] and several tests were designed to evaluate their performance. The best detector method was the algorithm proposed by Quellec et al. [11] that models the microaneurysms as 2D Gaussian functions and uses template matching in the wavelet domain. Nevertheless, one of the main conclusions of this challenge was the need for more research in this area since the performance of these automatic methodologies has not yet reached the level of accuracy of human experts.

Recently, Faust et al. [15] reviewed several algorithms for detecting microaneurysms and other lesions related with diabetic retinopathy.

In addition, there has recently been increasing interest in the development of computer-aided diagnosis systems for diabetic retinopathy diagnosis and screening. Abramoff et al. [16] and Sanchez et al. [17] evaluated systems for diabetic retinopathy detection and screening, respectively. These systems integrate several algorithms for detecting retinal structures as well as lesions. In the case of microaneurysms, their detection is based on the algorithms proposed by Niemeijer et al. [8]. In addition, Cunha-Vaz et al. [18] presented a commercial computer-aided system aimed at diabetic retinopathy screening that is able to detect microaneurysms and compute their turnover over time.

6.3 Methodology

In this section, we describe a complete methodology for computing the microaneurysm turnover rate from retinal images. This methodology consists of three main stages. First, the microaneurysms are detected in two input images from the same patient and eye. These images are then registered using the vessel tree as the reference, with the aim of computing the microaneurysm formation rate. Finally, the fovea is automatically detected in order to analyze possible vision damage.

6.3.1 Microaneurysm Detection

Microaneurysms are small circular red dots located within the retina. The image pixels within the microaneurysm are darker than the pixels in the surrounding area. On account of this, a simple methodology can be developed using size, shape, and intensity features [19]. First, all of the candidate microaneurysms are located within the image, and then they are filtered using domain knowledge in order to discard false lesions.

In the first stage of this methodology, the candidate microaneurysms can be detected by template matching using a circular kernel of the appropriate size. Figure 6.2 shows two kinds of kernels that can be used to this end: a circle-shaped kernel and a Gaussian kernel, defined as follows:

$$k_{\text{circle}(x,y)} = \begin{cases} 0 & x^2 + y^2 \le r^2 \\ a & \text{otherwise} \end{cases}, \; k_{\text{Gaussian}}(x,y) = ae^{-(x^2+y^2)/2\sigma^2} \tag{6.1}$$

where a controls the depth of the kernel while r and σ set the radius of the circle.

In both cases, there are three parameters that depend on the image features. On one hand, the kernel size and the circle radius (represented by σ in the Gaussian function) depend on the image resolution. On the other hand, the depth of the kernel, that is, the difference in the intensity between pixels inside and outside the circle, depends on image color features. In addition, microaneurysm size is not homogeneous, so correlation with a kernel of fixed size could not detect all of the microaneurysms. To solve this problem, the outputs of several kernels can be combined in order to increase the coverage of the search space:

$$I_{\text{corr}}(x,y) = \max\{I_{\text{corr}}(x,y), 1 \le i \le n\} \tag{6.2}$$

where n is the number of kernels and $I_{\text{corr}}(x,y)$ is the output of the correlation algorithm with the ith kernel at position (x,y).

Finally, the correlation image I_{corr} is thresholded in order to identify the candidate microaneurysms. Figure 6.3 shows a 1280×1024 retinal image labeled by two experts from the Complexo Hospitalario Universitario de A Coruña (Spain). Note that, due to the difficulty of the task, the labeling does not match exactly: one of the experts marked 50 microaneurysms whereas the other marked only 31. The number of coincidences between both experts is 28. This figure also shows the output of the template-matching stage. First, three Gaussian templates were applied to the green channel of the retinal image using the parameters shown in Table 6.1. The template matching was performed by means of

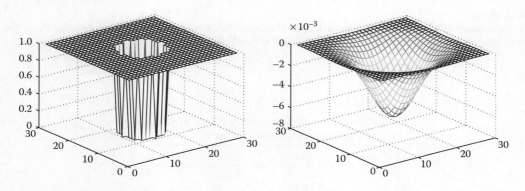

FIGURE 6.2
Templates for candidate microaneurysm detection. (*left*) 29×29 circular kernel with $r = 5$; (*right*) 29×29 Gaussian kernel with $r = 5$.

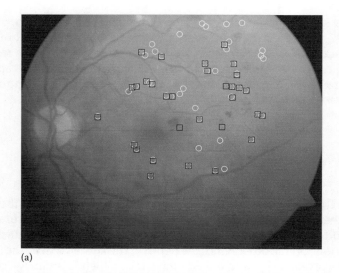

(a)

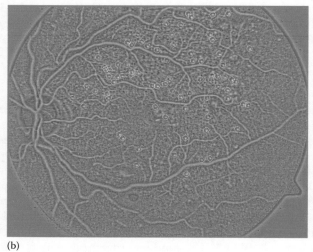

(b)

FIGURE 6.3
(a) Input image labeled by two experts; (b) output of the correlation with several Gaussian kernels. The circles mark the points with a correlation value larger than the threshold.

TABLE 6.1

Parameters of the Correlation Filters Applied
to the Retinal Image from Figure 6.3

	Size	σ	a
k_1	11×11	1.0	60
k_2	19×19	1.5	60
k_3	19×19	1.75	60

the normalized cross-correlation algorithm. Then, the outputs were combined using Equation 6.2. Finally, values higher than a threshold $t_{corr} = 0{:}5$ were chosen as candidate microaneurysms. In this example, all of the points selected by both experts are marked as candidate points.

Generally, all of the microaneurysms are detected by template matching, but several false positives are also achieved. In order to discard the incorrect points, several filters based on microaneurysm features are applied to the candidates:

6.3.1.1 Size

The microaneurysms are small, so those candidates whose area is larger than the threshold must be discarded. The template-matching procedure points out the pixels with a high correlation value but it does not define the boundaries of the region that surrounds the candidate point. To this end, a region-growing procedure is started from each candidate point. If several candidate points are connected, the pixel with the highest correlation is selected as the seed for the region-growing procedure. The following equation is used to compute the threshold that determines whether a connected pixel belongs to the candidate region:

$$t_{rg} = I_{seed} - \alpha \left(I_{seed} - I_{bg} \right) \tag{6.3}$$

where:
I_{seed} is the intensity at the seed coordinates
α is a weighting term
I_{bg} is the intensity of the background image computed from the input image by means of a median filter

Since the threshold is computed for each region, it does not depend on the image features. The growing process (more or less restrictive) is controlled by α.

Figure 6.4 (top) shows the output of the region-growing algorithm in black, with $\alpha = 0.5$. The size of the median filter is 41×41. White circles identify the regions that contain more than 65 pixels and that were discarded before further processing.

6.3.1.2 Shape

Microaneurysms are circular, so this property is checked in the remaining candidates using an equation that analyzes the circularity of a region:

$$C = \frac{p^2}{4\pi a} \tag{6.4}$$

where p represents the perimeter of the candidate region and a represents its area.

In order to smooth the boundaries of the candidate regions, a morphological closing is applied to the output of the region-growing procedure. Since the perimeter and the area are correlated, the circularity threshold does not depend on image features.

Figure 6.4 (bottom) shows in black the output of the morphological closing applied to the output of the region-growing algorithm. White circles point out regions with a circularity value lower than 0.5.

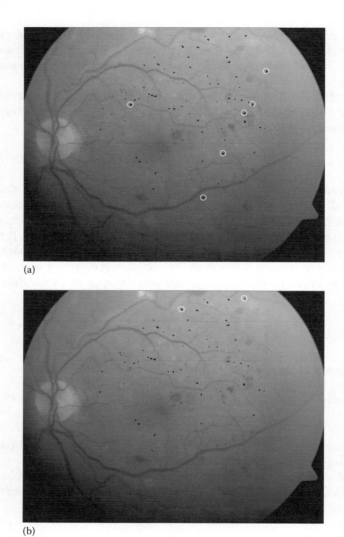

(a)

(b)

FIGURE 6.4
White circles indicate the candidate regions discarded due to their size (a) or shape (b). The black areas represent the output of the region-growing procedure (a) and its morphological closing (b).

6.3.1.3 Distance to Vessels

Template matching sometimes produces a high correlation coefficient inside retinal vessels. In order to discard these points, the skeleton of the vessel tree is computed using the MLSEC-ST operator [20] to discard the closest candidate points.

Figure 6.5 shows that the output of the MLSEC-ST operator (top) as well as the candidate region was discarded because it is located over a vessel.

6.3.1.4 Region Correlation

Not only is there a high correlation coefficient at the seed, but all of the pixels in the candidate region must also give a high enough correlation coefficient. To this end, we compute

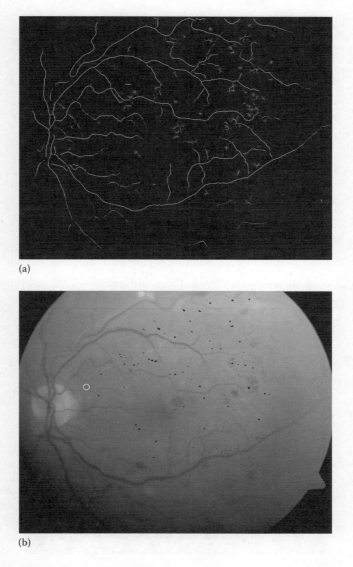

(a)

(b)

FIGURE 6.5
(a) Skeleton of the vessel tree computed by the MLSEC-ST operator; (b) the white circle indicates the candidate region discarded due to its distance from the vessel tree.

the mean correlation in the candidate region. If this value is larger than the threshold, the region is accepted as a microaneurysm.

Figure 6.6 shows the regions discarded because their mean correlation coefficient was lower than 0.4.

Finally, Figure 6.7 shows the output of the detection algorithm in the example image. Note that the algorithm was able to detect all of the microaneurysms detected by both experts.

In a data set of 75 images marked by an expert clinician, this methodology was able to correctly detect 70.7% of the lesions with a sensitivity of 0.785 [19].

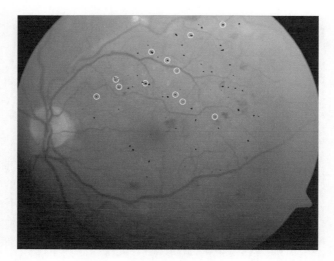

FIGURE 6.6
White circles indicate the candidate regions discarded because their mean region correlation is low.

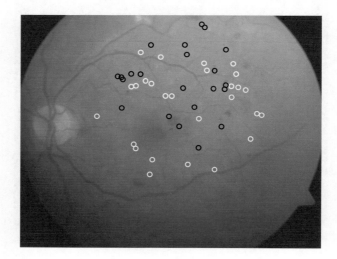

FIGURE 6.7
Output of the microaneurysm detector. White circles represent the coincidences of the described methodology with the labeling of two experts, whereas black circles stand for incorrect detections.

6.3.2 Turnover Analysis

Microaneurysm turnover is defined as the formation and disappearance rate of micro-aneurysms in images of the same patient taken at different times. Since the location of the retinal structures is different in each image due to the acquisition procedure, manual turnover computation is almost impossible. For this reason, an automatic registration and microaneurysm matching procedure is needed.

Marino et al. [21] described an automatic algorithm to register two images. This is based on the registration of the skeletons of the vessel tree, computed using the MLSEC-ST operator. One image is fixed (reference image) and the other one is transformed until a high correlation coefficient between both images is achieved. This task is time-consuming since it involves numerous image transformations. In order to reduce the computation times, a multiresolution approach is applied.

In the multiresolution approach, a pyramid of images is built for each skeleton image. Each pyramid level contains a half-resolution version of the image at the previous level. The process is repeated up to a minimum image size of 64 pixels in each axis. Then, an exhaustive search procedure is started at the top of the pyramid (smallest images) in the Fourier domain. The transformations with the highest correlation coefficients are the seeds for the search in the next pyramid level, where a Downhill Simplex algorithm is used to optimize the correlation. At the intermediate levels, the search finishes when the difference between the maximum and minimum values found in each neighboring transformation is lower than the threshold. Finally, the normalized cross-correlation coefficient is computed in the last level of the pyramid in order to find the best transformation and determine the quality of the overall process.

The output of the registration is a transformation matrix between the reference image and the other image. This transformation matrix is applied to the coordinates of the micro-aneurysms detected in the second image in order to set their position in the reference image. The coordinates of the microaneurysms are then compared in order to compute the statistics for the turnover analysis.

6.3.3 Fovea Location

The fovea is a region of the retina with a high concentration of cone photoreceptors and is responsible for sharp central vision and color perception. Any lesion near this region can cause significant vision loss. As a result, the location of lesions with respect to this structure is relevant.

In a retinal image, the fovea is seen as a dark circular spot similar to the optic disc in size. The distance to the optic disc is approximately two times the optic disc diameter, and no vessels go through it since it is located between the main vessel arcs. According to the morphology of the retina, a three-stage methodology can be developed in order to detect the fovea [22].

The first step of this methodology is the optic disc segmentation. The optic disc is a circular bright spot and is the entry point for the major vessels that irrigate the retina. Thus, one of most frequently studied procedures to locate this structure is the analysis of the crossing region of the main vessel arcs. To this end, a restrictive parameter configuration of the MLSEC-ST operator [20] can detect the thickest retinal vessels. After that, a third order polynomial fitting is performed in order to find the crossing region. Once the optic disc ROI is defined, the next step is the precise segmentation of its boundaries using one of the techniques proposed in the literature. Then, the main vessels are fitted to a parabola and a ROI for the fovea is defined inside this parabola at a distance of two optic disc diameters from the optic disc center. Finally, the fovea is detected within the ROI by template matching with a Gaussian kernel of the appropriate size. Figure 6.8 summarizes the steps of this procedure. Finally, the importance of each lesion can be weighted by computing its distance to the fovea.

The success rate of this methodology was 96% in a set of 50 images with different grades of diabetic retinopathy acquired at the Complexo Hospital Universitario de A Coruña (Spain).

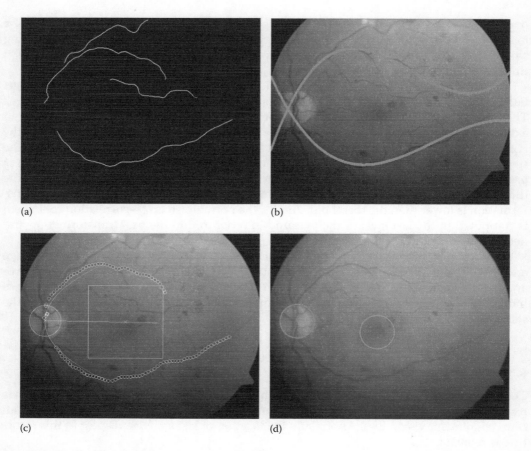

FIGURE 6.8
Fovea location: (a) output of the MLSEC-ST operator; (b) the crossing of the fitted third order polynomials points out the optic disc ROI; (c) the fovea ROI is detected after fitting the main vessels with a parabola; (d) the fovea is detected by template matching in the ROI.

6.4 Web-Based Framework for Retinal Analysis

Ortega et al. [23] presented the Sirius project, a web-based framework for processing retinal images. This project was built with two main objectives: the integration of several automatic image-processing methodologies with a user-friendly interface, and centralized data management accessible from different locations.

Sirius is a web application with a three-layer architecture summarized in Figure 6.9. From a functional point of view, the web application is accessed by authorized users over the Internet through a web browser. The web server manages the user requests. On one hand, medical histories and retinal images are stored in a relational database by means of web application forms. The application also generates reports summarizing the most relevant data for each patient. On the other hand, image-processing requests are launched from the web application and are executed in the image-processing server. This architecture distributes the workload across several computers in the intranet. In addition, users

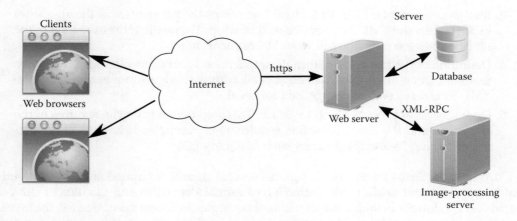

FIGURE 6.9
Overview of the Sirius framework. Several clients are connected to the web server where the application is running. The web application uses a relational database to store data and an image-processing server to process the retinal images.

are not affected by changes in the web application since they access the application via a web browser.

From a technical point of view, the web application was implemented in Java using the Model-View-Controller design pattern [24]. The View and Controller layers use the Apache Struts framework [25] and the JSTL library [26]. The database connections are managed using the JDBC library [27]. The web application runs in an Apache Tomcat web server [28] and data is stored in a PostgreSQL database [29]. Both programs run in a Debian Linux operating system. The image-processing server was implemented in C++ using the OpenCV libraries [30]. The communication protocol between the web application (Java) and the image-processing server (C++) is XML-RPC [31,32].

The integration of a new image-processing methodology into the Sirius framework entails three steps in the image-processing server:

1. Implementation and compilation of the algorithm as a C++ library
2. Definition of a new XML-RPC service that unwraps the input XML parameters, calls the appropriate functions in the C++ library, and returns the output of the algorithm wrapped in XML
3. Publication of the XML-RPC service in the XML-RPC server

The development of an interface for the image-processing algorithm in the web application comprises several steps:

1. Design of the domain objects using the Value Object design pattern [24]. For example, the class MicroaneurysmMethodVO stores the result of the execution of the microaneurysm detector (image, current date, list of detected microaneurysms, expert) whereas the class MicroaneurysmVO stores the coordinates of a microaneurysm in a given image.
2. Persistence of the domain objects in the relational database. This task requires the creation of the appropriate tables in the relational database and the implementation of a Data Access Object [24] to manage the data from the web application.

3. Implementation of a XML-RPC client that wraps the parameters of the algorithm in XML, calls the XML-RPC service, and unwraps the result. If the execution of the service takes too long, the call would be asynchronous.

4. Definition of the use cases within the application Front Controller [24]. Generally, there are three main use cases associated with each algorithm: execution of the XML-RPC service, data storage, and retrieval.

5. Design of an appropriate web interface. This step depends on the features of the algorithm and the user interaction requirements. Complex behaviors are implemented using JavaScript libraries, such as JQuery [33].

Currently, the Sirius framework integrates several algorithms aimed at processing retinal images with two main goals: extraction of retinal structures and calculus of clinical variables. The former includes automatic methodologies to detect the optic disc, the fovea, and the vessel tree structure. The latter consists of several methodologies to compute and monitor the arteriovenous ratio (AVR) [23] and the microaneurysm turnover.

In order to detect microaneurysms, the user selects an input image and the microaneurysm detection procedure. The web server receives the request and sends the data to the image-processing server. The image is automatically processed and its output, that is, the microaneurysm locations within the image, is sent back to the web server that generates the response shown in the browser.

Figure 6.10 shows a JavaScript tool developed for displaying the location of microaneurysms. This tool also allows user interaction in order to confirm or eliminate the candidate points.

In the case of microaneurysm turnover, the user selects two previously processed images of the same eye and starts the monitoring procedure in the web server. The web server sends the input images to the image-processing server and retrieves the transformation

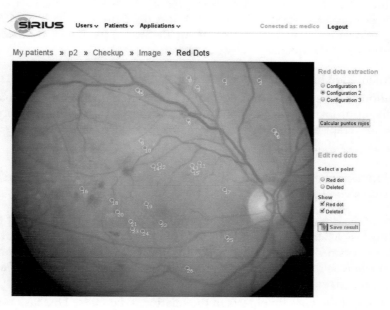

FIGURE 6.10
Detection of microaneurysms in the Sirius framework.

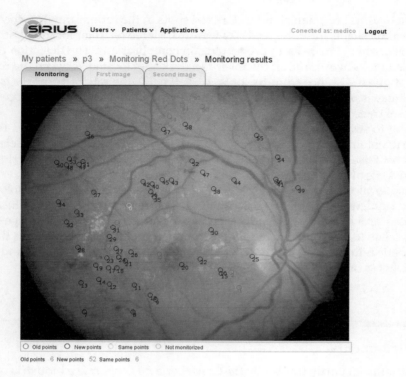

FIGURE 6.11
Turnover analysis in the Sirius framework.

matrix that aligns both images. The first image is used as the reference image. After that, the web server recomputes the microaneurysm locations in the reference image and generates the output for the browser.

Figure 6.11 shows the tool for displaying the results of the microaneurysm monitoring. Several colors represent microaneurysms detected in both images, in the first image only, or in the second image only. Moreover, another color represents the microaneurysms located outside the area covered by both images. Numeric data summarize the results of the monitoring.

6.5 Conclusions

Diabetic retinopathy is a significant complication of diabetes that causes vision loss. The prevalence of this pathology is continuously increasing, so automatic tools for diagnosis and screening are needed. Moreover, early diagnosis and treatment are required in order to minimize the adverse effects of this pathology.

This chapter describes a methodology for detecting microaneurysms from retinal images and computing their formation rate or turnover. Microaneurysms are the first signs of diabetic retinopathy and the study of their evolution is often used to evaluate the progress of the disease.

Microaneurysms are small circular dark red spots in the retina, and thus their detection can be based on shape, intensity, and size features. Moreover, their location with respect to the fovea is analyzed in order to prevent vision complications. The detection of the fovea is also based on known features: the fovea is a dark spot located between the retinal main vessels at a given distance from the optic disc. Finally, the rate of turnover is computed from two images of the same patient and eye by means of a registration procedure based on the vessel tree.

According to several experts, the more lesions detected, the better. In this respect, it is preferable to obtain a low false negative rate than a false positive rate in the detection stage because most false positives are due to similar lesions, such as microhemorrhages, therefore, an analysis of their evolution would prove interesting.

This chapter also describes the integration of image-processing methodologies into a web-based framework aimed at retinal analysis. The web framework simplifies data management and provides a user-friendly interface for interaction with the image-processing algorithms. The use of this kind of tool for computer-aided diagnosis allows the monitoring of diabetic retinopathy in large population groups, thus reducing costs and increasing the effectiveness of treatment.

Acknowledgments

This work has been partly funded by the Consellería de Economía e Industria of the Xunta de Galicia through the research project 10TIC009CT.

References

1. Danaei, G., M.M. Finucane, Y. Lu, G.M. Singh, M.J. Cowan, C.J. Paciorek, J.K. Lin, et al. National, regional, and 29 global trends in fasting plasma glucose and diabetes prevalence since 1980: Systematic analysis of health examination surveys and epidemiological studies with 370 country-years and 2.7 million participants. *The Lancet*, 378(9785):31–40, 2011.
2. Aiello, L.M., J. Berrocal, M.D. Davis, F. Ederer, M.F. Goldberg, J.E. Harris, C.R. Klimt, et al. The diabetic retinopathy study. *Archives of Ophthalmology*, 90(5):347–348, 1973.
3. Early Treatment Diabetic Retinopathy Study Research Group. Early treatment diabetic retinopathy study design and baseline patient characteristics. ETDRS Report Number 7. *Ophtalmology*, 98:741–756, 1991.
4. Kohner, E.M., I.M. Stratton, S.J. Aldington, R.C. Turner, and D.R. Matthews. Microaneurysms in the development of diabetic retinopathy (UKPDS 42). *Diabetologia*, 42(9):1107–1112, 1999.
5. Nunes, S., I. Pires, A. Rosa, L. Duarte, R. Bernardes, and J. Cunha-Vaz. Microaneurysm turnover is a biomarker for diabetic retinopathy progression to clinically significant macular edema: Findings for type 2 diabetics with nonproliferative retinopathy. *Ophthalmologica*, 223(5):292–297, 2009.
6. Cree, M., J. Olson, K. McHardy, P. Sharp, and J. Forrester. A fully automated comparative microaneurysm digital detection system. *Eye*, 11:622–628, 1997.
7. Frame, A.J., P.E. Undrill, M.J. Cree, J.A. Olson, K.C. McHardy, P.F. Sharp, and J.V. Forrester. A comparison of computer based classification methods applied to the detection of microaneurysms in ophthalmic fluorescein angiograms. *Computers in Biology and Medicine*, 28(3):225–238, 1998.

8. Niemeijer, M., B. van Ginneken, J. Staal, M.S.A. Suttorp-Schulten, and M.D. Abramoff. Automatic detection of red lesions in digital color fundus photographs. *IEEE Transactions on Medical Imaging*, 24(5):584–592, 2005.

9. Walter, T., P. Massin, A. Erginay, R. Ordonez, C. Jeulin, and J.-C. Klein. Automatic detection of microaneurysms in color fundus images. *Medical Image Analysis*, 11(6):555–566, 2007.

10. Niemeijer, M., B. van Ginneken, M.J. Cree, A. Mizutani, G. Quellec, C.I. Sanchez, B. Zhang, et al. Retinopathy online challenge: Automatic detection of microaneurysms in digital color fundus photographs. *IEEE Transactions on Medical Imaging*, 29(1):185–195, 2010.

11. Quellec, G., M. Lamard, P.M. Josselin, G. Cazuguel, B. Cochener, and C. Roux. Optimal wavelet transform for the detection of microaneurysms in retina photographs. *IEEE Transactions on Medical Imaging*, 27(9):1230–1241, 2008.

12. Sanchez, C., R. Hornero, A. Mayo, M. Garcia, and M.I. Lopez. Mixture model-based clustering and logistic regression for automatic detection of microaneurysms in retinal images. In *SPIE Medical Imaging*, 7260:72601M, 2009.

13. Jelinek, H. J., M.J. Cree, D. Worsley, A. Luckie, and P. Nixon. An automated microaneurysm detector as a tool for identification of diabetic retinopathy in rural optometric practice. *Clinical and Experimental Optometry*, 89:299–305, 2006.

14. Zhang, B., X. Wu, J. You, Q. Li, and F. Karray. Hierarchical detection of red lesions in retinal images by multiscale correlation filtering. In *SPIE Medical Imaging*, 7260:72601L, 2009.

15. Faust, O., U.R. Acharya, E.Y. Ng, K.-H. Ng, and J.S. Suri. Algorithms for the automated detection of diabetic retinopathy using digital fundus images: A review. *Journal of Medical Systems*, 36(1):145–157, 2012.

16. Abrámoff, M.D., M. Niemeijer, M.S.A. Suttorp-Schulten, M.A. Viergever, S.R. Russell, and B. van Ginneken. Evaluation of a system for automatic detection of diabetic retinopathy from color fundus photographs in a large population of patients with diabetes. *Diabetes Care*, 31(8):e64, 2008.

17. Sánchez, C.I., M. Niemeijer, A.V. Dumitrescu, M.S.A. Suttorp-Schulten, M.D. Abrámoff, and B. van Ginneken. Evaluation of a computer-aided diagnosis system for diabetic retinopathy screening on public data. *Investigative Ophthalmology and Visual Science*, 52(7):4866–4871, 2011.

18. Cunha-Vaz, J., R. Bernardes, T. Santos, C. Oliveira, C. Lobo, I. Pires, and L. Ribeiro. Computer-aided detection of diabetic retinopathy progression. In Yogesan, K., L. Goldschmidt, and J. Cuadros (eds), *Digital Teleretinal Screening*, pp. 59–66. Springer, Berlin, Heidelberg, 2012.

19. Marino, C., J. Novo, N. Barreira, and M.G. Penedo. Preventing diabetic retinopathy: Red lesions detection in early stages. *Diabetic Retinopathy*, pp. 249–270. Intech Open Access Publisher, Rijeka, Croatia, 2012.

20. López, A.M., D. Lloret, J. Serrat, and J.J. Villanueva. Multilocal creaseness based on the level-set extrinsic curvature. *Computer Vision and Image Understanding*, 77(2):111–144, 2000.

21. Marino, C., M. Penas, M.G. Penedo, J.M. Barja, V. Leborán, M.J. Carreira, and F. Gómez-Ulla. Methodology for the registration of whole SLO sequences. In *ICPR* (1), 779–783, 2002.

22. Marino, C., M.G. Penedo, S.P. Placer, and F. González. Crest line and correlation filter based location of the macula in digital retinal images. In *Biosignals* (2)'08, 521–527, 2008.

23. Ortega, M., N. Barreira, J. Novo, M.G. Penedo, A. Pose-Reino, and F. Gómez-Ulla. Sirius: A web-based system for retinal image analysis. *International Journal of Medical Informatics*, 79(10):722–732, 2010.

24. Fowler, M. *Patterns of Enterprise Application Architecture*. Addison-Wesley Longman, Boston, MA, 2002.

25. The Apache Software Foundation. Apache Struts framework. Available at http://struts.apache.org/ (accessed September 2012).

26. Oracle Corporation. JSP Standard Tag Library. Available at http://www.oracle.com/technetwork/java/jstl-137486.html (accessed September 2012).

27. Oracle Corporation. Java Database Connectivity. Available at http://www.oracle.com/technetwork/java/javase/jdbc/index.html (accessed September 2012).

28. The Apache Software Foundation. Apache Tomcat web server. Available at http://tomcat.apache.org/ (accessed September 2012).
29. The PostgreSQL Global Development Group. PostgreSQL Relational Database. Available at http://www.postgresql.org/ (accessed September 2012).
30. Bradski, G. and A. Kaehler. *Learning OpenCV: Computer Vision with the OpenCV Library,* O'Reilly Media, Sebastopol, CA, 2008.
31. The Apache Software Foundation. Apache XML-RPC for Java. Available at http://ws.apache.org/xmlrpc/ (accessed September 2012).
32. XML-RPC for C and C++. Available at http://xmlrpc-c.sourceforge.net/ (accessed September 2012).
33. The JQuery Foundation. JQuery JavaScript Library. Available at http://jquery.com/ (accessed September 2012).

7

A-Levelset-Based Automatic Cup-to-Disc Ratio Measurement for Glaucoma Diagnosis from Fundus Image

Jiang Liu, Fengshou Yin, Damon Wing Kee Wong, Zhuo Zhang, Ngan Meng Tan, Carol Cheung, Mani Baskaran, Tin Aung, and Tien Yin Wong

CONTENTS

To boost the performance of level set algorithms, we propose the A-Levelset algorithm, which cascades the level set and active shape model (ASM). The A-Levelset-based ARGALI system is built to automatically segment the optic cup and optic disc from 2D digital fundus images. The ARGALI system further calculates the cup-to-disc ratio (CDR), which is an important indicator in glaucoma assessment and diagnosis. The ARGALI system was tested on a large clinical image collection of 2616 patients in order to estimate the CDR values. The extensive experimental results clearly show that ARGALI outperforms the level set-based approach by reducing the mean absolute error rate of CDR measurement from 0.349 to 0.21 and the mean square error rate from 0.156 to 0.07. ARGALI demonstrates for the first time the capability of automatic CDR measurement in a large clinical data set. It paves the way for automatic objective glaucoma diagnosis and screening using widely available fundus images.

7.1 Introduction of Glaucoma Diagnosis

7.1.1 Glaucoma Is an Irreversible Blinding Optic Neuropathy

Glaucoma is the second leading cause of blindness, with an estimated 60 million cases globally in 2010 [1]. Glaucoma is a chronic and irreversible neurodegenerative disease in which the optic nerve is progressively damaged, leading to deterioration of vision and quality of life [1]. If undetected and untreated, glaucoma may first result in loss of peripheral vision, encroaching toward the central vision as the condition progressively worsens. At advanced stages, patients may complain of "tunnel vision" (the total loss of peripheral vision with the central vision remaining). Glaucoma is usually asymptomatic and patients are commonly unaware of the disease until noticeable visual loss occurs at a later stage. Due to its insidious nature, glaucoma is often termed the "silent thief of sight."

7.1.2 Early Detection of Glaucoma Is Important

Glaucoma is generally asymptomatic during the early stages and leads to irreversible blindness if left untreated. Without treatment, a substantial number of patients will experience significant progression of the disease. Several studies have demonstrated that the estimated progression of optic nerve fiber loss in glaucoma can be in the order of 9%–63% over a five-year period [2–4]. In view of this, early detection of glaucomatous changes is crucial to allow for early treatment prior to the onset of functional visual loss. However, despite the threat that glaucoma poses, studies in Singapore and other countries have shown that 60%–90% of glaucoma cases in the population remain undetected and untreated [5–10].

Timely treatment (e.g., lowering the intraocular pressure by medication, laser, or surgery) can halt or slow down the progression of the disease in the early stages. Hence, early detection is critical in preventing visual loss and blindness. The American Academy of Ophthalmology strongly recommends screening for glaucoma as part of a comprehensive adult medical eye evaluation, with the frequency depending on an individual's age and other risk factors for glaucoma. Due to the irreversible nature of the disease, early detection of glaucomatous changes is crucial to allow for early treatment prior to the onset of functional visual loss.

7.1.3 Glaucoma Is the Leading Cause of Irreversible Blindness

Glaucoma is the leading cause of surgically irremediable blindness worldwide. Late diagnosis can lead to irreversible damage to the optic nerve and loss of sight. While there is currently no cure for glaucoma, early detection and treatment can help prevent further damage to vision. Without treatment, glaucoma can cause total and permanent blindness within a few years.

The lowering of intraocular pressure (IOP) (e.g., by eye drops, laser, or surgery) is the only therapeutic approach that can reduce the risk of glaucoma development and slow down the rate of disease progression. However, a substantial proportion of glaucoma patients do not have IOP elevated above the normal range and therefore such strategies for lowering IOP do not prevent progressive vision loss in some glaucoma patients.

7.1.4 Currently There Are No Effective Tools for Glaucoma Screening

Despite early detection and treatment being essential in the prevention of glaucoma and the onset of vision loss, current tools for glaucoma screening remain limited. Glaucoma screening in the general population has been challenging, mainly due to the lack of simple and cost-effective screening methods. Existing glaucoma screening methods include the measurement of IOP (tonometry), visual field examination, and the use of optic nerve head imaging devices to determine optic nerve head structural damage or thinning of the retinal nerve fiber layer. Nonetheless, these methods have their limitations.

Measurement of IOP was reported to have poor sensitivity (~50%) as glaucoma may also occur when eye pressure is normal. This is typically true in cases of normal tension glaucoma. Visual field examination is often time-consuming and unreliable due to patient fatigue and the learning effect. Advanced optic nerve head imaging devices such as Heidelberg Retinal Tomography (HRT) and Optical Coherence Tomography (OCT) are very costly and normally only available at tertiary hospitals, and thus may not be feasible for wider application as a glaucoma screening tool.

7.1.5 Medical Cost of Glaucoma Management Is Substantial

The costs of glaucoma vary with patient age, disease severity, and response to treatment. Rein et al. estimated annual costs per glaucoma patient aged 40–64 years to be US$2546 for outpatient and inpatient services, and US$806 for pharmaceuticals (a total of US$3352; year 2004 values) [11]. For older patients, the costs of inpatient and outpatient services were US$5537 and pharmaceuticals were US$60, totaling US$5597 annually per patient. Average direct costs of treatment ranged from US$623 per patient per year for early stage (i.e., suspected glaucoma or early glaucoma diagnosis) to US$2511 for end-stage disease (year 2004 values) [12]. Furthermore, the above figures on glaucoma-related health-care costs may be an underestimate of the true societal and economic costs incurred by glaucoma. Costs for glaucoma are lower when the disease is in its earlier stages, suggesting that effective screening methods and early interventions could be potentially cost-saving.

7.1.6 A Sensitive, Reproducible, and Effective Tool for Screening Glaucoma Is Needed

An objective, fast, sensitive, reproducible, and effective method for detecting glaucomatous optic nerve damage for glaucoma screening is urgently needed in order to improve early detection of glaucoma and thus allow proper and timely treatment. With early detection and treatment glaucoma can almost always be controlled and vision can be preserved. Unfortunately, as addressed earlier, routine screening for glaucoma with current tests, such as tonometry, visual field testing, and retinal fiber layer imaging, may not be cost effective across the whole population, and is limited by their poor sensitivity and specificity. None of these tests, either alone or in combination, have been shown to be suitably efficient or cost effective for use as standardized screening tools for glaucoma [13]. However, the assessment of the optic nerve seems to have the most promise in terms of accuracy.

We aim to develop a novel, effective screening tool for glaucoma using automatic CDR measurement software. Such a system can be integrated into the existing fundus cameras, making the screening tool sustainable in the long term.

7.1.7 Glaucoma Is Highly Prevalent, Particularly in Asia

Glaucoma affected 60 million people worldwide in 2010 and it is estimated that this number will increase to 80 million by 2020 [1]. The disease is responsible for approximately 5.2 million cases of blindness (15% of the total burden of world blindness) [14]. The burden of the disease is heavier in Asia, where approximately half of the world's glaucoma cases can be found. Studies have reported that the prevalence of glaucoma is 2.1%–5% across Asian countries and race/ethnic groups [5,7,15]. Likewise, population-based studies in Singapore have reported that glaucoma is a major cause of visual impairment and blindness. In the Tanjong Pagar Study, the prevalence of glaucoma is 3%–4% and glaucoma contributes to 60% of bilateral blindness [15]. Glaucoma is also one of the leading causes of visual impairment in Singaporean Malay adults [5]. It is worth noting that, as ageing is one of the key risk factors of glaucoma, glaucoma morbidity will continue to rise in line with the ageing population.

7.1.8 The Economic Cost and Societal Burdens of Glaucoma Are Substantial

The public health burden and management of glaucoma contribute to significant health care costs, including both direct medical costs (ocular hypotensive medications, physician and hospital visits, glaucoma-related procedures, etc.) and indirect costs (lost productivity in patients and caregivers) [16]. In the United States, the direct cost estimate is US$2.9 billion [11] and in Australia it is AUS$144.2 million [17]. However, these figures probably underestimate the true costs if all sufferers were to be treated, since more than 50% of patients with glaucoma are undetected [5–10]. As addressed above, the health care cost of glaucoma increases as the disease severity increases. Furthermore, owing to the rapidly ageing population, the prevalence of glaucoma is increasing. Therefore, early case detection by an appropriate glaucoma screening program may not only reduce the individual burden of the disease, but also may minimize personal and societal economic burdens.

Current glaucoma detection and diagnosis require examination by a glaucoma specialist (ophthalmologists with specialized glaucoma training) with expensive equipment such as OCT and HRT, which are not widely available in public and private clinics. In contrast, the 2D fundus camera is less costly and widely used by optometrists, general ophthalmologists, and other medical professionals in primary health care for ocular disease monitoring, diagnosis, and screening. The irreversibility of vision loss, a shortage of glaucoma specialists, and lack of patient awareness (50%–90% [1,5,18]) demand an economic and objective automatic glaucoma early diagnosis system based on widely available image modalities such as fundus images.

The retinal optic CDR [18] (Figure 7.1) is widely regarded as an important indicator of the risk factor for glaucoma diagnosis. Most fundus image researchers [19–24] examine the optic nerve head to segment the optic disc using either fundus images or stereo images. Recently, some researchers [25–27] have reported the use of fundus images to directly measure both the optic disc and optic cup boundaries.

The ARGALI system [26] makes use of level set techniques in order to derive the boundaries of the optic cup and disc. It calculates the CDR from 2D fundus images and provides an objective and consistent measurement with potential for glaucoma screening. However, level set-based ARGALI was tested on only 104 images and the CDR error rates are still high. The A-Levelset medical image segmentation algorithm proposed in this

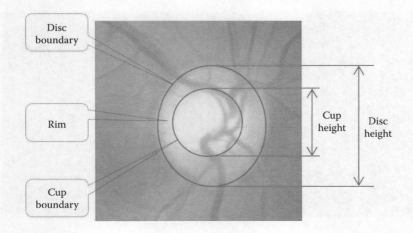

FIGURE 7.1
The optic disc (disc) is the circular area where ganglion cell axons exit the retina to form the optic nerve. The optic cup (cup) is the depression in the center of the optic disc. The area between the optic disc and cup is the optic neuroretinal rim, where the optical nerve resides. CDR = cup height/disc height.

chapter further boosts the CDR accuracy in comparison with the level set-based approach. The ARGALI system based on A-Levelset is tested on a large data set of 2616 images and achieves better experimental results. It demonstrates the capability of using fundus images to automatically measure CDR for glaucoma diagnosis.

7.2 A-Levelset Algorithm and the ARGALI System

7.2.1 ASM and Level Set for Fundus Image Segmentation

Parametric deformable ASM [28] uses an explicit parametric representation of the curve to fit the target object. The ASM is compact and able to handle images with noise and boundary gaps by constraining the boundaries to be smooth. It has been applied to optic disc boundary detection [22,23]. However, ASM's weakness in handling splitting and in situations where the object target is away from the initial contour [28] restricts its direct application to cup segmentation (as shown in Figure 7.2).

The level set [29] based ARGALI system [26] directly segments the optic disc and optic cup from 2D fundus images. It optimizes the optic disc/cup shapes globally to handle topological changes. Like ASM approaches, it can handle optic disc segmentation well. However, it is not robust to cup boundary gaps and cup local deformation, and often leaks from the temporal side of the cup during segmentation.

7.2.2 A-Levelset Algorithm

When the target object varies significantly in intensity and shape in different images, a gradient-based level set approach often fails to deal accurately with the inherent cup variability. Model-based algorithms such as ASM use a prior model of the image shape and adjust the model to find the best match to the new input image. The model is established

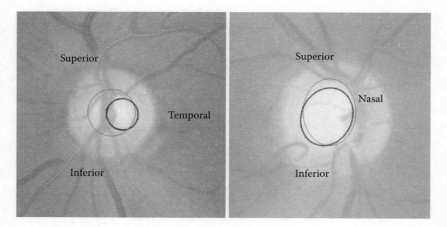

FIGURE 7.2
The first image shows ASM's difficulty in handling cup splitting into a few parts due to the blood vessels, which happens often. ASM misses the left part of the cup. The second image shows ASM falling into a local minimum when the initial contour is far from the global minimum. For large glaucomatous cups in particular, ASM is unable to segment the superior boundary (the black boundary denotes the ASM result and the gray boundary denotes the actual optic cup boundary).

through training with annotated sample images with landmark points, which can supplement the weakness of the level set in locations where the gradient change is not distinct.

To overcome the limitations of the level set-based algorithm in image segmentation, A-Levelset is proposed, which cascades the level set with the ASM algorithm and uses ASM to fine-tune the outcome of the level set algorithm. The A-Levelset algorithm includes the following three steps:

- First Step: Run level set algorithm over the image, obtain the segmented object
- Second Step: Register the level set segmented object with the ASM mean shape
- Third Step: Run ASM with the registered mean shape as the initial contour to get the fine-tuned segmented object

7.2.3 ARGALI System for Fundus Image Segmentation

In the following sections, A-Levelset is discussed in a specific application system: ARGALI. An A-Levelset-based ARGALI system is built to automatically segment the optic cup and optic disc from the 2D digital fundus images and further calculate the CDR for glaucoma diagnosis. Optic disc segmentation is not as complex as optic cup segmentation, and experimental results show that segmented optic discs from ASM, level set, and A-Levelset algorithms are comparable. For ease of discussion, from here on we focus on optic cup segmentation. Optic cup segmentation is challenging due to the condition of the decreased visibility of the boundary between the optic cup and the optic rim (as shown in Figure 7.1), and the condition is often further compounded by the high density of vascular architecture near the optic cup region.

We use $D(x, y)$ and $C(x, y)$ to represent optical disc and cup contours respectively. Disc area Da and Cup area Ca are defined as the regions enclosed by the $D(x, y)$ and $C(x, y)$. Finding the $C(x, y)$ can be understood as a fundus image segmentation issue, in which the optic cup segmentation is to find the closed contour (boundary) between the optic rim and the central cupping depression. A signed distance function $f_c(x, y)$ is used to determine the closeness of a given point (x, y) in the disc region Da to $C(x, y)$, where a positive value indicates that (x, y) is inside Ca, value zero indicates (x, y) is part of $C(x, y)$, and a negative value indicates (x, y) located outside of Ca. Using infimum function to denote the distance, we have:

$$f_c(x, y) = \begin{cases} \inf((x, y), Da) & \text{if } (x, y) \in Da \\ 0 & \text{if } (x, y) \in D \\ -\inf((x, y), Da) & \text{if } (x, y) \notin Da \end{cases} \qquad (7.1)$$

The cup segmentation becomes finding the solution for $f_c(x, y) = 0$, while satisfying the constraint C inside D.

7.2.4 The First Step in ARGALI: Level Set-Based Optic Cup Segmentation

In the ARGALI system, the optic cup is considered as the zero level set of a level set function. The segmentation of the optic cup is transferred to find the zero level set $F_{lc} = \{(x, y) \mid \phi(t, x, y) = 0\}$ of the level set function $\phi(t, x, y)$. The optic cup is thus a contracting evolution process from $D(x, y)$. Following the variational level set principle [30], the ARGALI system calculates the energy function, which keeps the level set function $\phi(t, x, y)$ close to $f_c(x, y)$. This results in a gradient flow which minimizes the overall energy of the level set function. The cup evolution can be expressed as:

$$\frac{\partial \phi}{\partial t} = \mu \left[\Delta \phi - \text{div}\left(\frac{\nabla \phi}{|\nabla \phi|} \right) \right] + \lambda \partial(\phi) \text{div}\left[g \frac{\nabla \phi}{|\nabla \phi|} \right] + vg\partial(\phi) \qquad (7.2)$$

In the above equations, μ determines the deviation of ϕ from $f_c(x, y)$ and λ and v are the coefficients of the weighted length of the zero level optical cup curve $F_{lc}(t)$ and the weighted area enclosed by $F_{lc}(t)$, respectively.

The edge indicator function is represented by g.

From ϕ, we can get the level set segmentation optic cup contour when the contour becomes stable:

$$F_{lc} = \{(x, y) \mid \phi(t, x, y) = 0\} \qquad (7.3)$$

7.2.5 The Second Step in ARGALI: Register the Level Set Segmented Cup with the ASM Mean Shape

In the second step, ARGALI calculates the ASM mean cup C_m (X_m, Y_m), which is often used as the initial contour, from the training samples. To integrate the level set-based segmentation result and provide a better estimate of the cup contour, ARGALI combines C_m and F_{lc} to form a new registered mean cup C_{rm}:

$$C_{rm} = \text{Reg}(C_m, S, \theta, h, k) \qquad (7.4)$$

$$X_{rm} = S\left(X_m \cos\theta + Y_m \sin\theta\right) + h \tag{7.5}$$

$$Y_{rm} = S\left(-X_m \sin\theta + Y_m \cos\theta\right) + k \tag{7.6}$$

where:
  S is the scaling factor
  θ is the rotational factor and
  (h, k) is the location translational difference between $C_{rm}(X_{rm}, Y_{rm})$ and $C_m(X_m, Y_m)$

The above parameters can be determined by matching N control points in F_{lc} and $C_m(X_m, Y_m)$ along the two cup boundaries. While parameters (h, k) are determined by centroid mapping, the parameters s and θ are calculated by:

$$S = \sqrt{\left(\sum_{i=1}^{N} \frac{X_m(i) Y_{rm}(i) - Y_m(i) X_{rm}(i)}{X_m^{\,2}}\right) + \left(\frac{X_m \cdot X_{rm}}{X_m^{\,2}}\right)^2} \tag{7.7}$$

$$\theta = \operatorname{atan} \sum_{i=1}^{N} \frac{X_m(i) Y_{rm}(i) - Y_m(i) X_{rm}(i)}{X_m \cdot X_{rm}} \tag{7.8}$$

In the ARGALI system, the scaled, rotated, and center-translated new mean shape C_{rm} is used as the initial contour for the ASM algorithm fine-tuning in the third step.

7.2.6 The Third Step in ARGALI: Run ASM with the New Registered Mean Shape as the Initial Contour

In ARGALI, the ASM landmark point set is represented by:

$$LM_c = \left(x_1, \ldots x_i, \ldots x_n, y_1, \ldots y_i, \ldots y_n\right) \tag{7.9}$$

where:
  (x_i, y_i) denotes the ith landmark point and
  LM_c is a $2n$ dimensional vector.

PCA is applied first to reduce dimensions and prevent overfitting, thus LM_c can be further described as:

$$LM_c = T\left(h, k, S, \theta\right)\left(\operatorname{Mean}\left(LM_c(i) + Ev\right)\right) \tag{7.10}$$

where:
  T is the translation factor (similar to the definitions in Equations 7.4 through 7.6 in the second step
  E is the eigenvectors of the covariance matrix
  Mean is the average function and
  v is a vector defining shape variation

Step 3 of ARGALI can be described as:

C1. Initialization:

For all landmark points: $LM_c(i)$ = Landmark point (x_i, y_i) in C_{rm}; construct cup boundary from those landmark points:

Let $C_{al} = C_{al}(LM_c)$.

C2. Update landmark points:

For all landmark points, find the best nearby match $New\text{-}LM_c(i)$ by looking along profiles normal to the model boundary.

Let: $LM_c = New\text{-}LM_c$; $C_{al} = C_{al}(LM_c)$.

C3. Apply constraint to parameter v to make sure that cup boundary does not deviate too far away from C_{rm}:

C_{al} = Constraint (C_{al}, C_{rm}).

C4. Repeat C2 to C3 until C_{rm} converges or the maximum iteration is reached.

C5. Smooth the cup boundary using ellipse fitting:

Get the final cup boundary of ARGALI:

$C(x, y)$ = Ellipse-fit (C_{al}).

7.3 Results

7.3.1 Data Sets Used for ARGALI System Evaluation

The 2616 images used for evaluation are from three sources: an RVGSS data set of 291 cases collected from a national eye center with 66 confirmed glaucoma cases and 225 non-glaucoma cases; a Chinese eye population study SCES [31] data set with 75 glaucoma cases and 1600 non-glaucoma cases of ethnic Chinese; and an ORIGA light [32] data set of 650 cases collected from a Malay eye population study [33] with 165 glaucoma cases and 485 non-glaucoma cases of ethnic Malays (some samples are shown in Figure 7.3). The images were taken using slightly different camera settings. This is the largest fundus data set ever used for automatic CDR measurement testing; the number of images ARGALI [26] used is only 104 from SIMES [33].

7.3.2 ARGALI Experimental Results and Analysis

The optic cup ASM model is trained using 325 ground truth fundus images from data set ORIGA light. Empirically, 4 control points are used in the A-Levelset second step; 20

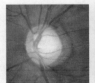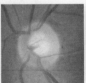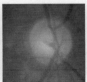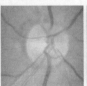

FIGURE 7.3
Sample images from left to right are: one glaucoma case and one non-glaucoma case from RVGSS; one glaucoma case and one non-glaucoma case from the Chinese eye study; two cases from ORIGA light database with ground truth optic disc and optic cup boundary marked.

landmark points evenly distributed at 15° each; and 0.2 CDR maximum variations are used as the constraints in Step 3. Parameters h and k are decided by the distance between the centroids of the initial ASM cup mean shape and the level set segmented cup in both the second and third step.

In the experiment, the ARGALI system is run on a Dell Precision T3500V Workstation with Intel Xeon CPU W3503 2.4 GHz (Duo-Core) processor and 4 GB of RAM. The average time to obtain the CDR value from a fundus image is 7.4 s. This is an acceptable patient waiting time in a clinical setting. Figure 7.4 illustrates ARGALI's leaking prevention compared with the level set-based approach.

We use the outputs of the first step of ARGALI as the level set cup boundary results and compare the CDRs of the two approaches. As the structure of the optic disc is relatively distinctive, the disc segmentation results from ASM, level set, and A-Levelset algorithms are rather similar. To make the comparison objective (in case both optic disc and optic cup are wrongly segmented but still get good CDR ratio), we use the ASM segmented disc as the common disc to compare CDRs for both level set- and A-Levelset-based algorithms. So, CDR-LS = Cup height (level set)/Disc height (ASM) and CDR-ARGALI = Cup height (ARGALI)/Disc height (ASM).

Table 7.1 compares ARGALI and level set-based approaches using the mean square error (MSE) and mean absolute error (MAE) for the CDR. Figure 7.5 shows four sets of image comparison of the level set approach and ARGALI cup segmentation results. The experimental results clearly demonstrate that A-Levelset is able to boost the performance of level set across most of the sub data sets, with or without glaucoma pathology. The exception is

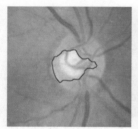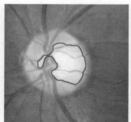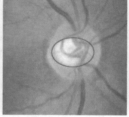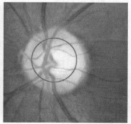

FIGURE 7.4

The first two images are the output of level set algorithm and the last two images are the ARGALI's results, where the leakings of the first two are prevented at the temporal side.

TABLE 7.1

ARGALI and Level Set-Based Approach in CDR Measurement (Numbers of Subsample Size in Brackets)

		RVGSS (291)			ORIGA (650)			SCES (1675)			Combined (2616)		
		Norm (225)	Glau (66)	All (291)	Norm (485)	Glau (165)	All (650)	Norm (1600)	Glau (75)	All (1675)	Norm (2310)	Glau (306)	All (2616)
CDR-LS	MSE	0.215	0.013	0.169	0.089	0.021	0.072	0.194	0.027	0.187	0.174	0.021	0.156
	MAE	0.438	0.090	0.359	0.264	0.119	0.227	0.407	0.140	0.395	0.380	0.118	0.349
CDR-ARGALI	MSE	0.079	0.026	0.067	0.030	0.014	0.026	0.091	0.024	0.088	0.077	0.019	0.070
	MAE	0.236	0.133	0.212	0.133	0.096	0.123	0.249	0.119	0.244	0.224	0.110	0.210

Note: SCES glaucoma patient with large CDR. ORIGA normal patient with medium CDR.

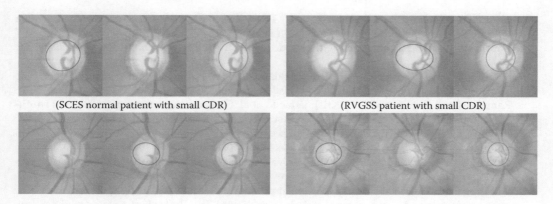

(SCES normal patient with small CDR)   (RVGSS patient with small CDR)

FIGURE 7.5
Each triplet consists of one original image, one level set cup segmentation result, and one ARGALI cup segmentation result. ARGALI is able to give better estimates of the cup boundaries in all four cases.

the RVGSS glaucoma subset with a few complex multiple pathologies. It also shows that ARGALI outperforms the level set-based approach by reducing the CDR measurement MAE from 0.349 to 0.21 and MSE from 0.156 to 0.07. As expected, ARGALI performs better in the ORIGA data set than in others due to the relatively clearer images and training. Furthermore, ARGALI's MAE is close to the inter- and intraobserver variability rates of the glaucoma specialist, which stand at 0.2 [34] and 0.15, respectively [35]. This demonstrates that ARGALI's CDR measurement is still far from perfect, but is comparable with clinical measurements.

7.4 Conclusions

A-Levelset was proposed as a general principle to boost the performance of level set algorithms. Its effectiveness was demonstrated by the ARGALI system, which automatically segmented the optic cup and disc from widely available 2D digital fundus images. Even though the results are still far from perfect, exhaustive testing using a large collection of 2616 clinical fundus images from various races and sources demonstrated ARGALI's capability in providing reasonably accurate CDR values for objective glaucoma diagnosis and screening from fundus images.

References

1. Quigley HA, Broman AT. The number of people with glaucoma worldwide in 2010 and 2020. *Br J Ophthalmol* 2006;90:262–267.
2. Kass MA, Heuer DK, Higginbotham EJ, et al. The ocular hypertension treatment study: A randomized trial determines that topical ocular hypotensive medication delays or prevents the onset of primary open-angle glaucoma. *Arch Ophthalmol* 2002;120:701–713; discussion 829–730.

3. Komulainen R, Tuulonen A, Airaksinen PJ. The follow-up of patients screened for glaucoma with non-mydriatic fundus photography. *Int Ophthalmol* 1992;16:465–469.
4. Caprioli J. Clinical evaluation of the optic nerve in glaucoma. *Trans Am Ophthalmol Soc* 1994;92:589–641.
5. Shen SY, Wong TY, Foster PJ, et al. The prevalence and types of glaucoma in Malay people: The Singapore Malay eye study. *Invest Ophthalmol Vis Sci* 2008;49:3846–3851.
6. Ramakrishnan R, Nirmalan PK, Krishnadas R, et al. Glaucoma in a rural population of southern India: The Aravind comprehensive eye survey. *Ophthalmology* 2003;110:1484–1490.
7. Vijaya L, George R, Paul PG, et al. Prevalence of open-angle glaucoma in a rural south Indian population. *Invest Ophthalmol Vis Sci* 2005;46:4461–4467.
8. Varma R, Ying-Lai M, Francis BA, et al. Prevalence of open-angle glaucoma and ocular hypertension in Latinos: The Los Angeles Latino eye study. *Ophthalmology* 2004;111:1439–1448.
9. De Voogd S, Ikram MK, Wolfs RC, Jansonius NM, Hofman A, de Jong PT. Incidence of open-angle glaucoma in a general elderly population: The Rotterdam study. *Ophthalmology* 2005;112:1487–1493.
10. Tielsch JM, Sommer A, Katz J, Royall RM, Quigley HA, Javitt J. Racial variations in the prevalence of primary open-angle glaucoma. The Baltimore eye survey. *JAMA* 1991;266:369–374.
11. Rein DB, Zhang P, Wirth KE, et al. The economic burden of major adult visual disorders in the United States. *Arch Ophthalmol* 2006;124:1754–1760.
12. Fiscella RG, Lee J, Davis EJ, Walt J. Cost of illness of glaucoma: A critical and systematic review. *Pharmaco Economics* 2009;27:189–198.
13. Tielsch JM, Katz J, Singh K, et al. A population-based evaluation of glaucoma screening: The Baltimore eye survey. *Am J Epidemiol* 1991;134:1102–1110.
14. Thylefors B, Negrel AD. The global impact of glaucoma. *Bull World Health Organ* 1994;72:323–326.
15. Foster PJ, Oen FT, Machin D, et al. The prevalence of glaucoma in Chinese residents of Singapore: A cross-sectional population survey of the Tanjong Pagar district. *Arch Ophthalmol* 2000;118:1105–1111.
16. Varma R, Lee PP, Goldberg I, Kotak S. An assessment of the health and economic burdens of glaucoma. *Am J Ophthalmol* 2011;152:515–522.
17. Taylor HR, Pezzullo ML, Keeffe JE. The economic impact and cost of visual impairment in Australia. *Br J Ophthalmol* 2006;90:272–275.
18. Jonas JB, Bergua A, Schmitz-Valckenberg P, et al. Ranking of optic disc variables for detection of glaucomatous optic nerve damage. *Invest Ophthalmol Vis Sci* 2000;41:1764–1773.
19. Hoover A, Goldbaum M. Locating the optic nerve in a retinal image using the fuzzy convergence of the blood vessels. *IEEE T Med Imaging* 2003;22:951–958.
20. Niemeijer M, Abràmoff MD, van Ginneken B, et al. Segmentation of the optic disc, macula and vascular arch in fundus photographs. *IEEE T Med Imaging* 2007;26:116–127.
21. Zhu X, Rangayyan RM. Detection of the optic disc in images of the retina using the Hough transform. *Conf Proc IEEE Eng Med Biol Soc* 2008: 3546–3549.
22. Li H, Chutatape O. Boundary detection of optic disk by a modified ASM method. *Pattern Recogn* 2003;36:2093–2104.
23. Xu J, Chutatape O, Sung E, et al. Optic disk feature extraction via modified deformable model technique for glaucoma analysis. *Pattern Recogn* 2007;40:2063–2076.
24. Abramoff MD, Alward WLM, Greenlee EC, et al. Automated segmentation of the optic disc from stereo color photographs using physiologically plausible features. *Invest Ophthalmol Vis Sci* 2007;48:1665–1673.
25. Joshi GD, Sivaswamy J, Karan K, et al. Vessel bend-based cup segmentation in retinal images. In: International Conference on Pattern Recognition (ICPR), Hyderabad, India, 2010.
26. Liu J, Wong DWK, Lim JH, et al. ARGALI: An automatic cup-to-disc ratio measurement system for glaucoma analysis using level-set image processing. *IFMBE Proc* 2009;23:559–562.
27. Wong DWK, Liu J, Lim JH, et al. Automated detection of kinks from blood vessels for optic cup segmentation in retinal images. *Conf Proc SPIE Med Imaging* 2009: 72601J.

28. Cootes TF, Cooper D, Taylor CJ, et al. Active shape models: Their training and application. *Comput Vis Image Und* 1995;61:38–59.

29. Osher S, Sethian JA. Fronts propagating with curvature dependent speed: Algorithms based on Hamilton-Jacobi formulations. *J Comput Phys* 1988;79:12–49.

30. Li C, Xu C, Gui C, et al. Level set evolution without re-initialization: A new variational formulation. In: *IEEE Computer Society Conference on Computer Vision and Pattern Recognition*, vol. 1, pp. 430–436, 2005.

31. Lavanya R, Wu R, Wong WL, et al. Methodology of the Singapore Indian Chinese Cohort (SICC) eye study: Quantifying ethnic variations in the epidemiology of eye diseases in Asians. *Ophthalmic Epidemiol* 2009;16:325–336.

32. Zhang Z, Yin FS, Liu J, et al. ORIGA(-light): An online retinal fundus image database for glaucoma analysis and research. *Conf Proc IEEE Eng Med Biol Soc* 2010;2010:3065–3068.

33. Foong AW, Saw SM, Loo JL, et al. Rationale and methodology for a population-based study of eye diseases in Malay people: The Singapore Malay Eye Study (SiMES). *Ophthalmic Epidemiol* 2007;14:25–35.

34. Varma R, Spaeth GL, Steinmann WC, et al. Agreement between clinicians and an image analyzer in estimating cup-to-disc ratios. *Arch Ophthalmol* 1989;107:526–529.

35. Stamper RL, Lieberman MF, Drake MV. Diagnosis and Therapy of the Glaucomas, 7th edn. St. Louis, MO: Mosby, 1999.

8

The Singapore Eye Vessel Assessment System

Qiangfeng Peter Lau, Mong Li Lee, Wynne Hsu, and Tien Yin Wong

CONTENTS

8.1 Introduction

Images of the retina provide one of the few avenues to observe human microcirculation in a noninvasive manner. A variety of measurements have been proposed over the years[1] to quantify multiple aspects of retinal vascular morphology. Many of these measures have been found through population studies to have good diagnostic capabilities for diseases as cardiovascular risk factors,[2–9] while other measures are actively being investigated in large-scale population studies.

These population studies make use of computer-assisted semiautomated systems to take measurements from retinal images. Such real-world applications use image-processing techniques to reduce the time taken for manual editing (grading) and limit human error, producing reliable results for large studies. After the diagnostic capabilities of particular measurements have been verified, the systems can continue to be used for extracting these measurements from patients as routine risk indicators. The importance of such systems for medical research and possible clinical applications therefore serve as strong motivators for their development.

Over the years a variety of computer systems for retinal image analysis have been developed. The most widely used system was developed by Hubbard et al.[10] and measures summaries of retinal vascular caliber over a specific area in the retinal image. Apart from systems that primarily measure vessel caliber, systems also exist that perform other specialized measurements, for example, for the tortuosity[9] and the fractal dimension[11] of blood vessels. The development of these systems often requires the integration of multiple image-processing techniques together with methods from artificial intelligence (AI) literature. Often these methods do not provide near-perfect accuracy on all retinal images. Hence they may require a certain amount of manual intervention.

This chapter describes the capabilities and architecture of the semiautomated Singapore Eye Vessel Assessment (SIVA) system, which has been used in several clinical studies.[9,12–15] SIVA is capable of providing a large number of measurements that relate to vascular caliber, tortuosity, fractal dimension, and vascular branching, among others. SIVA identifies important landmarks in the retina such as the optic disc and blood vessels using image-processing techniques. Further AI techniques are used to differentiate between blood vessels that stem from the same vessel segments, to label vessels as arteries or veins, and to select reliable samples for measuring vessel caliber. In addition to these automated techniques, we describe how user intervention may be carried out at various stages to correct inaccuracies. The result (see Figure 8.1) produced from a retinal image is a model of the

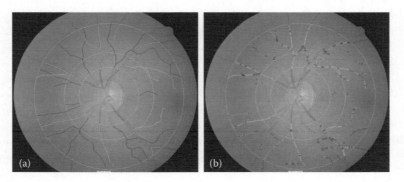

FIGURE 8.1
Example of detection and editing results using SIVA: (a) vessel center lines and (b) sampled vessel diameters.

vascular structure as seen in the retinal image. This vascular structure model may be stored and queried for a large number of measurements. Finally, we describe the measurements of individual vessels that SIVA exports as well as image-level summaries for further statistical analysis.

The rest of the chapter is organized as follows. First, Section 8.2 describes preliminary concepts such as the vascular model and areas of measurement. Next, Section 8.3 details the system architecture and its various functions. Then, Section 8.4 defines the various measurements that SIVA provides. Finally, Section 8.5 concludes with some future directions.

8.2 Preliminaries

Figure 8.2 shows a typical retinal image. The region marked by the innermost circle is the optic disc with radius *r*. Retinal vessels in the images originate outwards from the optic disc, perpendicularly to the plane of the image, before bending to lie on the plane. We can define two zones relative to the optic disc center as follows:

1. *Zone B* is the ring area of the retinal image formed by subtracting the circle of radius 2*r* from a circle of radius 3*r* with both circles centered at the optic disc center.

2. *Zone C* is the ring area of the retinal image formed by subtracting the circle of radius 2*r* from a circle of radius 5*r* with both circles centered at the optic disc center. Note that Zone C includes Zone B.

These zones control the extent of grading for various retinal images. Subsequently, measurements of retinal vessels are computed with respect to these zones. These measurements have been used in numerous studies.[2,9,10,12]

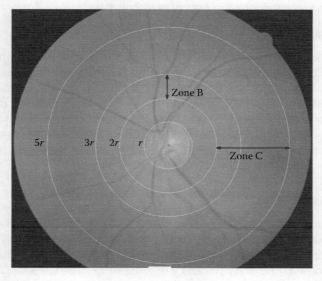

FIGURE 8.2
Optic disc (innermost circle), its center (cross), corresponding radii, and the zones.

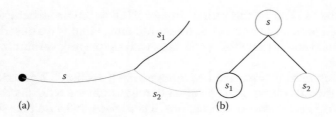

FIGURE 8.3
A vessel consisting of three segments: root segment (dark gray), and daughter segments (black and light gray) as well as the root point (black circle): (a) vessel and (b) vessel tree.

We use a forest of binary trees to model the vascular structure of a retinal image. Each *vessel, v,* is a binary tree with the property that each node has exactly zero or two child nodes. Figure 8.3 shows the centerline of a vessel with three segments s, s_1, and s_2. The binary tree that corresponds to this vessel is shown in Figure 8.3. Each node in the binary tree is a *segment*.

The segment at the root node of a vessel is called the *root segment*, denoted as root(v), and the first point in the segment at the root node is the *root point*. The segments, s_1 and s_2, which are the child nodes of a node with segment s, are called the *daughter segments* of s. Every point in the vessel or segment has a corresponding *width* value that refers to the diameter of the vessel at that point as measured from the retinal image. A vessel may be labeled as an artery or a vein.

We use the terms diameter, caliber, and width of a vessel or segment interchangeably. Note that measurements are not computed for parts of segments within $2r$ of the optic disc center in order to minimize the influence of distortion in a 2-dimensional retinal image. Hence the root points of vessels start outside $2r$.

8.3 System Overview

Figure 8.4 shows a screenshot of the SIVA system. Starting from an input retinal image, SIVA first detects the optic disc and uses its radius to define the measurement zones. Next, a vessel segmentation procedure is performed to obtain the centerline of the vascular structure. Vessel identification is carried out to separate and construct the tree structures representing the vessels. Once the vessel trees have been constructed, they are automatically labeled as arteries or veins. Finally, the system computes the vessel widths among other measurements for each vessel. Figure 8.5 summarizes the work flow of the system. The following subsections describe the details of each step.

8.3.1 Optic Disc Detection

There are numerous automated optic disc detection methods in the literature.[16–22] These methods can be easily incorporated into our modular SIVA system. For large population studies, we found the template-fitting approach described in Pallawala et al.[16] to be efficient and robust, and thus refined it for the optic disc detection in SIVA. We use Daubechies wavelet transformation in combination with vessel segmentation to quickly locate the optic disc region. The wavelet transformation highlights the bright region in

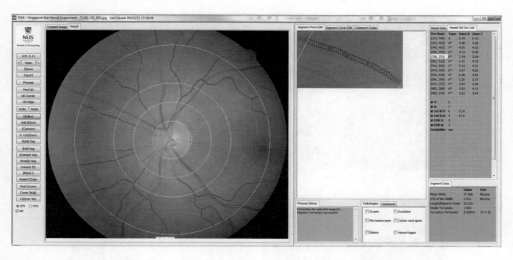

FIGURE 8.4
Screenshot of the SIVA system.

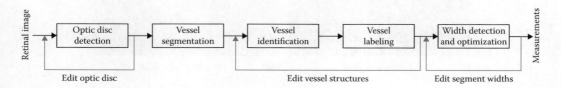

FIGURE 8.5
Work flow of the main processes in SIVA.

the retinal image, which usually corresponds to the cup in the optic disc. This location is further confirmed by the presence of a confluence of blood vessels.

Figure 8.6a shows the green channel of a retina image. First, the wavelet transform is performed. The resulting wavelet coefficients are thresholded via a high pass in the horizontal and vertical directions. Then, an inverse wavelet transform maps the image back to its original space as shown in Figure 8.6b. Next, we position an ellipse template over the bright region that is located by the wavelet transform and further confirmed by a confluence of blood vessels. Figure 8.6c shows the template used to find the best-fitting ellipse. The template consists of three parts. The coordinates of the ellipse center vary within the inner square. The ellipse's minor and major radii are allowed to vary within the ring area between the two circles. The smaller of the two circles is meant to cover the optic cup to prevent its edge pixels from affecting the result. Next, we score ellipses using an objective function directly proportional to high pixel intensity at the circumference but inversely proportional to circumference size. Figure 8.6d shows the optimal ellipse that has been fitted to the optic disc.

8.3.2 Vessel Segmentation

The segmentation of blood vessels from retinal images is a well-studied problem. These techniques can be categorized into two main approaches. The first approach segments each vessel individually by tracking along the path of the vessels from some start points.[23–27] The second approach processes the entire image to separate vessel pixels usually with

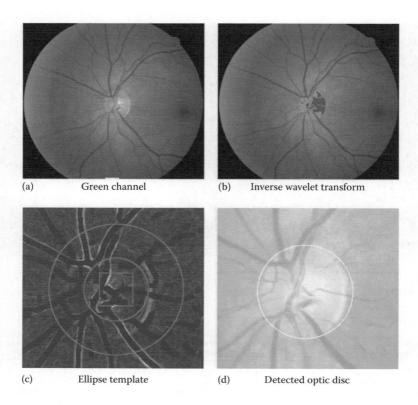

(a)   Green channel   (b)   Inverse wavelet transform

(c)   Ellipse template   (d)   Detected optic disc

FIGURE 8.6
The various steps to find the optic disc: (a) the initial green channel, (b) finding the likely location of the optic disc, and (c,d) template fitting to find the optic disc.

some form of thresholding on a transformed image.[28–30] SIVA uses a variation of the second approach to find the *centerlines* of vessels. These centerlines compactly represent the vascular structure for vessel identification in the next step.

We find the centerlines of the vessels by applying a modified unsupervised trench detection algorithm given in Garg et al.[31] The trench detection algorithm computes the surface tangent derivative (STD) for every pixel in the image. The STD quantifies the bend in the surface of the image along a particular direction. After the STD is computed, a procedure distinguishes *trench* pixels using a threshold to give the *thresholded STD image*. A higher threshold will capture larger vessels while ignoring smaller vessels and noise, while a lower threshold captures smaller vessels but with increasing noise. We bias the threshold toward larger vessels as most measurements of interest usually require aggregation of the larger retinal vessels. Figure 8.7b shows the result of applying the STD algorithm on the retinal image in Figure 8.7a.

We also carry out postprocessing on the thresholded STD image to improve the connectivity of the centerlines (see Figure 8.7c). Small broken lines are removed, as are those outside Zone C. The final output is shown in Figure 8.7d.

8.3.3 Vessel Identification

After vessel segmentation, the next operation is vessel identification. Vessel identification is the process of grouping line segments that belong to the same vessel. Figure 8.8a shows

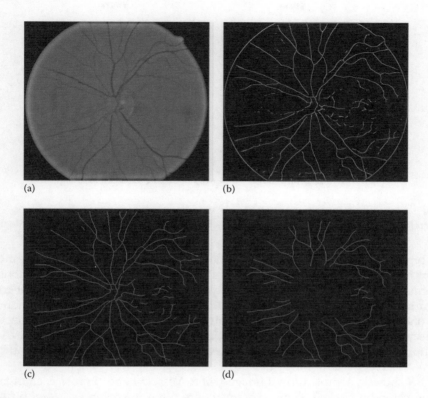

FIGURE 8.7
Various steps performed for vessel centerline segmentation. (a) Illumination corrected image, (b) thresholded STD image, (c) reconnect broken lines, and (d) crop and line smoothing.

the line segments obtained from the vessel centerlines. These line segments are grouped to form individual vessels. Each vessel is denoted by either black or white in Figure 8.8b.

Existing vessel identification methods combine the identification of individual vessels simultaneously with segmentation.[23–27] This approach usually leads to the wrong identification of vessels because of ambiguities caused by vessel bifurcations and crossovers.

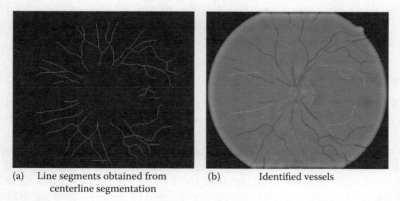

(a) Line segments obtained from   (b)   Identified vessels
         centerline segmentation

FIGURE 8.8
Grouping of line segments to form individual vessels: (a) line segments obtained from centerline segmentation and (b) identified vessels.

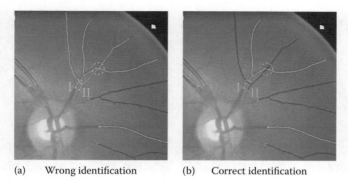

(a)   Wrong identification   (b)   Correct identification

FIGURE 8.9
Vessels I and II crossing each other twice at gray circles: (a) wrong identification and (b) correct identification.

Another branch of methods treat identification as a postprocessing step to segmentation. However, they either identify vessels one at a time without taking into account other vessels' orientations and locations[32] or they only resolve local crossovers without constructing the entire vessel trees.[33,34] This may result in less robustness to segmentation noise as errors in one location are not taken into account when dealing with other connected parts in the vascular structure, leading to suboptimal identification. In contrast, SIVA utilizes global information[35] from the segmented centerlines to simultaneously identify all the vessels.

Figure 8.9 shows a sample retinal image where Vessels I and II cross each other at two places (indicated by circles). These crossovers are often mistaken as vessel bifurcations, leading to I and II being regarded as one single vessel, as shown in Figure 8.9a. Figure 8.9b shows the correctly identified vessel structures for Vessels I and II marked in white and black, respectively. Note that there may be cases where a line segment is shared by two vessels as shown by the crossing in Figure 8.13b.

By first segmenting the vascular structure, we can use information of other vessels to help disambiguate between the bifurcation of a vessel and the crossover of two vessels, and better determine the linkage of vessels at crossovers. We model the segmented vascular structure as a vessel segment graph, and transform the problem of identifying true vessels to that of finding an optimal forest in the graph. We design objective functions to score forests based on pixel intensity and angular information. Our solution employs candidate generation and expert knowledge to prune the search space.

8.3.4 Vessel Classification

Vessel classification is the problem of determining if a vessel should be labeled as an artery or a vein. This is important as measurements based on different vessel types may be related to the risk of different diseases.

We employ an unsupervised approach to classify vessels by clustering vessels into two clusters based on their pixel intensity values. This is because retinal images of various patients may not have consistent contrast in their pixel intensity values. Reasons for this include the use of different fundus cameras, presence of disease, and natural differences in patients of different backgrounds. Hence a supervised approach will need to take these factors into account while unsupervised clustering will find the best clusters in the locality of the current retinal image.

We cluster entire vessels based on the well-known expectation–maximization algorithm to approximate a mixture model of two Gaussian components. The data points used are the mean intensity values of the root segment for each vessel. After the mixture model is computed, vessels are assigned to their most probable Gaussian component. Then, the vessels from the Gaussian component with a lower mean value are labeled as veins while those from the other component are labeled as arteries.

8.3.5 Vessel Width Detection

The last step in producing the vessel structures for measurements is to find the width of the vessel segments. The width of the blood vessel is used in several measurements of interest described in Section 8.4. Hence it is important to have reliable samples of the width.

The width of the vessel segments is automatically detected by first finding the orientation at each point of the vessel segment from the centerlines. Then, the cross-sectional intensity of the vessel is analyzed in the direction that is perpendicular to each point's orientation. This process yields the left and right vessel edge limits (points).

Often it is the case where, due to poor contrast, artifacts, or retinopathy, the detected width samples may be inaccurate. SIVA utilizes an optimization procedure to automatically discard unreliable width samples by minimizing a cost function.

Each width sample in a segment is treated as a binary variable where 0 indicates it will be discarded and 1 otherwise. We term the discarded width samples as *covered* and the retained width samples as *uncovered*. We find the lowest cost assignment of values to the binary variables such that the overall cost of the segment is minimized. Figure 8.10b demonstrates the effect of applying this procedure to a segment in Figure 8.10a.

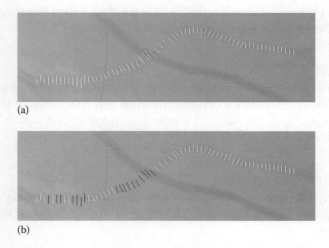

(a)

(b)

FIGURE 8.10
(a) Width samples from a vessel segment. (b) After optimization, black width samples are covered (discarded).

8.4 Extracted Measurements

The SIVA system extracts a multitude of summary measurements from a retinal image in addition to individual vessel measurements. This section describes the three categories of measurements that SIVA outputs.

8.4.1 Line Segment Measurements

We begin by describing the measurements of individual line segments. As a vessel is a tree of such segments, these are the basic building blocks for vessel-level summaries and image-level aggregation.

8.4.1.1 Mean Width ω(s)

Sample widths of the vessel segment, s, are taken at fixed intervals. The mean width of s is the average of the sample uncovered widths. We subscript ω with $\omega_B(s)$ and $\omega_C(s)$ to denote averages of samples within Zones B and C, respectively, that is, samples outside the zones are discarded.

8.4.1.2 Standard Deviation of Width Samples σ(s)

The standard deviation of the width samples of s is calculated from the same sample widths as the mean. $\sigma_B(s)$ and $\sigma_C(s)$ denote the standard deviations of sampled diameters within Zones B and C, respectively.

8.4.1.3 Length λ(s)

The length of s is computed as the sum of the pairwise Euclidean distance between two adjacent points on the centerline of s, that is, it is the arc of the centerline of the segment. $\lambda_B(s)$ and $\lambda_C(s)$ denote the lengths within Zones B and C, respectively.

8.4.1.4 Simple Tortuosity τ(s)

Simple tortuosity is calculated as the arc–chord ratio, $\tau(s) = \lambda(s)/C(s)$ where C is the chord of s, that is, the Euclidean distance between the first and last points of the centerline of s. Similarly, $\tau_C(s) = \lambda_C(s)/C_C(s)$, for Zone C, where the chord within Zones B and C is measured using the first and last points of the centerline of s within them.

8.4.1.5 Curvature Tortuosity ζ(s)

This is computed from the centerline of segment s using the formula τ_4 given in Hart et al.[36] Since the points on the centerline of s are discrete, the integral is estimated using summation to give

$$\varsigma(s) = \frac{1}{\gamma^2} \frac{1}{\lambda(s)} \sum_{i=1}^{|s|} \frac{\left[x'(t_i) y''(t_i) - x''(t_i) y'(t_i) \right]^2}{\left[y'(i_i)^2 + x'(t_i)^2 \right]^3},$$

where:

t_i is the ith point on the centerline of s

$|s|$ is the number of points on the centerline of s

γ is the scale factor of the image for normalizing over different absolute image sizes

The first-order parametric differentials are estimated using

$$f'(t_i) = f(t_{i+1}) - f(t_{i-1}),$$

and the second order is estimated using

$$f''(t_i) = f'(t_{i+1}) - f'(t_{i-1}),$$

where f is the parametric function x or y. The tortuosity within Zone C, $\zeta_C(s)$, is similarly defined on the points within the zone.

8.4.2 Vessel Measurements

The line segment measurements in the previous section are used to produce the vessel measurements listed below.

8.4.2.1 Zone B Mean Width $w_B(v)$ and Standard Deviation $sd_B(v)$

These are obtained from mean width and standard deviation of the sampled width of the root segment.

8.4.2.2 Zone C Mean Width $w_C(v)$ and Standard Deviation $sd_C(v)$

The Zone C mean width and standard deviation of a vessel is a recursive combination of the root segment and its descendants. Intuitively this measure estimates the average combined width of the parent and daughter segments of a vessel weighted by their respective line segment lengths.

8.4.2.3 Simple Tortuosity $st(v)$ and Curvature Tortuosity $ct(v)$

These are computed using an average of the line segments' simple and curvature tortuosity weighted by their respective lengths.

8.4.2.4 Branching Coefficient

The following measurements involve bifurcations (branching) in a vessel and are only defined if the bifurcations exist.

The branching coefficient of a vessel is given by the area ratio[37]

$$bc(v) = \frac{\omega(s_1)^2 + \omega(s_2)^2}{\omega(s)^2},$$

where s is the root segment of vessel v and s_1 and s_2 are daughters of s.

8.4.2.5 Asymmetry Ratio ar(v)

The asymmetry ratio[37] is defined as

$$ar(v) = \left(\frac{\min\{\omega(s_1), \omega(s_2)\}}{\max\{\omega(s_1), \omega(s_2)\}} \right)^2,$$

where s_1 and s_2 are the daughters of the root segment of v.

8.4.2.6 Junctional Exponent je(v)

The junctional exponent[38] is calculated by solving for x in the equation

$$s^x = s_1^x + s_2^x,$$

where s is the root segment of v with daughter segments s_1 and s_2. Numerical fixed-point iterative methods such as the Newton–Raphson or Halley's method can be used.

8.4.2.7 Junctional Exponent Deviation jed(v)

The junctional exponent deviation[1] expresses the deviation from the theoretical optimal value of 3 and is defined as

$$jed(v) = \frac{\sqrt[3]{\left| \omega(s)^3 - \omega(s_1)^3 - \omega(s_2)^3 \right|}}{\omega(s)},$$

where s_1 and s_2 are the daughters of the root segment s of v. This measurement avoids the problem of a lack of solution when using numerical methods for finding $je(v)$.

8.4.2.8 Branching Angle ba(v)

The branching angle cite[37] of the vessel is computed by measuring the angles between the centerline of the root segment s of v and its daughter segments s_1 and s_2 near the branching point.

8.4.2.9 Angular Asymmetry aa(v)

This measures the absolute difference in the daughter angles of the first-order branch given by $|\theta_1 - \theta_2|$, where θ_1 and θ_2 are measured in the same way as for the branching angle.

8.4.2.10 Length Diameter Ratio ldr(v)

This measure is the ratio of the length of the segment s to its average diameter[39], $\lambda_C(s)/\omega_C(s)$, that is, where s is the segment between the first- and second-degree branch of v (see Figure 8.11).

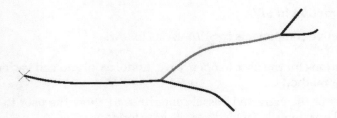

FIGURE 8.11
Example of a segment, in gray, between the first- and second-degree branches of a vessel. The gray cross indicates the root point.

8.4.3 Image-Level Measurements

This set of measurements summarizes the vascular structure of the entire image and, consequently, the patient. They have either been shown to be useful as risk factors for certain diseases or are currently under investigation with respect to other diseases.

8.4.3.1 Zone B Central Retinal Artery/Vein Equivalent

The central retinal artery/vein equivalent (CRAE and CRVE) for Zone B summarizes the six largest artery and veins as originally described in Hubbard et al.[10] and Parr and Spears,[40,41] respectively. We used the revised formulas given in Knudtson et al.[42] The six largest arteries and veins are referred to as the *big 6*. The calculation involves iteratively joining consecutive pairs of Zone B vessel mean widths, $w_B(v)$, which are sorted in descending order, using:

$$\text{arteries: } \hat{w} = 0.88 \cdot \sqrt{\left(w_1^2 + w_2^2\right)},$$

$$\text{veins: } \hat{w} = 0.95 \cdot \sqrt{\left(w_1^2 + w_2^2\right)},$$

where w_1, w_2 is a pair of width values and $\hat{w}$ is the new combined width value for the next iteration. This is performed until a single value is obtained, which is the estimated width for the central retinal artery or vein.

8.4.3.2 Zone B Arteriovenous Ratio (AVR)

This value is the ratio given by the Zone B CRAE divided by the Zone B CRVE.

8.4.3.3 Zone C CRAE/CRVE/AVR

These measurements in Zone C are similarly computed as in Zone B by using the Zone C mean width $w_C(v)$.

8.4.3.4 Big 6 Bifurcation Measurements

These measurements take the average of branching coefficient, branching angle, angular asymmetry, asymmetry ratio, and the junction exponent deviation of the six largest arteries and the six largest veins.

8.4.4 User Interaction in SIVA

The main interactive components in SIVA are as follows:

1. A list of buttons for the user to open, save, undo, redo, and call various processing and editing methods.
2. The display of the extracted vessel centerlines to allow the user to edit the lines and relabel erroneously labeled vessels as arteries or veins.
3. The display of a selected line segment to allow the user to discard unreliable samples and adjust the sampled widths.
4. The display of a list of measurements output by SIVA. Vessels with suspiciously high standard deviations of width are highlighted in red for the user's attention.

The SIVA system provides an initial detection of the vascular structure in a retina image. It allows the user to intervene at the following three points:

1. If the detected optic disc is inaccurate, the user may intervene. This may occur due to the presence of retinopathy in the retinal images, for example, cotton wool spots or laser scars. A sample retinal image is shown in Figure 8.12a. In this situation, the user may directly indicate the region where the true optic disc lies by using a resizable black circle to cover the optic cup as shown in Figure 8.12b. Template fitting is performed with the disc center restricted to the vicinity of the black circle. Figure 8.12c shows the detected optic disc.
2. If the vascular structure extracted is not accurate or the vessels are labeled wrongly as arteries or veins, the user can intervene to edit the vessel structures or reassign vessel labels. The user can directly add or remove a line segment, connect two line segments, mark vessel crossovers, and toggle the vessel type. The system will reidentify the vessels after the user edits, except for the toggling of vessel type. Figure 8.13b shows the identified vessels after the user marks a crossover in Figure 8.13a.
3. If the detection of vessel widths varies too much from the acceptable standard deviation, the user can adjust the detected width samples as desired. For example, Figure 8.14a shows some width samples erroneously detected due to the presence

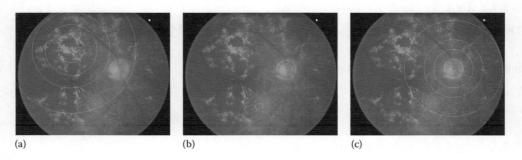

(a) (b) (c)

FIGURE 8.12
A circle is used to cover the optic cup area as a user heuristic. The template is limited to the position of the circle. (a) Wrong optic disc and zones, (b) user heuristic covers the disc cup, and (c) correct optic disc and zones.

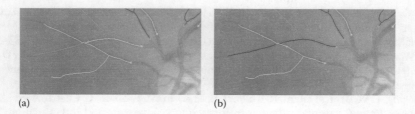

(a) (b)

FIGURE 8.13
(a) An erroneous vessel identification due to a misidentified crossover and (b) reidentified vessels after the user has marked the crossover.

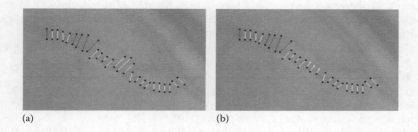

(a) (b)

FIGURE 8.14
Editing width samples directly. The shifted points are shown in gray in (b). (a) Bad width samples and (b) edited width samples.

of a nearby vessel. Figure 8.14b shows three points in gray adjusted by the user to the correct edge points.

8.5 Conclusion

In conclusion, we have described a real-world retinal analysis system, SIVA, that quantifies retinal vascular morphology. SIVA is implemented in C++ and currently supports major Windows platforms (e.g., Windows XP, Vista, 7, and 8). Where applicable, SIVA makes use of multiple CPU cores for computationally intensive operations. Automated techniques are used to construct a representative of the vascular structure. Then, trained graders may edit these structures at various stages. This act of *grading* yields highly accurate vascular structures. Grading each image can typically be accomplished in less than 15 minutes. Once this is done, a large variety of measurements are exported by the system, which are used for population studies involving thousands of patients[9,12–15] and continue to be used in ongoing studies seeking new discoveries.

References

1. N. Patton, T. M. Aslam, T. MacGillivray, I. J. Deary, B. Dhillon, R. H. Eikelboom, K. Yogesan, and I. J. Constable. Retinal image analysis: Concepts, applications and potential. *Prog Retinal Eye Res*, 25:99–127, 2006.

2. T. Y. Wong, M. D. Knudtson, R. Klein, B. E. K. Klein, S. M. Meuer, and L. D. Hubbard. Computer-assisted measurement of retinal vessel diameters in the beaver dam eye study: Methodology, correlation between eyes, and effect of refractive errors. *Ophthalmology*, 111(6):1183–1190, 2004.

3. T. Y. Wong, R. Klein, A. R. Sharrett, B. B. Duncan, D. J. Couper, B. E. K. Klein, L. D. Hubbard, F. J. Nieto, and Atherosclerosis Risk in Communities Study. Retinal arteriolar diameter and risk for hypertension. *Ann Intern Med*, 140(4):248–255, 2004.

4. T. Y. Wong, F. M. Amirul Islam, R. Klein, B. E. K. Klein, M. F. Cotch, C. Castro, A. R. Sharrett, and E. Shahar. Retinal vascular caliber, cardiovascular risk factors, and inflammation: The multi-ethnic study of atherosclerosis (mesa). *Invest Ophthalmol Vis Sci*, 47(6):2341–2350, 2006.

5. T. Y. Wong, A. Kamineni, R. Klein, A. R. Sharrett, B. E. Klein, D. S. Siscovick, M. Cushman, and B. B. Duncan. Quantitative retinal venular caliber and risk of cardiovascular disease in older persons: The cardiovascular health study. *Arch Intern Med*, 166(21):2388–2394, 2006.

6. G. Liew, A. R. Sharrett, J. J. Wang, R. Klein, B. E. K. Klein, P. Mitchell, and T. Y. Wong. Relative importance of systemic determinants of retinal arteriolar and venular caliber: The atherosclerosis risk in communities study. *Arch Ophthalmol*, 126(10):1404–1410, 2008.

7. K. McGeechan, G. Liew, P. Macaskill, L. Irwig, R. Klein, B. E. K. Klein, J. J. Wang, et al. Meta-analysis: Retinal vessel caliber and risk for coronary heart disease. *Ann Intern Med*, 151(6):404–413, 2009.

8. K. McGeechan, G. Liew, P. Macaskill, L. Irwig, R. Klein, B. E. K. Klein, J. J. Wang, et al. Prediction of incident stroke events based on retinal vessel caliber: A systematic review and individual-participant meta-analysis. *Am J Epidemiol*, 170(11):1323–1332, 2009.

9. C. Y. Cheung, Y. Zheng, W. Hsu, M. L. Lee, Q. P. Lau, P. Mitchell, J. J. Wang, R. Klein, and T. Y. Wong. Retinal vascular tortuosity, blood pressure, and cardiovascular risk factors. *Ophthalmology*, 118:812–818, 2011.

10. L. D. Hubbard, R. J. Brothers, W. N. King, L. X. Clegg, R. Klein, L. S. Cooper, A. R. Sharrett, M. D. Davis, and J. Cai. Methods for evaluation of retinal microvascular abnormalities associated with hypertension/sclerosis in the atherosclerosis risk in communities study. *Ophthalmology*, 106(12):2269–2280, 1999.

11. V. F. Cosatto, G. Liew, E. Rochtchina, A. Wainwright, Y. P. Zhang, W. Hsu, M. L. Lee, et al. Retinal vascular fractal dimension measurement and its influence from imaging variation: Results of two segmentation methods. *Curr Eye Res*, 35(9):850–856, 2010.

12. C. Y. Cheung, W. Hsu, M. L. Lee, J. J. Wang, P. Mitchell, Q. P. Lau, H. Hamzah, M. Ho, and T. Y. Wong. A new method to measure peripheral retinal vascular caliber over an extended area. *Microcirculation*, 17:1–9, 2010.

13. C. Y. Cheung, W. T. Tay, P. Mitchell, J. J. Wang, W. Hsu, M. L. Lee, Q. P. Lau, et al. Quantitative and qualitative retinal microvascular characteristics and blood pressure. *J Hypertension*, 29(7):1380–1391, 2011.

14. P. Benitez-Aguirre, M. E. Craig, M. B. Sasongko, A. J. Jenkins, T. Y. Wong, J. J. Wang, N. Cheung, and K. C. Donaghue. Retinal vascular geometry predicts incident retinopathy in young people with type 1 diabetes: A prospective cohort study from adolescence. *Diabetes Care*, 34(7):1622–1627, 2011.

15. M. B. Sasongko, T. Y. Wong, K. C. Donaghue, N. Cheung, A. J. Jenkins, P. Benitez-Aguirre, and J. J. Wang. Retinal arteriolar tortuosity is associated with retinopathy and early kidney dysfunction in type 1 diabetes. *Am J Ophthalmol*, 153:176–183, 2011.

16. P. Pallawala, W. Hsu, M. Lee, and K.-G. Eong. Automated optic disc localization and contour detection using ellipse fitting and wavelet transform. In T. Pajdla and J. Matas (eds), *Computer Vision -ECCV 2004*, volume 3022 of *Lecture Notes in Computer Science*, pp. 139–151. Springer, Prague, Czech Republic, 2004.

17. M. D. Abramoff and M. Niemeijer. The automatic detection of the optic disc location in retinal images using optic disc location regression. In *Proceedings of 28th Annual International Conference of the IEEE Engineering in Medicine and Biology Society (EMBS)*, pp. 4432–4435. New York, 2006.

18. M. Park, J. S. Jin, and S. Luo. Locating the optic disc in retinal images. In *Proceedings of International Computer Graphics, Imaging and Visualisation Conference*, pp. 141–145. Sydney, Australia, 2006.

19. X. Zhu and R. M. Rangayyan. Detection of the optic disc in images of the retina using the Hough transform. In *Proceedings of 30th Annual International Conferene of the IEEE Engineering in Medicine and Biology Society (EMBS)*, pp. 3546–3549. Vancouver, Canada, 2008.

20. A. A.-H. Abdel-Razik Youssif, A. Z. Ghalwash, and A. A. S. Abdel-Rahman Ghoneim. Optic disc detection from normalized digital fundus images by means of a vessels' direction matched filter. *IEEE Trans Med Imaging*, 27(1):11–18, 2008.

21. S. Lu. Accurate and efficient optic disc detection and segmentation by a circular transformation. *IEEE Trans Med Imaging*, 30(12):2126–2133, 2011.

22. A. Giachetti, K. S. Chin, E. Trucco, C. Cobb, and P. J. Wilson. Multiresolution localization and segmentation of the optical disc in fundus images using inpainted background and vessel information. In *Proceedings of 18th IEEE International Conference on Image Processing (ICIP)*, pp. 2145–2148. Brussels, Belgium, 2011.

23. Y. A. Tolias and S. M. Panas. A fuzzy vessel tracking algorithm for retinal images based on fuzzy clustering. *IEEE Trans Med Imaging*, 17(2):263–273, 1998.

24. H. Li, W. Hsu, M. L. Lee, and T. Y. Wong. Automatic grading of retinal vessel caliber. *IEEE Trans Biomed Eng*, 52(7):1352–1355, 2005.

25. E. Grisan, A. Pesce, A. Giani, M. Foracchia, and A. Ruggeri. A new tracking system for the robust extraction of retinal vessel structure. In *Proceedings of 26th Annual International Conference of the IEEE Engineering in Medicine and Biology Society (EMBS)*, Vol. 1, pp. 1620–1623. San Francisco, 2004.

26. M. E. Martinez-Perez, A. D. Highes, A. V. Stanton, S. A. Thorn, N. Chapman, A. A. Bharath, and K. H. Parker. Retinal vascular tree morphology: A semi-automatic quantification. *IEEE Trans Biomed Eng*, 49(8):912–917, 2002.

27. Y. Yin, M. Adel, M. Guillaume, and S. Bourennane. A probabilistic based method for tracking vessels in retinal images. In *Proceedings of 17th IEEE International Conference on Image Processing (ICIP)*, pp. 4081–4084. Hong Kong, 2010.

28. A. D. Hoover, V. Kouznetsova, and M. Goldbaum. Locating blood vessels in retinal images by piecewise threshold probing of a matched filter response. *IEEE Trans Med Imaging*, 19(3):203–210, 2000.

29. J. Staal, M.D. Abramoff, M. Niemeijer, M.A. Viergever, and B. van Ginneken. Ridge-based vessel segmentation in color images of the retina. *IEEE Trans Med Imaging*, 23(4):501–509, 2004.

30. E. Ricci and R. Perfetti. Retinal blood vessel segmentation using line operators and support vector classification. *IEEE Trans Med Imaging*, 26(10):1357–1365, 2007.

31. S. Garg, J. Sivaswamy, and S. Chandra. Unsupervised curvature-based retinal vessel segmentation. In *Proceedings of 4th IEEE International Symposium on Biomedical Imaging: From Nano to Macro*, pp. 344–347. Arlington, 2007.

32. V. S. Joshi, M. K. Garvin, J. M. Reinhardt, and M. D. Abramoff. Automated method for the identification and analysis of vascular tree structures in retinal vessel network. volume 7963, page 79630 I. SPIE, 2011.

33. B. Al-Diri, A. Hunter, D. Steel, and M. Habib. Joining retinal vessel segments. In *Proceedings of 8th IEEE International Conference on Bioinformatics and Bioengineering (BIBE)*, pp. 1–6. Athens, Greece, 2008.

34. B. Al-Diri, A. Hunter, D. Steel, and M. Habib. Automated analysis of retinal vascular network connectivity. *Comput Med Imaging Graphics*, 34(6):462–470, 2010.

35. Q. P. Lau, M. L. Lee, W. Hsu, and T. Y. Wong. Simultaneously identifying all true vessels from segmented retinal images. *IEEE Trans Biomed Eng*, 60(7):1851–1858, 2013.

36. W. E. Hart, M. Goldbaum, P. Kube, and M. R. Nelson. Automated measurement of retinal vascular tortuosity. In *Proceedings of the AMIA Fall Conference*, pp. 459–463. Nashville, 1997.

37. M. Zamir, J. A. Medeiros, and T. K. Cunningham. Arterial bifurcations in the human retina. *J Gen Physiol*, 74(4):537–548, 1979.

38. N. Patton, R. Maini, T. MacGillivary, T. M. Aslam, I. J. Deary, and B. Dhillon. Effect of axial length on retinal vascular network geometry. *Am J Ophthalmol*, 140(4):648–653, 2005.

39. N. Witt, T. Y. Wong, A. D. Hughes, N. Chaturvedi, B. E. Klein, R. Evans, M. McNamara, S. A. McG Thom, and R. Klein. Abnormalities of retinal microvascular structure and risk of mortality from ischemic heart disease and stroke. *Hypertension*, 47(5):975–981, 2006.

40. J. C. Parr and G. F. Spears. General caliber of the retinal arteries expressed as the equivalent width of the central retinal artery. *Am J Ophthalmol*, 77(4):472–477, 1974.

41. J. C. Parr and G. F. Spears. Mathematic relationships between the width of a retinal artery and the widths of its branches. *Am J Ophthalmol*, 77(4):478–483, 1974.

42. M. D. Knudtson, K. E. Lee, L. D. Hubbard, T. Y. Wong, R. Klein, and B. E. K. Klein. Revised formulas for summarizing retinal vessel diameters. *Curr Eye Res*, 27(3):143–149, 2003.

9

Quantification of Diabetic Retinopathy Using Digital Fundus Images

Hasan Mir, Hasan Al-Nashash, and U. Rajendra Acharya

CONTENTS

9.1 Introduction

An average meal usually contains carbohydrates, proteins, and fat. The carbohydrates absorbed from the gastrointestinal tract are then converted to glucose. Much of the absorbed glucose is catabolized by body cells to carbon dioxide and water to provide the body with essential energy. The blood glucose level (BGL) in healthy humans is usually maintained within the normal range of 4–8 mM or 70–120 mg/dL [1]. This level is elevated following a meal, but in healthy subjects it should return to the normal range within 3 h. If the BGL remains elevated above the normal level after the 3 h period or during fasting, this is referred to as hyperglycemia. In cases of hyperglycemia, the BGL may reach as high as 300–700 mg/100 ml. On the other hand, if the BGL drops below the normal level, a state referred to as hypoglycemia, the subject or patient may experience fainting, coma, or even death. The BGL in a hypoglycemic patient can fall as low as 30 mg/100 ml. If hyperglycemia or hypoglycemia conditions persist due to impaired physiological function, then the subject is diagnosed as having diabetes mellitus. Nondiabetic pregnant women or patients suffering from certain medical stresses may also temporarily exhibit symptoms of diabetes caused by irregular hormone levels in the blood.

The BGL is regulated by insulin and glucagon hormones secreted by the pancreas, with insulin considered to be the most important controller of organic metabolism. The actions of insulin are generally divided into two main categories: (a) metabolic effects on carbohydrate, lipid, and protein synthesis and (b) growth effects on DNA cell division, differentiation, and DNA synthesis [2]. An increase in plasma insulin in the blood circulation leads to rapid uptake or consumption of glucose by the various organs and tissues of the body. Also, increased insulin leads to enhanced uptake of glucose for glycogen synthesis in the liver and muscles. The surplus glucose is converted to fatty acids and stored in adipose tissues. There are other physiological functions of insulin, including enhanced amino acid uptake and protein synthesis. The major controlling factor for insulin secretion is BGL. An increase in BGL stimulates insulin secretion, and a decrease in BGL inhibits the secretion of insulin. The physiological role of the glucagon hormone is opposite to that of insulin, as it mobilizes glucose, fatty acids, and amino acids from stores into the blood circulation and increases BGL. Insulin and glucagon work together to maintain the BGL within the normal range.

In people who have diabetes, the pancreas either does not produce any or enough insulin, or it is unable to effectively use the insulin it produces [2]. As a result, glucose builds up in the bloodstream, potentially leading to serious health problems such as retinopathy and blindness, heart disease, kidney failure, susceptibility to infection, amputation, and nerve damage. Clinically, diabetes is divided into Types 1 and 2. In patients with Type 1 diabetes, insulin is completely (or almost completely) absent from the plasma. As a result, these patients need to take insulin every day. Type 1 diabetes is an autoimmune disease, wherein the immune system will act to destroy the cells that produce insulin. Type 2 diabetes usually affects adults for whom the insulin produced does not lead to or accelerate the absorption of glucose by body tissue cells. This situation is termed "insulin resistance," wherein the target cells do not respond to circulating insulin because of physiological alterations to insulin receptors or an intracellular process following receptor activation [2]. Most patients with Type 2 diabetes also develop a defect in their ability to secrete insulin in response to increased BGL. Patients with Type 2 diabetes can maintain normal BGLs by reducing their weight, living a healthy lifestyle, undertaking physical activity, healthy eating, and taking the correct medicine. Type 2 diabetes is a progressive disease, and over time patients may need to use insulin to regulate their BGLs.

According to the statistics published in 2011 by the International Diabetes Federation, there are more than 366 million people around the world with diabetes. This total is expected to rise to 552 million within 20 years [3]. Diabetes is one of the major health concerns of the United Arab Emirates (UAE). Published statistics show that UAE ranks second in the world in terms of the proportion of the population suffering from diabetes [4,5]. The Imperial College London Diabetes Centre (ICLDC) presented important figures that illustrate the seriousness of the rapid increase in diabetes among the UAE population. The ICLDC states that about 19.5% of the UAE population is diabetic, with one in every five individuals aged from 20 to 79 living with diabetes [4]. There are many factors influencing the large number of diabetics in UAE, including obesity, unhealthy eating habits, and inactive lifestyle. Vast amounts of money are being spent on treating and raising awareness of diabetes. However, this has not stopped the continuous increase in the number of diabetic people in the UAE and the Gulf region. According to the National Health Insurance Company, AED 15,000 is spent on each diabetic patient per year. It is projected that by the year 2020, the UAE government will have spent AED 10 billion on diabetes [6].

Visual impairment and blindness are major complications associated with diabetes [7]. The excess blood glucose in diabetic patients leads to what is called diabetic retinopathy (DR). This refers to damage to blood vessels inside the light-sensitive retinal tissue at the back of the eye. Damage of this nature causes the blood vessels to leak fluid onto the retina, leading to the formation of retinal lesions. The longer a person has diabetes, the higher their chances of developing DR. The different stages of DR are [8]:

- Mild, nonproliferative: early changes, with minor swelling to areas of the retinal blood vessels

- Moderate, preproliferative: some of the blood vessels that feed the retina are blocked
- Severe, preproliferative: several areas of the retina are deprived of blood supply, leading to the growth of new retinal blood vessels
- Proliferative retinopathy: further growth of abnormal and fragile blood vessels

Exudates are a visible type of lesion which result from DR. Exudates are a major cause of vision loss, and are manifested as yellow patches on the retina with variable size, shape, and position, as shown in the DR-affected eye in Figure 9.1.

If DR is identified at an early stage, then laser photocoagulation can be used to slow down the progression of the disease. Without regular screening, a patient may only become aware of the severity of his or her condition when the extent of the retinal lesions has rendered effective treatment almost impossible. To ensure that treatment is received in time, the eye fundus of diabetic patients needs to be examined at least once a year [9]. High examination costs coupled with a lack of access to ophthalmologists obstruct regular examinations of diabetic patients [10]. In order to encourage regular screenings for patients with DR, cost-effective automated detection of anomalous retinal features using digital fundus images have been studied in the existing literature. In a study by Ward et al. [11], exudates were detected from a fundus image in which shade variations were reduced in order to facilitate detection based on a gray-level threshold. Coarse segmentation by fuzzy C-means clustering and fine segmentation by morphological reconstruction for automated exudate detection were proposed by Sopharak and Uyyanonvara [12]. Pixel-level exudate recognition was used by both Osareh [13] and Wang [14] to classify each pixel as lesion or nonlesion. In a study by Acharya [15], a robust exudate detection method based on morphological operations was employed.

While most of the existing work has focused on the detection of lesions, an additional important aspect in the context of exudate detection is their location relative to the fovea (see Figure 9.1). The fovea is the region of the eye that is responsible for high-sensitivity color vision [16]. Knowledge of the fovea location and shape can aid in providing a more detailed assessment of the patient's condition, since exudates located far from the fovea are not considered to be an immediate threat to visual function and may disappear spontaneously [13].

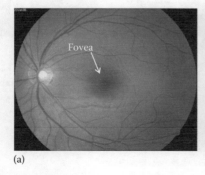

(a)

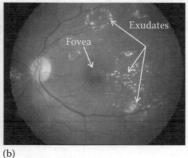

(b)

FIGURE 9.1
(a) Normal eye; (b) DR-affected eye.

9.2 Detection and Assessment of Diabetic Retinopathy

In this section, a framework is developed to aid in the detection of features relevant to DR using digital fundus images. Whereas diagnosis using digital fundus images is unlikely to completely replace current screening modalities, it does offer a more objective and economical method of diagnosis.

A block diagram of the assessment process is shown in Figure 9.2. Beginning with the fundus image, standard contrast enhancement is performed in order to improve the separation of features of interest from the image background. The next step is the extraction of the red channel, the green channel, and the grayscale intensity. The red channel and the grayscale image are useful in the localization of the fovea [16]. In particular, the red channel is useful in isolating the image background, with the features of interest being relatively obscured. On the other hand, the grayscale image exhibits the fovea as a relatively darker region against a light background. Fovea detection may therefore be achieved by subtracting the complement of the red channel from the grayscale intensity image since this will preserve the foveal region while suppressing the background. The local contrast of darker regions can be further improved using contrast-limited adaptive histogram equalization (CLAHE), which will result in enhanced foveal detection performance [17].

As noted by Acharya [15], the green channel provides the best contrast between exudates and the image background, while the blue and red channels provide moderate and poor contrast, respectively. Based on the results obtained by Acharya [15], an octagonal structuring element is used to perform morphological closing on the green channel in order to enhance the differentiation between the exudates and the background. Postprocessing is

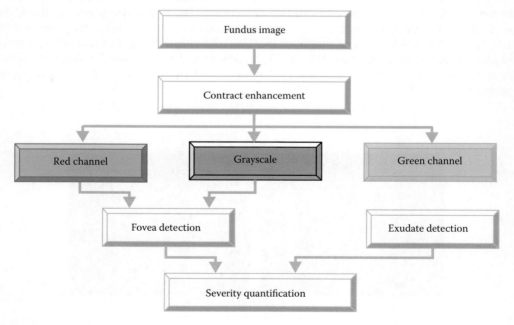

FIGURE 9.2
Block diagram of the assessment process of DR.

then performed to remove the optic disc, based on *a priori* knowledge of its size and position. This sequence of operations results in a binary image with lighted pixels only at the exudate locations.

With the fovea and exudates extracted from the fundus image, the last stage of the assessment process is to develop a measure that can quantify the severity of the DR. As noted in the Introduction, exudates that are in close proximity to the fovea pose a greater threat to visual function than those that are farther away. As such, it is desirable to develop a measure of DR severity that takes account of not only the total amount of exudate buildup, but also of the location of the exudate formation relative to the fovea.

In order to develop such a measure, let F denote the set of all coordinates (x_f, y_f) on the fovea boundary, and let E denote the set of all exudate coordinates (x_e, y_e). Note that all exudate locations are of interest, whereas only the fovea boundary locations are of interest since locations internal to the fovea indicate that visual acuity has already been severely compromised.

Each exudate coordinate $(x_e, y_e) \in E$ will be associated with a measure $d(x_e, y_e)$ which represents the minimum distance of the exudate coordinate to any location on the fovea boundary. This may be mathematically expressed as:

$$d(x_e, y_e) = min_{(x_f, y_f) \in F} \sqrt{(x_e - y_e)^2 + (x_f - y_f)^2} \quad (9.1)$$

Furthermore, an additional set S_δ will be defined as a set of all exudate locations whose minimum distance to the fovea boundary (as defined in (9.1)) is less than a distance of δ. This can be expressed mathematically as:

$$S_\delta = \{(x_e, y_e) \in E : d(x_e, y_e) \leq \delta\} \quad (9.2)$$

The measure that will be adopted here to quantify the DR severity is the area of the exudate formations whose minimum distance to the fovea boundary does not exceed δ. This measure, which will be denoted as a_δ, can be mathematically expressed as:

$$a_\delta = \sum \sum_{(x,y) \in S_\delta} \Delta A = |S_\delta| \Delta A \quad (9.3)$$

A curve of a_δ versus δ can thus be developed in order to provide a quantitative evaluation of the imminency of the threat that the exudate formations pose to visual function.

9.3 Example of Detection and Assessment of Diabetic Retinopathy Using Fundus Images

Digital fundus images from DR-affected patients were obtained courtesy of the National University Hospital, Singapore. The images were taken with a Ziess Visucamlite fundus camera, which generated 24-bit JPEG format images.

Figures 9.3 through 9.5 show examples of the output at various stages from the framework in Figure 9.2, with each image containing examples from two patients: the left column corresponds to a patient who has been diagnosed by a qualified ophthalmologist as

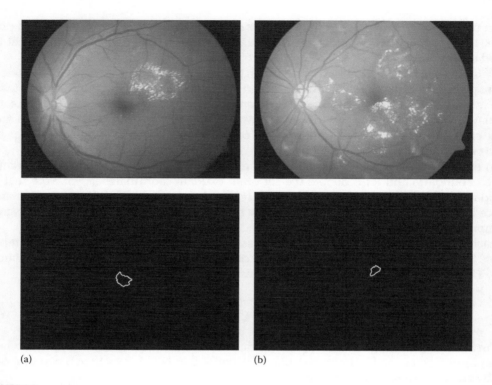

FIGURE 9.3
(a) Fundus image and extracted foveal region for mild DR; (b) fundus image and extracted foveal region for moderate DR.

having mild DR, whereas the right column corresponds to a patient who has been diagnosed as suffering from moderate DR.

Figure 9.3 demonstrates the foveal region extraction from the fundus image. It can be seen that the result is a binary image of the fovea boundary, with all other features suppressed. Figure 9.4 demonstrates the exudate formation extraction from the fundus image. While the exudate extraction also results in a binary image, it can be seen that the entire exudate formation (as opposed to just the boundary) is captured, since the total exudate formation area is of interest. Finally, Figure 9.5 shows the results of applying the severity assessment metric described in Figures 9.1 through 9.3 (which use the extracted foveal boundary and exudate formations in Figures 9.3 and 9.4) for various values of δ.

While there are a number of features that ophthalmologists may use when assigning a category to an observed stage of DR, the severity assessment curves in Figure 9.5 can provide a useful quantitative complement to the ophthalmological assessment. For example, Osareh [13] has stated that only exudates located less than 0.5 mm from the fovea should be considered to be an immediate threat to visual function. It can be seen that for the mild DR case in Figure 9.5a, the curve for a_δ at $\delta = 0.5$ mm has a value of less than 0.01 mm^2, while for the moderate DR case in Figure 9.5b, the curve for a_δ at $\delta = 0.5$ mm has a significantly larger value of around 0.4 mm^2. Therefore, curves such as those in Figure 9.5 can be used to develop an index for the imminency of the impairment to visual function posed by the exudate formations close to the fovea.

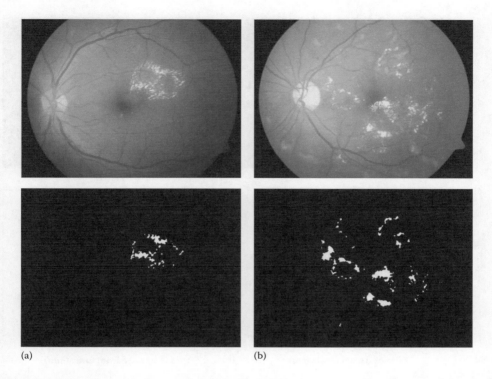

(a)   (b)

FIGURE 9.4
(a) Fundus image and extracted exudates for mild DR; (b) fundus image and extracted exudates for moderate DR.

It should be noted that adiagnosis of mild DR is often complicated by the presence of microaneurysms rather than exudates. Still, pathological formations close to the fovea may be of concern, and such formations can be detected and quantified using the proposed framework. Future work could concentrate on the statistical properties of the severity assessment curve from a wider sample of patients. This would be useful in order to establish the relationship between the typical range for a particular index and the corresponding stage of DR.

9.4 Summary

A significant and growing portion of the human population suffers from diabetes. DR is a common complication that results in impaired visual function. In order to encourage regular screenings, low-cost automated detection and assessment of DR is an invaluable tool. This work discussed a methodology for assessing the severity of DR using digital fundus images. The methodology uses the foveal region and exudates (which are a visible sign of retinal damage) in order to quantify the severity of DR. Results on example digital fundus images were used to demonstrate the performance of the methodology as well as its potential role as a complement to standard ophthalmological assessments.

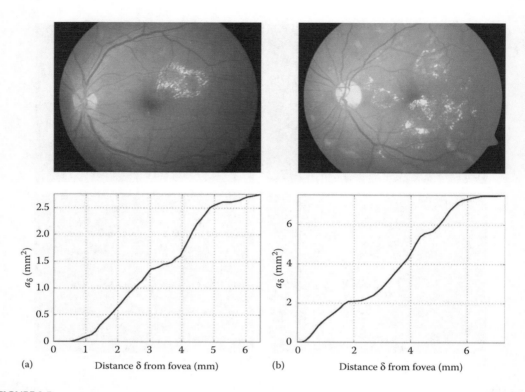

FIGURE 9.5

(a) Fundus image and severity assessment curves for mild DR; (b) fundus image and severity assessment curves for moderate DR.

References

1. Webster J., (ed.) *Medical Instrumentation: Application and Design*, 4th edn. Wiley: Hoboken, NJ, 2009.
2. Vander A., Sherman J., and Luciano D., *Human Physiology: The Mechanisms of Body Function*, 9th edn. McGraw-Hill: Boston, 2004.
3. International Diabetes Federation, The global burden, http://www.idf.org/diabetesatlas/5e/the-global-burden. International Diabetes Federation Report: Brussels, 2011.
4. El-Shammaa D., Diabetes is growing problem in UAE. *Gulf News*, http://gulfnews.com/news/gulf/uae/health/diabetes-is-a-growing-problem-in-uae-experts-1.84110.
5. Barakat M., Frequently asked questions, Imperial College London Diabetes Centre, UAE, http://www.icldc.ae/faq.html, 2009.
6. El-Shammaa D., Diabetes likely to cost UAE Dh10b by 2020. *Gulf News*, http://www.gulfnews.com/Nation/Health/10258900.html, November 12, 2008.
7. Resnikoff S., et al., Global data on visual impairment in the year 2002. *B World Health Organ* 82:844, 2004.
8. Frank RN., Diabetic retinopathy. *Prog Retin Eye Res* 14:2361–2392, 1995.
9. Fong DS., Aiello L., Gardner TW., King GL., Blankenship G., Cavallerano JD., Ferris FL., and Klein R., Diabetic retinopathy. *Diabetes Care* 26:1226–1229, 2003.

10. Javitt J., Canner J., and Sommer A., Cost-effectiveness of current approaches to the control of retinopathy in type I diabetics. *Ophthalmology* 96:255–264, 1989.
11. Ward N., Tomlinson S., and Taylor C., Image analysis of fundus photographs. *Ophthalmology* 96:80–86, 1989.
12. Sopharak A. and Uyyanonvara B., Automatic exudates detection from diabetic retinopathy retinal image using fuzzy c-means and morphological methods. In: Proceedings of the Third IASTED, pp. 359–364, April 2007.
13. Osareh A., Automated identification of diabetic retinal exudates and the optic disc. Doctoral Dissertation, University of Bristol, January 2004.
14. Wang H., Hsu W., Kheng G.G., and Lee M.L., An effective approach to detect lesions in color retinal images. *Proc IEEE Conf Comp Vis Pat Recog* 2:181–186, 2000.
15. Acharya U., Computer-based detection of diabetes retinopathy stages using digital fundus images. *Proc Inst Mech Eng H* 223:545–553, 2009.
16. Kolb H., Simple anatomy of the retina. *Webvision*, University of Utah. http://webvision.med.utah.edu/book/part-i-foundations/simple-anatomy-of-the-retina/, 2011.
17. Singh J. and Sivaswamy J., Fundus foveal localization based on image relative subtraction-IReS approach. In: Proceedings of National Conference Communications. February 2008, Mumbai.

10

Diagnostic Instruments for Glaucoma Detection

Teik-Cheng Lim, U. Rajendra Acharya, Subhagata Chattopadhyay, Jasjit S. Suri, and Eddie Y. K. Ng

CONTENTS

10.1 Introduction

Glaucoma is a dreaded eye disease wherein the optic nerve is incrementally damaged. The instruments for diagnosis of glaucoma reviewed in this chapter can be broadly categorized into primarily mechanics-based and primarily optics-based instruments.

10.2 Mechanics-Based Instruments

Tonometry is the only mechanics-based glaucoma detection procedure. The following sub-sections review the various types of tonometry instruments employed in practice.

10.2.1 Noncontact (Air-Puff) Tonometry

Noncontact tonometry measures intraocular pressure by obtaining corneal deflection as a result of an air puff, that is, a sudden release of pressurized air to the cornea, as shown in Figure 10.1. An example of a commercial noncontact tonometer is the Pulsair tonometer, which has a compressor that is connected to a hand-held air gun. When placed perpendicularly to and an appropriate distance from the cornea surface, the tonometer shoots an air impulse. It measures the amount of pressure that is needed to depress the cornea within a small circular area of 3 mm in diameter [1,2].

10.2.2 Applanation Tonometry

Applanation tonometry quantifies the intraocular pressure by obtaining the amount of pressure that is needed to flatten a small area of the cornea, as shown in Figure 10.2. The most famous applanation tonometer is the Goldmann tonometer [3,4], which obtains the pressure necessary to flatten a circular area of 3.06 mm in diameter. Although there are other types of applanation tonometers (see, for example, [5–10]), the Goldmann tonometer sets the reference standard, as most intraocular pressure readings of newly developed tonometers are compared with its readings.

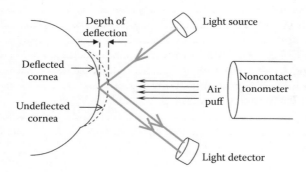

FIGURE 10.1
Generic noncontact tonometry.

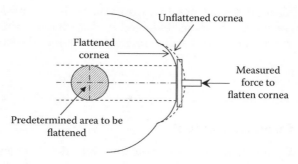

FIGURE 10.2
Generic applanation tonometry.

10.2.3 Indentation Tonometry

In indentation tonometry, intraocular pressure is measured by imposing pressure directly on the cornea, as illustrated in Figure 10.3. It obtains the depth of indentation by means of a predetermined force. A well-known indentation tonometer is the Schiotz tonometer [11,12], which employs a plunger to slowly depress the cornea. The intraocular pressure is ascertained by measuring the force that is applied to flatten the cornea. Indentation tonometers are also known as impression tonometers.

10.2.4 Rebound Tonometry

In rebound tonometry, an induction coil magnetizes a metallic probe with a polymer tip (see Figure 10.4). When magnetized, the probe hits the cornea and then bounces back. An induction current is generated when the probe travels back into the device. The generated induction current allows the intraocular pressure to be quantified [13].

10.2.5 Pneumatonometry

In pneumatonometry, a regulated flow of air goes into a piston that floats on an air bearing, as illustrated in Figure 10.5. A fenestrated membrane at the edge of the piston is exposed

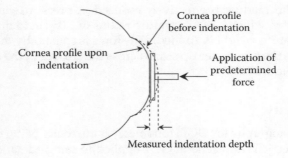

FIGURE 10.3
Generic indentation tonometry.

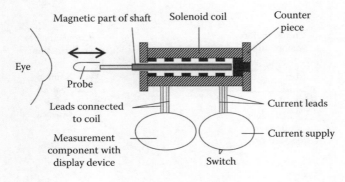

FIGURE 10.4
Generic rebound tonometry.

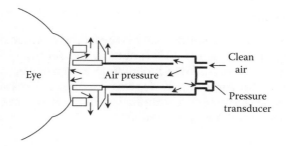

FIGURE 10.5
Generic pneumatonometry.

to forces arising from the air flow and the cornea. The intraocular pressure is measured at force equilibrium [14,15].

10.2.6 Dynamic Contour Tonometry

Dynamic contour tonometry (DCT) [16–18] uses the principle of profile- or contour-matching rather than simply flattening a region of the cornea. As a result, the effect of cornea stiffness on the intraocular reading is effectively reduced. A pressure sensor is embedded at the tip of the tonometer, which has a curvature radius of 1.05 cm to match the cornea curvature when a force of 1 g weight is applied. This force is constantly maintained by means of control feedback as the tonometer tip scans across the surface of the cornea. A schematic of DCT is shown in Figure 10.6.

10.2.7 OCT Tonometry

Optical coherence tomography (or OCT) tonometry is currently being developed as a form of noncontact tonometry. While general OCT applied to image-detailed retinal tissues in other fields of ophthalmology, or any other biological tissues, OCT tonometry obtains the change in cornea curvature arising from sound waves or air pressure. The working principle of OCT tonometry is similar to that of conventional OCT.

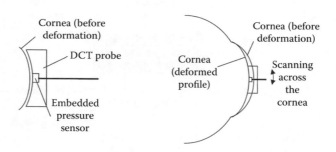

FIGURE 10.6
Generic DCT: Closed-up view before deformation (*left*) and zoomed-out view during deformation of cornea (*right*).

10.3 Optics-Based Instruments

10.3.1 Gonioscopy

The principle of gonioscopy is the visual evaluation of the anterior chamber of the eye [19–21], specifically the iridocorneal angle, by means of a mirror or prism (see Figure 10.7). As a result, ophthalmologists may evaluate whether the drainage angle is open or closed. The buildup of intraocular pressure takes place with a closed drainage angle.

In direct (or Koeppe) gonioscopy, the goniolens is placed on the patient's cornea, with an application of lubricating fluid to prevent damage to the cornea. The patient lies down during this procedure. In indirect (or Goldmann) gonioscopy, the eye-care provider uses a mirror to direct light from the iridocorneal angle to the observer's view. The patient is seated upright during this procedure. In Zeiss gonioscopy, prisms are used instead of mirrors to direct the light. The use of four prisms in Zeiss gonioscopy permits the four quadrants of the patient's iridocorneal angle to be observed.

10.3.2 Optical Coherence Tomography

Optical coherence tomography (or OCT) is an optical method that can be used to construct 3D images of biological tissues [22–24]. Its applications include imaging of the retina in

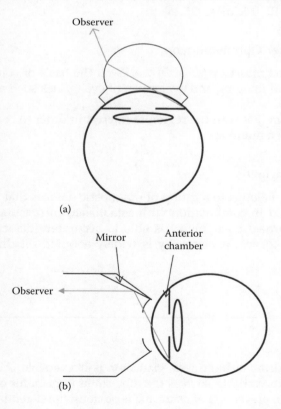

FIGURE 10.7
Generic goniolenses: (a) Koeppe goniolens and (b) Goldmann goniolens.

order to observe nerve damage. General OCT is an established medical imaging technique that gained prominence because it entails no harmful radiation and does not need sample preparation, so measurements can be done *in vivo*. Furthermore, this technique provides instant imaging.

The working principle of OCT is based on optical coherence, whereby a beam emitting from a coherent light source is split into two, so that one beam is reflected by the tissue to be imaged while the other is reflected by a reference mirror. As such, the scattered light from the tissue is removed. The interference of the recombined light during scanning enables a 3D image to be constructed.

10.3.3 Scanning Laser Polarimetry

Scanning laser polarimetry (or SLP) uses a polarized laser to measure the thickness of the retinal nerve fiber layer (RNFL) in order to detect glaucoma. SLP measures the RNFL by means of the polarized change retardation that takes place when a light beam passes through materials with birefringent properties. The birefringent property in RNFL arises from the parallel array of microtubules inside the axon bundles.

The polarized light in SLP is split into two before entering the eye. This light is then projected onto the surface of the retina and double-crosses the RNFL. A retardation (or phase shift) takes place when both parts of the split light move at different speeds. The amount of retardation is in proportion to the thickness of the RNFL, as confirmed by microscopic measurements of RNFL thickness [25,26].

10.3.4 Scanning Laser Ophthalmoscopy

Scanning laser ophthalmoscopy (or SLO) works on the basis of confocal laser scanning microscopy for optical imaging and evaluation of eye tissues such as the cornea and the retina.

SLO utilizes mirrors that scan the region of interest in order to construct raster images that can be seen from a monitor.

10.3.5 Corneal Pachymetry

Corneal pachymetry belongs to a group of diagnostic devices that measure the corneal thickness. When used in combination with established intraocular pressure measurement techniques, corneal pachymetry is able to accurately detect the early stages of glaucoma. As such, corneal pachymetry is widely adopted for diagnosing early-stage glaucoma.

10.4 Conclusions

Unlike some other forms of blindness, glaucoma is irreversible. Although a number of glaucoma implants are available, such as the tube-shunt implant for ocular liquid drainage of a glaucomatous eye, prevention of glaucoma is obviously preferential. Several mechanics-based and optics-based instruments for early detection of glaucoma have been surveyed in this chapter. Tissue-imaging methods enable the generation of highly accurate evidence for the occurrence of glaucoma through the observation of damaged tissues. On the other hand, the more indirect techniques possess the potential for detecting the early signs of glaucoma buildup before retinal damage takes place.

References

1. L. Bonomi, S. Baravelli, C. Cobbe, and L. Tomazzoli, Evaluation of Keeler Pulsair non-contact tonometry: Reliability and reproducibility, *Graefe's Arch. Clin. Exp. Ophthalmol.* **229**, 210–212 (1991).
2. T.A. Armstrong, Evaluation of the Tono-Pen and the Pulsair tonometers, *Am. J. Ophthalmol.* **109**, 716–720 (1990).
3. H. Goldmann and T. Schmidt, Über Applanationstonometrie, *Ophthalmologica* **134**, 221–242 (1957).
4. M.J. Moseley, N.M. Evans, and A.R. Fielder, Comparison of a new non-contact tonometer with Goldmann applanation, *Eye* **3**, 332–337 (1989).
5. A. Posner, An evaluation of the Maklakov applanation tonometer, *Eye Ear Nose Throat* **41**, 377–378 (1962).
6. W.G. Kett, Tonometry: A case for the Maklakov tonometer, *Aust. J. Optometry* **33**, 107–108 (1961).
7. B.R. Hammond and P. Bhattacherjee, Calibration of the Alcon applanation pneumatonograph and Perkins tonometer for use in rabbits and cats, *Curr. Eye Res.* **3**, 1155–1159 (1984).
8. J. Wallace and H.G. Lovell, Perkins hand-held applanation tonometer. A clinical evaluation, *British Med. J.* **52**, 568–572 (1968).
9. A. Posner and R. Inglima, The tonomat applanation tomometer, *Eye Ear Nose Throat* **46**, 996–1000 (1967).
10. A. Posner and R. Inglima, The tonomat applanation tonometer: A comparison with the Goldmann applanation tonometer and the applanometer, *Eye Ear Nose Throat* **48**, 189–194 (1969).
11. M.F. Armaly, Schiötz tonometer calibration and applanation tonometry, *Arch. Ophthalmol.* **64**, 426–432 (1960).
12. R.A. Moses, Theory of the Schiotz tonometer and its empirical calibration, *Trans. Am. Ophthalmol. Soc.* **69**, 494–562 (1971).
13. L.N. Davies, H. Bartlett, E.A.H. Mallen, and J.S. Wolffsohn, Clinical evaluation of rebound tonometer, *Acta Ophthalmol.* **84**, 206–209 (2006).
14. S. Wittenberg, Evaluation of the pneuma-tonometer, *Am. J. Optom. Physiol. Opt.* **55**, 337–347 (1978).
15. A.J. Morgan, J. Harper, S.L. Hosking, and B. Gilmartin, The effect of corneal thickness and corneal curvature on pneumatonometer measurements, *Curr. Eye Res.* **25**, 107–112 (2002).
16. H.E. Kanngiesser, C. Kniestedt, and Y. Robert, Dynamic contour tonometry: Presentation of a new tonometer, *J. Glaucoma* **14**, 344–350 (2005).
17. O.S. Punjabi, C. Kniestedt, R.L. Stamper, and S.C. Lin, Dynamic contour tonometry: Principle and use, *Clin. Exp. Ophthalmol.* **34**, 837–840 (2006).
18. C. Kniestedt, M. Nee, and R.L. Stamper, Dynamic contour tonometry: A comparative study on human cadaver eyes, *Acta Ophthalmol.* **122**, 1287–1293 (2004).
19. J. Rourke, M. Lal, and W. Kalwat, Weightless Koeppe gonioscopy, *Arch. Ophthalmol.* **99**, 1646 (1981).
20. R.N. Shaffer and R.L. Tour, A comparative study of gonioscopic methods, *Trans. Am. Ophthalmol. Soc.* **53**, 189–208 (1955).
21. P.L. Kaufman, M.W. Neider, and W.H. Pankonin, Slitlamp mount for Zeiss gonioscopy lens, *Arch. Ophthalmol.* **99**, 1455 (1981).

22. J.G. Fujimoto, Optical coherence tomography, *Comptes Rendus de l'Académie des Sciences Series IV Physics* **2**, 1099–1111 (2001).
23. A.F. Fercher, W. Drexler, C.K. Hitzenberger, and T. Lasser, Optical coherence tomography: Principles and applications, *Rep. Prog. Phys.* **66**, 239–303 (2003).
24. A.G. Podoleanu, Optical coherence tomography, *Br. J. Radiol.* **78**, 976–988 (2005).
25. R.N. Weinreb, A.W. Dreher, A. Coleman, H. Quigley, B. Shaw, and K. Reiter, Histopathologic validation of Fourier-ellipsometry measurements of retinal nerve fiber layer thickness, *Arch. Ophthalmol.* **108**, 557–560 (1990).
26. J.E. Morgan, A. Waldock, G. Jeffrey, and A. Cowey, Retinal nerve fibre layer polarimetry: Histological and clinical comparison, *Br. J. Ophthalmol.* **82**, 684–690 (1998).

11

Automated Cup-to-Disc Ratio Estimation for Glaucoma Diagnosis in Retinal Fundus Images

Irene Fondón, Carmen Serrano, Begoña Acha, and Soledad Jiménez

CONTENTS

11.1 Introduction

Glaucoma diagnosis and treatment constitutes one of the challenges of the twenty-first century. According to the World Health Organization (WHO) [1], the number of people suffering from vision loss due to glaucoma is rising as a result of increased life expectancy and population growth. It is also one of the top three causes of visual impairment and blindness. The WHO estimates that 80 million people are currently affected by glaucoma and approximately six million are blind due to the disease, accounting for over 12.3% of all blindness cases [1].

Glaucoma refers to a group of diseases characterized by damage of the optic disc (OD), the area where the optic nerve and blood vessels enter the retina, detected by pathological cupping of the OD that leads to a loss of field of vision. Glaucoma cannot be cured, but when detected early and treated, blindness due to glaucoma can be prevented.

Accurate measurement of the intraocular pressure is not enough to detect glaucoma because a relationship between the two does not exist. By contrast, the appearance of the OD might be related to the visual damage [2]. Cupping of the optic nerve is a classic sign of glaucoma.

Thus, one of the main indicators of glaucoma adopted in clinical practice is the cup-to-disc-ratio (CDR). While the OD contains nerve fibers, the cup is an area within it with no fibers at all (see Figure 11.1). As glaucoma advances, the cup enlarges due to increased ganglion cell death until it occupies most of the disc area. Therefore, if the relation between the area of the physiological cup and the area of the OD, the CDR, exceeds a certain value, or a difference in ratio between the two eyes is encountered as well as a progressive enlargement of the cup with time, glaucoma may be suspected. The CDR is either manually estimated by ophthalmologists or computed with high-priced systems using retinal tomography. Therefore, mass screening programs are very expensive and time-consuming. Besides, as has been proved, manual estimation of the CDR is highly dependent on the experience and skill of the clinicians, and differentiation between glaucomatous and nonglaucomatous cupping can be difficult even for experienced observers [3]. Hence, the use of a fully automatic and robust CAD tool based on retinal fundus image analysis could help to overcome these problems.

A wide variety of methods for the detection of the OD have been proposed in the past, but significantly fewer methods have been presented for CDR estimation due to the difficulty in encountering an accurate edge of the cup area, which is usually diffuse and occluded by blood vessels. Moreover, human perception adaptation, something that is always desirable when trying to emulate a human operator, is usually forgotten and gray-level images or color images represented in nonuniform color spaces are adopted. In this chapter we will review state-of-the-art CDR calculation in detail. Then, the research application of CDR estimation will be presented. Finally, discussion of existing methods and

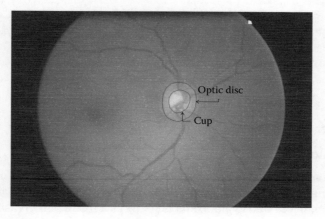

FIGURE 11.1
An example of a retinal color fundus image with the ground truth of the areas corresponding to the optic disc and cup manually marked by an expert ophthalmologist.

databases that facilitate the research, comparison of results among researchers, and some future lines of research are presented.

11.2 Computer-Aided Image Analysis in CDR Calculation Research

11.2.1 Imaging Techniques and Image Databases

Retinal imaging has developed rapidly during the last 160 years and is a now a mainstay of the clinical care and management of patients with retinal as well as systemic diseases [4]. Three broad groups of image acquisition methods are the focus of research in medical imaging of the retina: retinal fundus imaging, optical coherence tomography (OCT), and Heidelberg retinal tomography (HRT). The former provides a 2D representation of the retina, where a 3D anatomical structure is projected into the image plane using reflected light. Of all the imaging techniques belonging to this group (fundus imaging, hyperspectral imaging, stereo fundus photography, scanning laser ophthalmoscopy, adaptive optics, etc.), color fundus imaging is prevalent in mass screening programs for the early detection of glaucoma and other diseases due to its capability for noninvasive acquisition and the lower cost of equipment [5]. In color fundus photography three wavebands are used (reflected light corresponding to R, G, and B), resulting in a color image. OCT is also a noninvasive imaging technique capable of producing 3D volumetric or high-resolution transversal cuts, tomograms, similar to the histological cuts *in vivo*. HRT uses a confocal scanning laser for the acquisition of 3D images of the retina. However, the detection of glaucoma through OCT or HRT is expensive [6] when compared with the cost of digital fundus images.

With regard to publicly available image databases, there are two that are commonly used: STARE [7] and DRIVE [8]. The former provides information about the OD center, while the latter is intended for blood vessel segmentation. Therefore, they do not provide enough information for the detection of glaucoma, that is, OD area, cup area, and CDR. Another database for vessel segmentation is ReviewDB [9]. ONHSD [10], Diaretdb0 [11], and Diaretdb1 [12] are other image benchmarks providing a few OD images with segmentation ground truth, sometimes with low resolution [13]. DRIONS-DB [14] is another database intended for OD segmentation. The data set comprises 110 images with two ground truth segmentations each. Recently, the RIM-ONE database was created. This is a public database with 169 images and 5 OD expert segmentations per image. The most complete image database for glaucoma is ORIGA–light [15] with 650 retinal color images along with ground truth for OD and cup segmentation. However, its web interface does not seem to be publicly available, so it is necessary to request permission from the author to download the database [13]. This lack of a publicly available database containing enough information for glaucoma algorithms makes a real quality comparison among different methods difficult. Accuracy measures are usually made on the basis of private databases and ground truth obtained by the authors themselves.

11.2.2 Anatomical Structure Detection for Glaucoma Diagnosis: Optic Disc and Cup

Of all the retinal structures that could exist on a retinography, our interest is focused on OD and cup detection because our final objective is to measure the CDR.

Existing techniques are mainly focused on OD detection because:

1. The OD is considered to be one of the main features of a retinal fundus image. OD detection is a key preprocessing component in many algorithms designed for the automatic extraction of retinal anatomical structures and lesions, and is thus an associated module of most retinopathy screening systems [16].

2. Accurate cup detection is a difficult task due to the blurred border between this area and the neuroretinal rim and the presence of blood vessels occluding the precise edge.

Therefore, there is a vast amount of literature relating to OD segmentation. In this chapter, we will review the most relevant techniques intended for glaucoma application from a point of view of color engineering. We will also present the most relevant methods for trying to isolate the OD region that are easily adaptable to glaucoma applications by adding a cup detection stage.

11.2.3 OD Detection Methods

Although the OD has well-defined features and characteristics, localizing it in an automatic and robust manner is not a straightforward process since its appearance may vary significantly due to retinal pathologies. State-of-the-art algorithms devoted to OD segmentation within retinographies can be classified with regard to the image representation selected. Although the study performed by Osareh et al. [17] demonstrated that CIE $L^*a^*b^*$ color space is the most suitable for this application. Gray-level-based techniques applied to the gray-level version of the color image itself or to a single plane of its color representation are numerous. The number of methods that make use of the complete color representation of the image is still low.

Methods based on gray-level image representation try to exploit the knowledge acquired by the use of well-known gray-level techniques developed in the past. An algorithm based on the gray-level version of the original image is presented by Chaichana et al. [18]. The method is a shape-based template matching in which the OD is modeled as a circular object by the preliminary detection of the main edges in the grayscale image and the search for circular areas with the Hough transform. This technique suffers from the drawbacks of classical edge detectors such as missing true edges, false edges detection, noise problems, etc. The minimum and maximum radius size for Hough transform has been experimentally fixed and could lead to erroneous results. Langroudi et al. [19] proposed an algorithm where the grayscale image is preprocessed to correct uneven illumination and improve contrast. Next, the OD region is found through morphological operations. Thresholding techniques are used by Kavitha and Shenbaga [20], where the OD is selected from the gray-level image thresholding it and keeping the brightest region containing the convergence point, that is, the location of the image where vessels converge. Another method that uses the general structure of vessels to detect the OD in the gray-level image was presented by Foracchia et al. [21]. It is based on a model of the geometrical directional pattern of the retinal vascular system that implicitly embeds the information on the OD position.

Other techniques are also utilized for OD detection in gray-level images, such as level set [22], tensor voting, graph-based segmentation [23], projection of features [24], and gradient vector flow [25].

All of these methods ignore the color information present in the retinographies, neglecting the *a priori* knowledge about OD appearance. Human perception adaptation is obviously not considered while the use of color in retinographies is limited. Many of the existing algorithms do not exploit the whole color image with its three-plane representation (RGB, HSV, etc.), only making use of a single plane that is treated in the same way as the gray-level image-based methods previously discussed. Sometimes two planes are used, but not combined, that is, some processing is done on one plane while the rest is done on the other. Only a few articles mention the use of three planes (usually RGB in combination with the grayscale image) but, once again, separately processed. The use of human-perception-related color space is generally forgotten and a minority of techniques are designed in CIE $L^*a^*b^*$ color space.

The majority of methods use a plane from the RGB color space since it is the easiest representation of the fundus image as it is stored in this format. The G plane of the RGB color space is the most widely adopted color plane. The reason claimed by the authors is its high contrast compared with the R and B channel images and the grayscale image. Thresholding is a frequently used technique [26,27], along with the use of Hough transform [26,28]. The approximately constant distance between the fovea and the OD is utilized by Xu et al. [29] and Kovacs et al. [30] to detect both regions at the same time. In their study, Vahabi et al. [31] introduced a new filtering approach in the wavelet domain for image preprocessing.

Another color space employed is that of the HSL family because intensity is separate from hue. The authors that adopt a luminance plane from the HSL color space, such as Walter et al. [32] and Lu et al. [33], claim that as the OD belongs to the brightest parts of the color image it is more reliable to work on the L channel of the HSL color space in order to localize it. More specifically, in Walter et al. [32] the OD is detected by means of morphological filtering techniques and the watershed transformation, while in Lu et al. [33] thresholding was adopted.

The RGB and HSL families are nonuniform color spaces, that is, the Euclidean distance between colors measured in them does not correspond to perceived differences. Therefore, a few approaches prefer the use of CIE $L^*a^*b^*$ uniform color space because of its correlation with human perception. For example, Shijian et al. [34] proposed a shape-based template-matching algorithm, while Yu et al. [35] adopted a level-set technique. Dynamic programming was the method selected by Abbas et al. [36].

Some methods combine two planes of a color space instead of using only one.

In Lee et al. [37] R and G color planes are combined to detect the OD using a technique based on intensity profiles building. Lu et al. [38] combined R and B instead. The methodology exploits color planes to maximize information extraction of features while keeping interference (blood vessels) to a minimum. A combination of several techniques, including scanning filters, thresholding, region growing, and a modified Chan–Vese (CV) model with a shape constraint, is used to segment the OD.

Methods that make use of the three planes of the selected color space are in the minority. The color space preferred is RGB along with the HSI family, for simplicity in the first case and intensity separation in the second. The methods proposed by Marrugo and Millan [39] and Venkatalakshmi et al. [40] are based on the processing of the R, G, and B planes of the RGB color space. Marrugo and Millan [39] proposed a system based on PCA analysis of each plane taken independently. In Venkatalakshmi et al. [40] color segmentation is carried out in the original RGB image with a statistical classification method used to detect the objects with a bright-yellowish color. A group of features are defined so the elements present in the retinal image map to nonintersecting classes in the feature space, and then can easily be identified with a classifier. Harangi et al. [41] presented the idea of detecting the OD by entropy filtering the HSI color space.

However, a few approaches make use of the CIE $L^*a^*b^*$ uniform color space. For instance, in Kande et al. [42] localization of the OD was accomplished by following three steps.

First the center of the OD was estimated by finding a point that has maximum local variance. The color morphology in CIE $L^*a^*b^*$ space is used in order to have a homogeneous OD region. The boundary of the OD was located using a geometric active contour with variational formulation. Sáez et al. [43] presented a method fully adapted to human perception wherein an edge-based level-set algorithm is applied. Its main contribution is the utilization of color information during the segmentation. Specifically, vector gradients in CIE $L^*a^*b^*$ are applied in the edge-based level-set algorithm and, instead of the Euclidean norm, CIE 94 color difference formula is applied to those vector gradients.

11.2.4 CDR Estimation Methods

As we have seen, approaches aimed at determining the OD and its boundaries have been widely reported. However, far fewer approaches have been developed to determine the contour of the cup area due to the difficulties in determining an accurate optic cup boundary. We present here some relevant research made in the field of CDR estimation.

11.2.4.1 OD Segmentation

With regard to image representation (gray-level or color), most of the systems in the literature for CDR computation are based on gray-level techniques. Sometimes the segmentation is performed along the grayscale representation of the original image. Madhusudhan et al. [44] used the gray-level version of the original color image to detect the OD region for two of the three different approaches presented: multithresholding and active contour without edges. A preprocessing step is performed on the gray-level image in order to correct uneven illumination. Vessels are removed with morphological closing before the segmentation process starts. With regard to the multithresholding technique, the thresholds are manually fixed and thus low quality results are obtained for some images.

The use of a single color space representation, usually R or G of the RGB color space, is the most common. Of all the existing techniques, the most famous set of methods based on the study of the R plane in the RGB representation of the original image is the ARGALI (Automatic cup-to-disc Ratio measurement system for Glaucoma detection and AnaLysIs) group [25,45–50]. The ARGALI is a CAD tool developed for the early detection of glaucoma. It comprises several steps for the determination of OD (in the R plane) and cup (in the G plane) in order to estimate the CDR. The R channel is used because the OD has its best visibility on it. The initial step in the system involves locating a region of interest (ROI) in the R plane based on the assumption that the OD generally occupies less than 5% of the pixels in a typical retinal fundus image. The retinal image is first subdivided into 64 regions. As the OD region is usually brighter than the surrounding retinal area, the system automatically selects 0.5% of the pixels of the image with the highest intensity. The region containing the highest number of these selected pixels is used as the center of the ROI that is finally built from this center as a square or circle of dimensions twice the size of the typical OD diameter. A preprocessing stage can be added to the system in order to avoid errors due to uneven illumination occurring at the edges of the retina. To this purpose Zhang et al. [51] searched for a trimming circle by the least square fitting method. The ROI obtained is used as the initial boundary for the OD segmentation with a variational level-set technique. It must be noted that the system does not remove blood vessels, thereby reducing the computational cost of the algorithm. However, the detected contour is often uneven due to the influence of the blood vessels across the boundary of the disc and therefore a final ellipse fitting step is added to the system. For this final step, two techniques have been proposed: the traditional direct least square fitting [25,45–48,50] and the convex-hull-based ellipse optimization [48]. In an attempt to improve the ARGALI system, the AGLAIA (Automatic GLaucoma Diagnosis and Its Genetic Association Study through Medical Image InformAtics) system was proposed [52]. Following the same procedure, the system is an expansion of ARGALI. The novelty introduced is the cascade of an improved level-set, A-levelset, and the variational level-set along with an active shape model.

Another technique based on the processing of the *R* plane of an RGB color image was proposed by Kavitha [53]. Blood vessels are detected and removed by means of mathematical morphology that is then used once more to obtain an initial ROI. The final detection of the OD is performed with the component-labeling algorithm.

In Joshi et al. [54] the *R* color plane is used again. Firstly the ROI is localized by thresholding the image with a fixed threshold value of 0.95 and selecting the largest group of connected pixels. The ROI is built as a square of fixed size around the detected location. Next, a vessel-free and smooth ROI image is obtained by the use of the bottom-hat transform. A region-based active contour procedure is performed on this image. However, in cases where the OD cannot be easily distinguished in terms of global statistics this technique may lead to an erroneous segmentation. To overcome this problem Joshi et al. proposed [55,56] a very interesting method based on region-based active contour improvement by including in the CV model image information at a support domain for each point of interest while not imposing any shape constraint. The method begins by detecting a rough OD. To this purpose vessels are detected using a curvature-based technique and are subsequently inpainted by the morphological closing operation in eight directions. Next, the edges are detected with a Canny detector and Hough transform is applied for fixed radius values. The OD center is considered to be the pixel with the highest accumulator value, while its radius is estimated with the nearby edges. The most interesting novelty introduced by this method is the inclusion of two texture features along with the selected color feature (the *R* value for each pixel). These texture characteristics are obtained by filtering the *R* image at different scales. A pixel will be described as a set of three values: two for texture and one for color. Finally, this vector-valued image is used in the improved region-based active contour technique.

The *G* channel is used by other algorithms. For instance, after detecting and inpainting the blood vessels, Chih-Yin [57] again uses the idea of creating an initial ROI by thresholding the image, here the *G* color plane image, and retaining the brightest connected pixels. Neighboring connected areas are merged if their intensity is under a certain threshold. The ROI is considered as the bounding box of the region thus obtained. Next, the histogram of the ROI is analyzed to find three peaks corresponding to the background, OD, and cup respectively. A circle is built with the pixels obtained for each peak. This circle is used as the initialization curve for an active contour procedure.

The gray-level image combined with the RGB color image is used by Madhusudhan et al. [44] and Hatanaka et al. [58,59]. The first two use the color planes separately for p-tile thresholding in order to detect the initial ROI. The area of the gray-level image corresponding to the ROI is used to extract edges with a Canny detector and join the result with spline interpolation. The third method of Madhusudhan et al. is a region-growing procedure where the seeds are extracted from the *G* plane while the growing is performed in the RGB color space with the Euclidean distance. The results obtained show that this method, although not adapted to human perception, gives better results than the two other proposed methods (already explained based on the gray-level image).

A method fully adapted to human perception is proposed by Valencia and Millan [60]. However, the technique is cumbersome and semiautomatic, and is not appropriate for practical applications. Nevertheless, several interesting points are introduced by the algorithm. Human perception of retinal images is emulated based on S-CIELAB. The images are preprocessed using a sharpening algorithm to smooth noise and sharpen edges. Subsequently, the ROI is manually selected and transformed to polar coordinates for OD boundary extraction. The CIEDE 2000 color distance, that is, an advanced color difference proposed to improve the uniformity of CIE $L^*a^*b^*$ color space, is calculated in all radial directions between neighboring pixels. Pixels with the highest color difference are used to extract the OD boundary. The algorithm assumes an almost circular shape and seeks local distortions of the contour.

11.2.4.2 Cup Segmentation

Color plane selection for the challenging task of cup region detection has been done on the basis of contrast between the cup area and the remaining retinal image. The more frequent selection is the G plane of the RGB color space. For instance, some of the ARGALI system algorithms detect cup region by a level-set procedure initialized by a threshold accounting for 66.7% of the pixels in the image. Similar to the OD detection stage, an ellipse fitting technique is applied to smooth and regulate the shape of the segmented cup [45,46,47]. Tan et al. [50] after detecting the OD region with the ARGALI method, processed the G channel of the ROI obtained with a Gaussian mixture model technique. The AGLAIA system uses the G channel to detect the cup region by adding the cascade of A-level set and active shape model to the level-set of ARGALI. The method proposed by Ho et al. [57], as has previously been explained, processes the G channel of the image looking for three peaks on the resultant image. The one corresponding to the cup area is used to obtain an initial curve to perform an active contour process that finally leads to the desired cup region. Kavitha et al. [53] use the G channel to perform a component analysis to isolate the cup region. In [44] three algorithms are compared. The first two use G color plane to obtain the cup region. For this purpose a high threshold is used in the multithreshold technique, while a region-based active contour procedure is used by the second proposed algorithm.

A few approaches make use of other color spaces, mainly B and R from the RGB color space. Hatanaka et al. [58,59] use intensity profiles in the B channel along with the zero-crossing technique and spline interpolation to obtain a smooth cup border.

In an interesting work presented by Joshi et al. [55,56], the appearance of the cup area in the R plane is combined with anatomical knowledge about vessels traversing the region. Therefore, the cup is modeled as a region enclosing the pallor region and defined by a boundary passing through a sparse set of vessel bends. However, in another approach [54] the color plane used by Joshi et al. is a^* from the CIE $L^*a^*b^*$ uniform color space. The reason stated by the authors is that the cup region appears continuous and well contrasted with respect to the background. Cup symmetry is used after thresholding to obtain a coarse OD segmentation. However, the use of a fixed threshold is not adequate for handling large intensity variations on the desired region.

A combination of color planes is adopted by some authors, although the processing is preformed separately on each color channel. For example, returning to the ARGALI group of algorithms, there are some proposed semiautomatic techniques, such as those presented by Liu and colleagues [25,46], where the user must first identify a point in the optic within the cup. Using the color intensity information from the chosen point, pixels in the three individual R, G, and B color channels are selected if their intensity values are all within the range of 25% from the selected pixel intensity. Once the pixels corresponding to the cup have been selected, direct ellipse fitting is applied to the detected area. A level-set technique in the G plane and thresholding in the R, G, and B planes are compared in Wong et al. [47], where the former achieves higher accuracy levels. In the work by Zhang and colleagues [48,49] a convex hull ellipse fitting is added to improve accuracy.

Four color planes are combined by Xu et al. [61]: G, B (RGB model) and H, S (HSV model). According to the authors, the R and V channels differ little between the OD and cup and are therefore discarded. This method is based on a machine-learning framework with sliding windows.

The third method proposed by Madhusudhan et al. [44], the region-growing technique, makes use of the vector nature of the color image using the RGB color image and Euclidean distance to make a decision on whether to include a new pixel in the grown region or not.

The method proposed by Valencia et al. [60] is, as occurred with the OD segmentation technique, fully adapted to human perception. It is based on image thresholding looking for the pixels with high luminance, low chrome, and yellow hue called seeds. The CIEDE 2000 color distance from all the pixels in the image to the previously selected seeds is calculated and a distance image is built. The cup region is obtained by the analysis of the histogram of this gray-level image.

11.3 Research Application of CDR Estimation

The algorithms described earlier focus on the CDR estimation from retinal fundus images. The presence of blood vessels occluding the cup boundary and the gradual transition between this region and the surrounding neuroretinal rim increase the difficulty of obtaining accurate results. Therefore, none of the presented methods provide a perfect result and the problem of automatic CDR calculation is still unsolved. Moreover, almost all of the published methods do not consider the whole color information, forgetting the vector nature of any pixel color and focusing on one or two color planes that are processed with gray-level image-processing techniques.

We present here an algorithm developed for use in an automated screening system for glaucoma diagnosis that is focused on adaptation to human perception [62]. In an attempt to take advantage of the color information that characterizes the cup inside the OD area, a uniform color space with an advance color distance is used.

11.3.1 OD Segmentation

The method adopted to isolate the OD area is the active contour technique, due to its autonomy and effectiveness. It is initialized with a square contour built from the OD center and applied on a vessel-free version of the original image.

11.3.1.1 OD Localization

Following a method based on the work presented by Sinthanayothin et al. [63], the algorithm makes use of the G channel of the RGB representation of the original image because this color plane possesses the highest contrast between structural information of retinal images and the retinal background, while contrast between background and abnormalities is kept low [64]. An example is shown in Figure 11.2a and b. Once the color plane has been selected, we make use of the concept of variance as a measure of contrast to localize the OD center. The OD area is the least homogeneous region in the retinography because of the dark blood

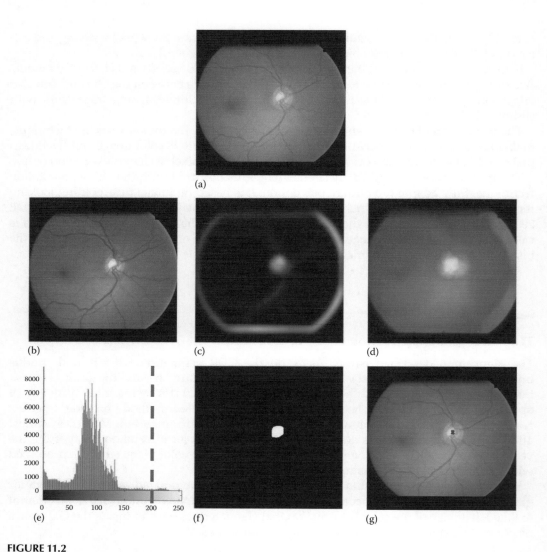

FIGURE 11.2
(a) Original color retinal image. (b) G color plane from RGB color space. (c) Variance image. Eyes edges could lead to false OD centers. (d) G plane blurred by anisotropic diffusion. (e) Histogram of the filtered image with the threshold marked with a dotted line. (f) Binary mask obtained after thresholding. (g) Final OD center superimposed on the original image.

vessels and bright cup area present within it. Therefore, these very different intensity levels make the OD region the one with highest variance in the image. The algorithm searches for the pixels with highest variance in the G channel. Taking a subimage W of size 21 × 21 centered in the pixel (i, j) the variance associated with this pixel is computed as:

$$v(i,j) = \left\langle G^2 \right\rangle_W - \left(\left\langle G \right\rangle_W \right)^2 \tag{11.1}$$

where the function $\left\langle G \right\rangle_W$ is defined as the average of the intensity of the G plane in the window W.

However, the eye edges, that is, the border of the eye and the black background, could lead to false centers outside the OD area (see Figure 11.2c). To avoid this error we apply an anisotropic diffusion filter to the G channel of the image [65], as in Figure 11.2d. Next, we threshold this image with a threshold value fixed to the maximum of the blurred image ponderated to 90%. An example of this thresholding is shown in Figure 11.2e. A binary mask is obtained (Figure 11.2f), wherein the white pixels correspond with candidate OD center pixels.

Finally, the center of the OD is considered to be the pixel with the highest average variance, discarding the ones not belonging to the mask (Figure 11.2g).

11.3.1.2 Vessel Detection and Removal

From the G channel of the RGB representation of the original image, the contrast is enhanced [66,67]. The image is high-pass filtered to highlight the details and a top-hat filter is used. This morphological filter removes lines from the input image, distinguishing between blood vessels (curve lines) and other elements usually present in the image with a rounded form (OD, microaneurysms, etc.). The filtered image is subtracted from the G plane one and the result is thresholded with an adaptive surface-based technique retaining only 10.5%, an experimentally fixed value for accounting for the vascular tree area, of the total surface of the image.

To remove the detected vascular tree, the algorithm applies a modified anisotropic diffusion operation [60] that assigns different diffusion coefficients depending on whether the pixel belongs to a vessel or not. The objective is to smooth inside the regions limited by edges, but not through them. Subsequently nonessential information such as the little and thin capillaries, hemorrhages, and microaneurysms are deleted while preserving the OD contour. Figure 11.3 shows an overview of the proposed method for vessels removal,

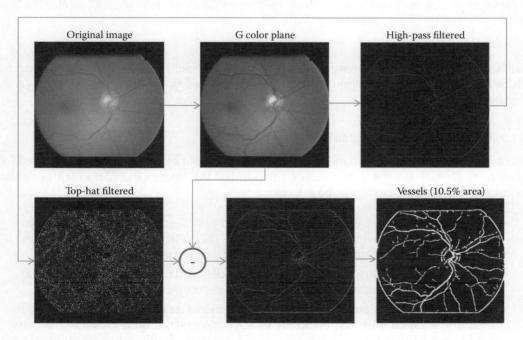

FIGURE 11.3
Proposed blood vessel removal method.

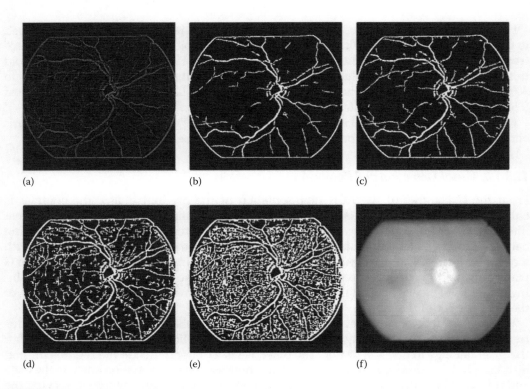

FIGURE 11.4
From the difference image obtained after subtracting the *G* channel of the original image and the top-hat fil-tered version (a), different vascular trees can be obtained depending on the threshold: (b) 8%, (c) 10.5%, (d) 20%, and (e) 50%. Final vessel-free image is shown in (f).

while in Figure 11.4 we present an example of how different thresholding values lead to different vascular tree detection results. The final vessel-free image can be observed in Figure 11.4f.

11.3.2 Active Contour Procedure

Active contours is an iterative method wherein local energies are iteratively calculated by moving the initial contour to minimize (or maximize) this energy. In order to achieve great accuracy, three parameters must be selected:

- Initial contour: This has been defined as a 100 pixels side-length square box cen-tered in the previously estimated OD center. This selection assures that the OD boundary is at least partially contained inside the initial contour.

- The localization radius: We assume a pseudo-elliptical form with a restricted size, and therefore the localization radius has been set empirically to 20 pixels.

- The number of iterations: This is strongly dependent on image size, initial contour size, and location with respect to the OD. An incorrect number of iterations may lead to over- or undersegmentation. In the present work this value has been set to 120 in order not to undersegment any image.

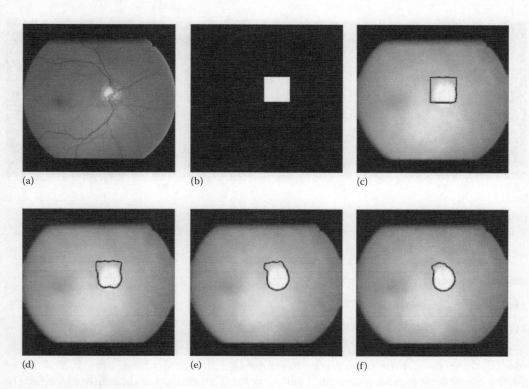

(a) (b) (c)

(d) (e) (f)

FIGURE 11.5
Active contour procedure is applied to the *G* channel of the original image (a), with the initial contour shown in the binary mask (b). Results obtained for (c) 5, (d) 30, (e) 80, and (f) 120 iterations.

An example of the evolution of the initial curve is shown in Figure 11.5. The result of this active contour procedure is a generally coarse and noisy OD and, occasionally, over-segmentation occurs (see Figures 11.5f and 11.6b). To overcome this issue, we perform a morphological opening operation with a disc as the structuring element. Its size is automatically estimated based on the coarse OD boundary in an iterative process as follows:

$$R_n = \left\lfloor \frac{1}{\alpha_n} \sqrt{\frac{A_{RFI}}{7\pi}} \right\rfloor; \quad \alpha_n = \alpha_{n-1} + 0.1; \quad \alpha_0 = 3; \quad n = 0, 1, \ldots, N \tag{11.2}$$

where:
R_n is the disc radius at the iteration n
A_{RFI} is the area of the retinal fundus image
α_n is the scaling factor in the iteration
n is an incremental factor
N is the number of iterations

This formula is based on physiological evidence that the OD radius is approximately 1/7 of the retinal radius. An initial value for the radius is assigned according to our database average OD radius size. Beginning from an experimentally fixed value, the algorithm performs as many area openings as needed until a non null value is obtained. After this multistep area opening, the accurate OD area is detected (Figure 11.6c).

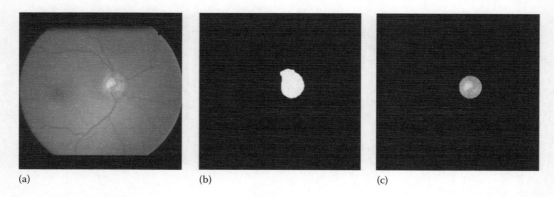

(a)   (b)   (c)

FIGURE 11.6
(a) Original image. (b) Active contour result. (c) Result obtained after multistep area opening.

11.4 Cup Segmentation

11.4.1 Perceptually Adapted *K*-Means Algorithm

In the OD area, every region is characterized by a precise color: Blood vessels have a dark reddish color, the neuroretinal rim is presented in different shades of orange, and, above all, the cup area possesses a saturated yellow color. Therefore, our algorithm identifies the cup area by searching for the brightest yellow pixels, considering the vector nature of each pixel color, and grouping them in the color space.

In this approach, due to its simplicity and effectiveness we have chosen a method based on the well-known *K*-means clustering technique, modifying this technique in order to use a uniform color space, that is, in the chosen color space, distance measures must be correlated with perceived color differences. In 1976, CIE proposed two color spaces that approximately possessed this property: CIE *L**a*b* and CIE *L**u*v*. The Euclidean distances in those spaces were believed to be approximately correlated with perceptual color differences. Later, it was shown that this goal was not strictly achieved. To improve the uniformity of color difference measurements in CIE *L**a*b*, an empirical modification of the Euclidean distance was proposed in 1995. This distance measure is abbreviated to CIE94 [68].

In this context, the codebook for *K*-means algorithm implementation, chosen to minimize the empirical quantization error, can be obtained through an optimization. Due to the nature of the CIE94 color distance formula, a heuristic method based on the direction of the gradient vector has been adopted in the proposed approach.

At each image pixel, the gradient vector points in the direction of largest possible function increase, corresponding its magnitude to the rate of change in that direction. The opposite one corresponds, then, to the direction of the function decrease and therefore it can be used to obtain its local minima. Hence, to find the location of the new codevectors, the algorithm moves from the old centroids in the opposite direction to the gradient. When moving along this direction, the function value will decrease until a local minimum is reached. In that particular moment, if the algorithm keeps moving the function will increase. This growth in the function's value is an indicator of the approximate location of the new codevector.

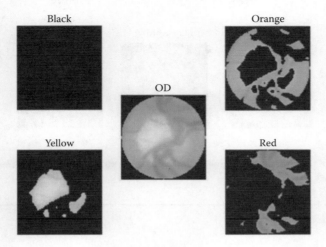

FIGURE 11.7
After automatically detecting the number of significant colors present in the OD window with Dunn, $K = 4$, the perceptually adapted K-means algorithm groups pixels according to their color (black, red, orange, and yellow).

As a result of this K-means procedure, every pixel in the OD area is assigned to one of the color centroids. Figure 11.7 shows an example of the groups obtained for $K = 4$. The cup group is the one closest to yellow. The K parameter is automatically obtained by computation of the Dunn coefficient [69].

11.4.2 Cup Boundary Smoothing

Following the general tendency to provide an ellipse as the result of cup segmentation [25,45–52], we have added the possibility of obtaining such a result from the segmented cup region [70]. Therefore, we propose two different methods:

- Ellipse fitting: An approximately round estimation of the cup boundary is obtained as the-best fitting least-square ellipse. The area enclosed within the ellipse will be considered as the cup surface when the CDR is calculated by means of this method.

- Gaussian smoothing: We make use of a morphological dilation technique in order to obtain a dilated cup boundary. Next a Gaussian smoothing of the dilated boundary is performed with the method described by Lee et al. [71], based on the classic curvature scale-space filtering idea [72].

The difference in the result obtained by each method can be seen in Figure 11.8.

11.4.3 CDR Estimation

Once the OD and cup surfaces have been estimated, the CDR is obtained as follows:

$$CDR = \frac{A_{CUP}}{A_{OD}} \tag{11.3}$$

where A_{CUP} is the cup surface calculated as the number of pixels enclosed by the cup boundary, regardless of which method has been performed, and A_{OD} is the OD surface calculated as the number of pixels enclosed by the OD boundary.

| OD | Ellipse fitting | Gaussian smoothing |

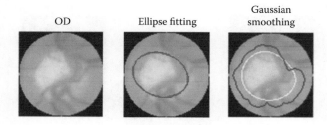

FIGURE 11.8
A smooth boundary of the cup can be obtained by two methods: ellipse fitting and Gaussian smoothing (final result marked in white).

11.5 Results

11.5.1 Data Set

We used a database consisting of 55 color fundus images in JPEG format taken by a TOPCON TRC 50-EX mydriatic retinograph provided by the University Hospital Puerta del Mar, Cádiz, Spain. The image size is 2544 × 1696 pixels. Our hardware research equipment consists of an HP Compaq dc7600 Convertible computer with 1 GB RAM and an Intel processor with 2.77 GHz. The software used was MATLAB software (2008a release).

To maintain a reasonable processing speed without diminishing the accuracy of the results, the images have been automatically resized to a 600 × 600 pixels resolution without distorting the original aspect ratio by adding two horizontal black bands in the top and the bottom of the original image and removing the vertical ones which belong to the black background.

11.5.2 Evaluation Measures

A common quantitative analysis has been performed to assess the overall performance of both the OD and cup segmentation methods. This evaluation is based on the error made by the algorithm, computed as the difference between the ground truth provided by two medical experts and the results provided by our algorithm. We compute the following quantities for both final rounding procedures, that is, ellipse fitting and Gaussian smoothing:

$$\mu(E) = \frac{1}{N} \sum_{i=1}^{N} E_i \tag{11.4}$$

$$\sigma(E) = \sqrt{\frac{1}{N} \sum_{i=1}^{N} \left(E_i - \mu(E)\right)^2} \tag{11.5}$$

$$E_i = \left| CDR_i - CDR_i^{GT} \right|, i = 1, 2, \ldots, N \tag{11.6}$$

where:
  N is the number of images
  CDR_i^{GT} is the CDR ground truth for image I
  $\mu(E)$ is the average error
  $\sigma(E)$ is the standard deviation of the error

11.5.3 Results

The mean error and standard deviation of the estimated error for both methods are shown in Table 11.1. The OD was satisfactorily localized on the complete image database. On the other hand, the OD border was accurately detected on 49 of the 55 images. However, on six images a high saturation of the *R* channel led to noticeable oversegmentation. The cup region was satisfactorily detected in all of the images in the database. An example of the final OD and cup region obtained is shown in Figure 11.9. The same example along with its ground truth is shown in Figure 11.10.

As shown in Table 11.2, with regard to observer variabilities, with the ellipse fitting method 39 images (70.91% of the whole set) were under the interobserver limit, while with Gaussian smoothing a correct diagnosis was achieved in 43 images (78.18% of the total set). With regard to intraobserver variability, the Gaussian smoothing method slightly outperforms the ellipse fitting method, with 35 images (63.64%) correctly classified against 34 images for ellipse. This algorithm obtains promising results, although there is a difficulty in comparing the obtained results due to the absence of public databases.

TABLE 11.1

Mean Error and Standard Deviation of the Estimated Error for Both Methods

	Ellipse Fitting Method	Proposed Method
$\mu(E)$	0.1400	0.1287
$\sigma(E)$	0.1166	0.1006

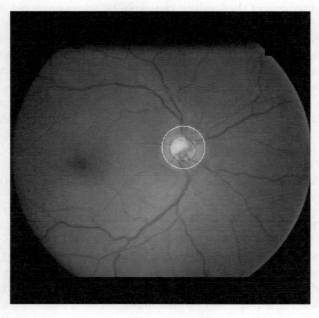

FIGURE 11.9
An example of the final OD and cup areas detected.

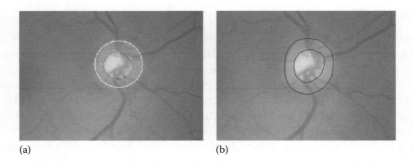

(a) 　　　　　　　　　　　　　　　　(b)

FIGURE 11.10
(a) The OD and cup areas of Figure 11.11, along with (b) the corresponding ground truth manually marked by two expert ophthalmologists.

TABLE 11.2

Classification of Error E in Ellipse Fitting Approach and Gaussian Smoothing Approach

E	Intraobserver Variability (<0.15 CDR units)	Interobserver Variability (<0.2 CDR units)	Out of Limit (>0.2 CDR units)
Ellipse fitting	34 (61.82%)	39 (70.91%)	16 (29.09%)
Gaussian smoothing	35 (63.64%)	43 (78.18%)	12 (21.82%)

11.6 Conclusion and Discussion

Glaucoma is currently one of the leading causes of blindness around the world. Ageing of population together with population growth is causing an increase in the number of vision loss cases due to glaucoma. However, investigations have shown that although glaucoma cannot be cured, its progression can be stopped if early detected and therefore blindness can be avoided. During glaucomatous progression the cup area within the OD enlarges due to the death of ganglion nerve cells. The relation between the cup and disc area, CDR, is thus a crucial indicator of this asymptomatic disease. Currently, CDR estimation requires the manual evaluation of retinal images by ophthalmologists. In order to reduce the time and costs incurred by mass screening programs an automatic and robust CAD tool must be developed.

Researchers are increasingly concerned with automated early diagnosis of glaucoma, and numerous techniques have been developed for the analysis of retinal structures in color fundus images, which are much more suitable for screening than OCT or HCT due to their lower equipment acquisition costs. The majority of the state of the art techniques are devoted to OD detection, mainly in the R plane of the RGB color space representation of the original image. A wide range of techniques have been successfully applied: shape-based template matching, active contours (gradient or regional based), level set, etc. Cup segmentation is usually a more challenging task as the cup boundary is diffuse and occluded by blood vessels. This is frequently carried out in the G plane of the RGB color space. Numerous techniques make use of thresholds to isolate this cup region once the OD has been detected. Active contours and level set are other frequently used echniques.

There is a lack of adaptation to human perception in the literature, where very few algorithms are developed on a uniform color space. Advanced color distances correlated with perceived color differences or color appearance models are mostly forgotten, with the consequent loss of relevant information.

There is also a need to establish publicly available databases of retinal fundus images along with the ground truth provided by medical experts about OD and cup areas and the estimated CDR for each of them. This kind of benchmark would reduce the variability among the quality assessments of different proposed techniques, leading to the development of better segmentation algorithms.

On the other hand, a CAD tool intended to decrease the workload of manual screening must detect abnormal OD and cup images, thus making the system really useful.

Finally, researchers in ophthalmology have published that measuring the CDR alone may not be enough for the clinical screening of glaucoma. Another sign that may help is the OD nerve pallor [73]. Thus, CAD tools for glaucoma screening should work on this basis.

References

1. World Health Organization. 2007. Vision2020 report.
2. Gloster, J. and Parry, D. G. 1974. Use of photographs measuring cupping in the optic disc. *British Journal of Ophtalmology* 58(850): 1–14.
3. Gupta, P. K., Asrani, S., Freedman, S., El-Dairi, M., and Bhatti, M. T. 2011. Differentiating glaucomatous from non-glaucomatous optic nerve cupping by optical coherence tomography. *The Open Neurology Journal* 5(5): 1–7.
4. Abràmoff, M. D., Garvin, M. K., and Sonka, M. 2010. Retinal imaging and image analysis. *IEEE Reviews on Biomedical Engineering* 3: 169–208.
5. Singer, D. E., Nathan, D., Fogel, H. A., and Schachat, A. P. 1992. Screening for diabetic retinopathy. *Annals of Internal Medicine* 116: 660–671.
6. Acharya, U. R., Ng, E. Y. K., and Suri, J. S. 2008. *Image Modeling of Human Eye.* Artech House: Norwood.
7. Hoover, A. and Goldbaum, M. 2003. Locating the optic nerve in a retinal image using the fuzzy convergence of the blood vessels. *IEEE Transactions on Medical Imaging* 22: 951–958.
8. Staal, J., Abràmoff, M. D., Niemeijer, M., Viergever, M. A., and Van Ginneken, B. 2004. Ridge-based vessel segmentation in color images of the retina. *IEEE Transactions on Medical Imaging* 23: 501–509.
9. Al-Diri, B., Hunter, A., Steel, D., Habib, M., Hudaib, T., and Berry, S. 2008. REVIEW: A reference data set for retinal vessel profiles. *Annual International Conference of the IEEE Engineering in Medicine and Biology Society* 2008: 2262–2265.
10. Lowell, J., Hunter, A., Steel, D., Basu, A., Ryder, R., Fletcher, E., and Kennedy, L. 2004. Optic nerve head segmentation. *IEEE Transactions on Medical Imaging* 23(2): 256–264.
11. Kauppi, T., Kalesnykiene, V., Kamarainen, J. K., Lensu, L., Sorri, I., Uusitalo, H., Kälviäinen, H., and Pietilä, J. 2006. DIARETDB0: Evaluation database and methodology for diabetic retinopathy algorithms. Technical report.
12. Kauppi, T., Kalesnykiene, V., Kamarainen, J.-K., Lensu, L., Sorri, I., Raninen, A., Voutilainen, R., Uusitalo, H., Kälviäinen, H., and Pietilä, J. 2007. DIARETDB1: Diabetic retinopathy database and evaluation protocol. Technical report.
13. Fumero, F., Alayon, S., Sanchez, J. L., Sigut, J., and Gonzalez-Hernandez, M. 2011. RIM-ONE: An open retinal image database for optic nerve evaluation. In: *Proceedings of the 24th International Symposium on Computer-Based Medical Sytems.* CBMS, Bristol, 2011, pp. 1–6.

14. Carmona, E. J., Rincón, M., García-Feijoo, J., and Martínez-de-la-Casa, J. M. 2008. Identification of the optic nerve head with genetic algorithms. *Artificial Intelligence in Medicine* 43(3): 243–259.

15. Zhang, Z., Yin, F. S., Liu, J., Wong, W. K., Tan, N. M., Lee, B. H., Cheng, J., and Wong, T. Y. 2010. ORIGA−light: An online retinal fundus image database for glaucoma analysis and research. *Proceedings of the IEEE Conference of the Engineering in Medicine and Biology Society* 2010: 1–4.

16. Aliaa, A. H., Abdel-Razik, Y., Atef Zaki, G., Amr Ahmed, S., and Abdel-Rahman, G. 2008. Optic disc detection from normalized digital fundus images by means of a vessels' direction matched filter. *IEEE Transactions on Medical Imaging* 27(1): 11–18.

17. Osareh, A., Mirmehdi, M., Thomas, B., and Markham, R. 2002. Comparison of colour spaces for optic disc localisation in retinal images. In: *Proceedings of the 16th International Conference on Pattern Recognition*, vol. 1. IEEE Computer Society, Quebec, pp. 743–746.

18. Chaichana, T., Yoowattana, S., Sun, Z., Tangjitkusolmun, S., Sookpotharom, S., and Sangworasil, M. 2008. Edge detection of the optic disc in retinal images based on identification of a round shape. In: *Proceedings of the International Symposium on Communications and Information Technologies*. ISCIT, Vientiane, Laos, 2008, pp. 670–674.

19. Langroudi, M. N. and Sadjedi, H. 2010. A new method for automatic detection and diagnosis of retinopathy diseases in colour fundus images based on morphology. In: *Proceedings of the International Conference on Bioinformatics and Biomedical Technology*. ICBBT, Chengdu, China, 2010, pp. 134–138.

20. Kavitha, D. and Shenbaga Devi, S. 2005. Automatic detection of optic disc and exudates in retinal images. In: *Proceedings of the International Conference on Intelligent Sensing and Information Processing*. Bangalore, India, January 2005, pp. 501–506.

21. Foracchia, M., Grisan, E., and Ruggeri, A. 2004. Detection of optic disc in retinal images by means of a geometrical model of vessel structure. *IEEE Transactions on Medical Imaging* 23(10): 1189–1195.

22. Echegaray, S., Soliz, P., and Luo, W. 2009. Automatic initialization of level set segmentation for application to optic disc margin identification. In: *Proceedings of the 22nd IEEE International Symposium on Computer-Based Medical Systems*. IEEE, New Mexico, August 2009, pp. 1–4.

23. Xu, X., Niemeijer, M., Song, Q., Sonka, M., Garvin, M. K., Reinhardt, J. M., and Abràmoff, M. D. 2011. Vessel boundary delineation on fundus images using graph-based approach. *IEEE Transactions on Medical Imaging* 30(6): 1184–1191.

24. Mahfouz, A. E. and Fahmy, A. S. 2010. Fast localization of the optic disc using projection of image features. *IEEE Transactions on Image Processing* 19(12): 3285–3289.

25. Liu, J., Wong, D. W. K., Lim, J. H., Jia, X., Yin, F., Li, H., Xiong, W., and Wong, T. Y. 2008. Optic cup and disk extraction from retinal fundus images for determination of cup-to-disc ratio. In: *Proceedings of the 3rd IEEE Conference on Industrial Electronics and Applications*. ICIEA, Singapore, 2008, pp. 1828–1832.

26. Mubbashar, M., Usman, A., and Akram, M. U. 2011. Automated system for macula detection in digital retinal images. In: *Proceedings of the International Conference on Information and Communication Technologies*. IEEE ICICT, Karachi, Pakistan, July 2011, pp. 1–5.

27. Siddalingaswamy, P. C. and Gopalakrishna Prabhu, K. 2010. Automatic grading of diabetic maculopathy severity levels. In: *Proceedings of 2010 International Conference on Systems in Medicine and Biology*. IIT, Kharagpur, India, pp. 331–334.

28. Aquino, A., Gegúndez-Arias, M. E., and Marín, D. 2010. Detecting the optic disc boundary in digital fundus images using morphological, edge detection, and feature extraction techniques. *IEEE Transactions on Medical Imaging* 29(11): 1860–1869.

29. Xu, X., Garvin, M. K., Abràmoff, M. D., and Reinhardt, J. M. 2010. Simultaneous automatic detection of the optic disc fovea on fundus photographs. *Medical Imaging* 7962: 79622T-1–79622T-7.

30. Kovacs, L., Qureshi, R. J., Nagy, B., Harangi, B., and Hajdu, A. 2010. Graph based detection of optic disc and fovea in retinal images. In: *Proceedings of the 4th IEEE International Workshop on Soft Computing Applications*. Arad, Romania, 2010, pp. 143–148.

31. Vahabi, Z., Vafadoost, M., and Gharibzadeh, S. 2010. The new approach to automatic detection of optic disc from non-dilated retinal images. In: *Proceedings of the Iranian Conference of Biomedical Engineering*. ICBME, Isfahan, 3–4 November, 2010, pp. 1–6.

32. Walter, T., Klein, J.-C., Massin, P., and Erginay, A. 2002. A contribution of image processing to the diagnosis of diabetic retinopathy detection of exudates in color fundus images of the human retina. *IEEE Transactions on Medical Imaging* 21(10): 1236–1243.

33. Lu, S. and Lim, J. H. 2010. Automatic optic disc detection through background estimation. In: *Proceedings of the IEEE 17th International Conference on Image Processing*. ICIP, Hong Kong, 26–29 September 2010, pp. 833–836.

34. Lu, S. and Lim, J. H. 2010. Automatic optic disc detection from retinal images by a line operator. *IEEE Transactions on Biomedical Engineering* 58(1): 88–94.

35. Yu, H., Barrigaa, S., Agurtoa, C., Echegaraya, S., Pattichisb, M., Zamoraa, G., Baumanc, W., and Soliza, P. 2011. Fast localization of optic disc and fovea in retinal images for eye disease screening. *Medical Imaging* 7963: 796317-1–796317-12.

36. Abbas, Q., Fondón, I., Jimenez, S., and Alemany, P. 2012. Automatic detection of optic disc from retinal fundus images using dynamic programming. *Lecture Notes in Computer Science* 7325: 416–423.

37. Lee, S. S., Rajeswari, M., Ramachandram, D., and Shaharuddin, B. 2006. Screening of diabetic retinopathy—Automatic segmentation of optic disc in colour fundus images. In: *Proceedings of the 2nd International Conference on Distributed Frameworks for Multimedia Applications*. IEEE, Pulau Pinang, Malaysia, 2006, pp. 1–7.

38. Lu, C.-K., Tang, T. B., Murray, A. F., Laude, A., and Dhillon, B. 2011. Automatic parapapillary atrophy shape detection and quantification in colour fundus images. In: *Proceedings of the IEEE Biomedical Circuits and Systems Conference*. BioCAS, Paphos, 3–5 November 2010, pp. 86–89.

39. Marrugo, A. G. and Millan, M. S. 2011. Retinal image analysis: Preprocessing and feature extraction. *Journal of Physics Conference Series* 274: 1–8.

40. Venkatalakshmi, B., Saravanan, V., and Niveditha, G. J. 2011. Graphical user interface for enhanced retinal image analysis for diagnosing diabetic retinopathy. In: *Proceedings of the IEEE 3rd International Conference on Communication Software and Networks*. ICCSN, Xi'an, China, 27–29 May 2011, pp. 610–613.

41. Harangi, B., Qureshi, R. J., Csutak, A., Peto, T., and Hajdu, A. 2010. Automatic detection of the optic disc using majority voting in a collection of optic disc detectors. In: *Proceedings of the IEEE International Symposium on Biomedical Imaging: From Nano to Macro*. IEEE Signal Processing Society, Rotterdam, 14–17 April 2010, pp. 1329–1332.

42. Kande, G. B., Venkata Subbaiah, P., and Satya Savithri, T. 2008. Segmentation of exudates and optic disk in retinal images. In: *Proceedings of the Sixth Indian Conference on Computer Vision, Graphics and Image Processing*. ICVGIP, Bhubaneswar, India, 16–19 December 2008, pp. 535–542.

43. Sáez, A., Fondón, I., Acha, B., Jiménez, S., Alemany, P., Abbas, Q., and Serrano, C. 2012. Optic disc segmentation based on level-set and colour gradients. In: *Proceedings of the Sixth European Conference on Colour in Graphics, Imaging, and MCS/10 Vision*. Society for Imaging Sciences and Technology, Amsterdam, pp. 121–125.

44. Madhusudhan, M., Malay, N., Nirmala, S. R., and Samerendra, D. 2011. Image processing techniques for glaucoma detection. *Advances in Computing and Communications* 192(3): 365–373.

45. Wong, D. W. K., Liu, J., Lim, J. H., Jia, X., Yin, F., Li, H., and Wong, T. Y. 2008. Level-set based automatic cup-to-disc ratio determination using retinal fundus images in ARGALI. In: *Proceedings of the 30th Annual International Conference of the IEEE Engineering in Medicine and Biology Society*. EMBS, Vancouver, BC, 20–25 August 2008, pp. 2266–2269.

46. Liu, J., Wong, D. W. K., Lim, J. H., Li, H., Tan, N. M., Zhang, Z., Wong, T. Y., and Lavanya, R. 2009. ARGALI: An automatic cup-to-disc ratio measurement system for glaucoma analysis using level-set image processing. In: *Proceedings of the 13th International Conference on Biomedical Engineering*, vol. 2. ICBME, Singapore, 3–6 December 2008, pp. 559–562.

47. Wong, D. W. K., Liu, J., Lim, J. H., Tan, N. M., Zhang, Z., Lu, S., Li, H., Teo, M. H., Chan, K. L., and Wong, T. Y. 2009. Intelligent fusion of cup-to-disc ratio determination methods for glaucoma detection in ARGALI. In: *Annual International Conference of the IEEE Engineering in Medicine and Biology Society*. EMBC, Minneapolis, MN, 3–6 September 2009, pp. 5777–5780.

48. Zhang, Z., Liu, J., Wong, W. K., Tan, N. M., Lim, J. H., Lu, S., Li, H., Liang, Z., and Wong, T. Y. 2009. Neuro-retinal optic cup detection in glaucoma diagnosis. In: *Proceedings of the 2nd International Conference on Biomedical Engineering and Informatics*. Tianjin, China, pp. 1–4.

49. Zhang, Z., Liu, J., Cherian, N.S., Sun, Y., Lim, J. H., Wong, W. K., Tan, N. M., Lu, S., Li, S., and Wong, T. Y. 2009. Convex hull based neuro-retinal optic cup ellipse optimization in glaucoma diagnosis. *Conference Proceedings of IEEE Engineering in Medicine and Biology Society* 2009: pp. 1441–1444.

50. Tan, N.M., Liu, J., Wong, D.W.K., Yin, F., Lim, J.H., and Wong, T.Y. 2010. Mixture model-based approach for optic cup segmentation. In: *Annual International Conference of the IEEE Engineering in Medicine and Biology Society*. EMBC, Buenos Aires, 31 August–4 September 2010, pp. 4817–4820.

51. Zhang, Z., Lee, B. H., Liu, J., Wong, D.W.K., Tan, N. M., Lim, J. H., Yin, F., Huang, W., Li, H., and Wong, T. Y. 2010. Optic disc region of interest localization in fundus image for Glaucoma detection in ARGALI. In: *Proceedings of the 5th IEEE Conference on Industrial Electronics and Applications*. ICIEA, Taichung, 15–17 June 2010, pp. 1686–1689.

52. Liu, J., Yin, F. S., Wong, D. W. K., Zhang, Z., Tan, N. M., Cheung, C. Y., Baskaran, M., Aung, T., and Wong, T. Y. 2011. Automatic glaucoma diagnosis from fundus image. *Conference Proceedings of the IEEE Engineering in Medicine and Biology Society* 2011: 3383–3386.

53. Kavitha, S., Karthikeyan, S., and Duraiswamy, K. 2010. Early detection of glaucoma in retinal images using cup to disc ratio. In: *Proceedings of the IEEE 2nd International Conference on Computing Communication and Networking Technologies*. Karur, India, pp. 1–5.

54. Joshi, G. D., Sivaswamy, J., Karan, K., and Krishnadas, S. R. 2010. Optic disk and cup boundary detection using regional information. In: *Proceedings of the IEEE International Symposium on Biomedical Imaging: From Nano to Macro*. CVIT, IIIT Hyderabad, India, 14–17 April 2010, pp. 948–951.

55. Joshi, G. D., Sivaswamy, J., Karan, K., and Krishnadas, S. R. 2010. Vessel bend-based cup segmentation in retinal images. In: *Proceedings of the International Conference on Pattern Recognition*. ICPR, Istanbul, 2010, pp. 2536–2539.

56. Joshi, G. D., Sivaswamy, J., and Krishnadas, S. R. 2011. Optic disk and cup segmentation from monocular color retinal images for glaucoma assessment. *IEEE Transactions on Medical Imaging* 30(6): 1192–1205.

57. Ho, C. Y., Pai, T. W., Chang, H. T., and Chen, H. Y. 2011. An atomatic fundus image analysis system for clinical diagnosis of glaucoma. In: *Proceedings of the International Conference on Complex, Intelligent and Software Intensive Systems*. CISIS, Seoul, 2011, pp. 559–564.

58. Hatanaka, Y., Noudo, A., Muramatsu, C., Sawada, A., Hara, T., Yamamoto, T., and Fujita, H. 2010. Automatic measurement of cup to disc ratio based on line profile analysis in retinal images. *Lecture Notes in Computer Science* 6165: 64–72.

59. Hatanaka, Y., Noudo, A., Muramatsu, C., Sawada, A., Hara, T., Yamamoto, T., and Fujita, H. 2011. Automatic measurement of cup to disc ratio based on line profile analysis in retinal images. In: *Proceedings of the Annual International Conference of the IEEE Engineering in Medicine and Biology Society*. EMBC, Boston, MA, August 30–September 3, pp. 3387–3390.

60. Valencia, E. and Millan, M. 2006. Color image analysis of the optic disc to assist diagnosis of glaucoma risk and evolution. In: *Proceedings of the 3rd European Conference on Colour in Graphics, Imaging, and Vision. Final Program and Proceedings*. CGIV, Leeds, pp. 298–301.

61. Xu, Y., Xu, D., Lin, S., Liu, J., Cheng, J., Cheung, C. Y., Aung, T., and Wong, T. Y. 2011. Sliding window and regression based cup detection in digital fundus images for glaucoma diagnosis. *Lecture Notes in Computer Science* 6893: 1–8.

62. Fondón, I., Núñez, F., Tirado, M., Jiménez, S., Alemany, P., Abbas, Q., Serrano, C., and Acha, B. 2012. Automatic cup-to-disc ratio estimation using active contours and color clustering in fundus images for glaucoma diagnosis. *Lecture Notes in Computer Science* 7325: 390–399.

63. Sinthanayothin, C., Boyce, J. A., Cook, H. L., and Williamson, T. H. 1999. Automated localization of the optic disc, fovea, and retinal blood vessels from digital colour fundus images. *British Journal of Ophthalmology* 83(8): 902–910.

64. Sanfilippo, P. G., Cardini, A., Hewitt, A. W., Crowston, J. G., and Mackey, D. A. 2009. Optic disc morphology: Rethinking shape. *Progress in Retinal and Eye Research* 28(4): 227–248.

65. Perona, P. and Malik, J. 1990. Scale space and edge detection using anisotropic diffusion. *IEEE Transactions on Pattern Recognition and Machine Intelligence* 12(7): 629–639.
66. Walter, T., Massin, P., Erginay, A., Ordoñez, R., Jeulin, C., and Klein, J. C. 2007. Automatic detection of microaneurysms in color fundus images. *Medical Image Analysis* 11(6): 555–566.
67. Jiménez, S, Alemany, P., Núñez, F., Fondón, I., Serrano, M. C., and Acha, B. 2010. A new method for automated CDR measurements in photographic retinal images. *European Glaucoma Society Congress* 9: 1–6.
68. McDonald, R. and Smith, K. J. 1995. CIE94: A new colour-difference formula. *Journal of the Society of Dyers and Colourists* 111: 376–379.
69. Maulik, U. and Bandyopadhyay, S. 2002. Performance evaluation of some clustering algorithms and validity indices. *IEEE Transaction on Pattern Analysis and Machine Intelligence* 24(12): 1650–1654.
70. Lee, K., McLean, D. I., and Atkins, M. S. 2003. Irregularity index: A new border irregularity measure for cutaneous melanocytic lesions. *Medical Image Analysis* 7(1): 47–64.
71. Mokhtarian, F. and Mackworth, A. 1986. Scale-based description and recognition of planar curves and two dimensional shapes. *IEEE Transactions on Pattern Analysis and Machine Intelligence* 8(1): 34–43.
72. Siebert, M., Gramer, E., and Leydhecker, W. 1989. Pallor of the optic papilla, an early sign of glaucoma. A clinical controlled study of the disk pallor and papillar cupping. *Klin Monbl Augenheilkd* 194(6): 433–436.

12

Arteriovenous Ratio Calculation Using Image-Processing Techniques

Manuel G. Penedo, Sonia González, Noelia Barreira, Marc Saez,
Antonio Pose-Reino, and María Rodríguez-Blanco

CONTENTS

12.1 Introduction

The eye fundus is a window to analyze the microvasculature *in vivo* since retinal vascular imaging techniques provide the means to observe the retinal structures and the retinal microcirculation in a noninvasive manner. The retinal vessel tree is affected by the same diseases as the rest of the vasculature, so that an analysis of retinal vascular changes helps in the diagnosis of several pathologies that affect the vasculature, such as hypertension or diabetes. The generalized use of nonmydriatic retinographs in hospitals and health-care centers allows the early detection of these microvascular abnormalities and the analysis of their evolution over time.

In the retina, the term *vascular abnormalities* usually refers to capillary occlusions (microaneurysms), retinal hemorrhages, the proliferation of new vessels, changes in the vascular structure (retinal tortuosity, pathological crossings, etc.), and changes in the retinal vessel widths. Figure 12.1 shows retinas with several vascular abnormalities.

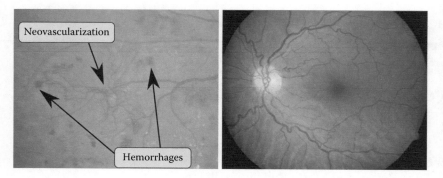

FIGURE 12.1
Vascular abnormalities. (*left*) Detail of a retina with several hemorrhages and neovascularization, both signs of diabetic retinopathy; (*right*) vascular tortuosity related to hypertension.

In particular, changes in the retinal vessel widths are one of the most studied vascular abnormalities, since arteriolar narrowing and venular widening have been associated with different pathologies. Cuspidi et al. presented a study that associated arteriolar narrowing with hypertension [1]. Wong et al. suggested that individuals that present with arteriovenous nicking, among other retinal abnormalities, were more likely to develop renal dysfunction [2]. Moreover, they also found that there was a relation between changes in the vessel widths and incident stroke [3], hypertension, and diabetes [4]. Furthermore, these changes can be seen as a risk factor for coronary heart disease [5] and some cerebrovascular diseases, such as cerebral atrophy [6] and lacunar stroke [7]. Table 12.1 summarizes the associations of the changes in the arteriolar and venular widths with other pathologies.

The conclusions of the aforementioned clinical studies stress the importance of measuring and monitoring the vessel widths over time. However, an analysis of isolated vessel widths makes the evaluation of the patient's condition complex for clinical practice. In this sense, because the arteriovenous ratio (AVR) is a variable that measures the relation between the artery and the vein widths, it is more suitable for screening purposes. The clinical guides define a procedure to compute the AVR that involves several steps. First, the vessel widths are measured at equidistant points from the optic disc center. The vessels are then classified as either arteries or veins and, finally, the AVR is calculated from a subset of the vessel widths, following a given formula [8]. However, performing these tasks manually from retinal images is not feasible, since they are time consuming, subjective, and nonrepeatable. For this reason, there is a growing need for the development of image-processing tools that are capable of computing the AVR in an objective and automatic

TABLE 12.1

Associations of Changes in Retinal Vessel Widths with Other Diseases

Retinal Arteriolar Narrowing	Retinal Venular Widening
Blood pressure	Impaired fasting glucose
Measures of atherosclerosis	Incident obesity
Incident hypertension	Cerebrovascular diseases
Incident diabetes	Carotid artery disease
Coronary heart disease	Hypertriglyceridemia

Source: Nguyen, T.T., Wang, J.J., and Wong, T.Y., *Diabetes Care*, 30, 2708–2715, 2007.

manner. Accordingly, screening tests could be performed easily, allowing the early diagnosis of coronary, brain, or other vascular diseases. Nevertheless, the development of an automatic methodology for computing the AVR is not straightforward. The complexity of this task lies not only in the stages of the AVR procedure, but also in the heterogeneity of the retinal images regarding lightness, contrast, and blurring, in addition to the inherent variability of the retinal structures. Thus, every automatic methodology for computing the AVR needs a combination of several procedures, namely, a contrast normalization technique, an algorithm for locating the optic disc, a procedure for segmenting and measuring vessels, and a classification technique for labeling the vessels as veins or arteries.

Due to the complexity of the procedure, there are few approaches in the literature that deal with the automatic computation of the AVR. Tramontan et al. [9] proposed a procedure for the automatic estimation of the AVR. First, the retinal image is preprocessed in order to normalize the image contrast. The vessel tree is then traced from a set of seed points. This procedure allows the extraction of the vessel center and width. Subsequently, the region of interest (ROI) where the measurements are performed is set by locating the optic disc. The optic disc is located where the vessel tree converges in the optic disc area. Tramontan et al. classified the vessels into arteries and veins by means of searching for the central reflex, which is only present in the arteries. Finally, the AVR is computed as the ratio of the central retinal artery equivalent (CRAE) and the central retinal vein equivalent (CRVE). This methodology obtained a correlation of 0.88 with respect to manual AVR computations. Nevertheless, since the vessel classification methodology relies on the detection of the central reflex, one of the limitations of this approach is that retinal images should have a large resolution.

Ortega et al. [10] describe a web-based framework for computing the AVR. In this framework, the user selects the optic disc center as well as the ROI where the measurements will be performed. The system then detects the vessels and measures their widths by means of specialized snakes. Finally, the user selects the vessels and classifies them as either an artery or a vein in order to compute the final AVR value. Recently, a procedure for the automatic classification of vessels was included in this framework [11]. This procedure combines a local classification stage based on color features and an unsupervised classifier (k-means) with a vessel tracking stage that ensures the vessel classes along the vessel tree. With this approach, the authors obtained a correlation of 0.856 with two different experts in a set of 58 images.

Muramatsu et al. [12] proposed an automatic methodology to compute the AVR. They used an active contour model to locate the optic disc and then to detect the ROI where the vessels were measured. The vessel segmentation was performed using morphological operators and a linear discriminant classifier was applied to group the arteries and veins. They also developed a strategy to select the major vessels for AVR computation. In the digital retinal images for vessel extraction (DRIVE) database, the average error in the AVR measurements was 0.11 in comparison with the experts. Even though this methodology achieved good results with low-resolution images, it only used the retinal main vessels and it was not tested with images that show arteriolar narrowing.

Niemeijer et al. [13] also proposed another methodology to measure the AVR. In their approach, they segmented the vessel tree using the filter outputs of a Gaussian filter bank as the input of a k-nearest neighbor (k-NN) classifier. They then detected the optic disc by means of analyzing the convergence of the vessel tree. The vessel measurement was performed from the segmented vessel tree, in the normal direction of the local vessel angle. This angle was computed from the vessel centerline obtained by thinning. Next, the vessels were classified as either arteries or veins using a supervised classifier. They also ensured the vessel class by analyzing all the vessel segments found along the same vessel in the ROI. Finally, they computed the AVR as the ratio between the CRAE and the CRVE. With this approach, they obtained a mean error of 0.06 in 40 images.

In this chapter, we describe the stages involved in the computation of the AVR and we explain how they can be implemented using image-processing techniques. We analyze the problems related to each stage and we propose solutions to overcome the limitations found. Moreover, we analyze the different approaches proposed in the literature with the aim of providing alternatives for developing an automatic methodology for the AVR computation.

This chapter is organized as follows. Section 12.2 briefly explains the main stages of the methodology. Section 12.3 describes the steps to locate the ROI where the vessel widths are measured. Section 12.4 explains how the vessel width can be computed. Section 12.5 summarizes the different approaches to classify the vessels into arteries and veins. Section 12.6 discusses several algorithms to select a set of vessels and compute the AVR value. Finally, Section 12.7 presents the conclusions of this chapter.

12.2 Methodology

Manually, the computation of the AVR is performed by measuring the vessel widths at several circumferences centered at the optic disc and applying a given equation. This task seems easy at first glance but it is actually time consuming, very subjective, and nonrepeatable. For this reason, some efforts have been made to develop an automatic procedure to provide a reliable and accurate AVR measure. According to the experts, a procedure to compute the AVR must involve several stages, as shown in Figure 12.2. First, the optic disc is located in order to select the ROIs where the vessel widths will be measured. These regions lie on several circumferences centered at the optic disc. Subsequently, the vessels are segmented within these regions and are classified into either arteries or veins. Finally,

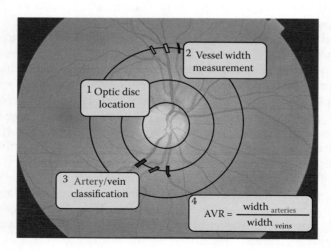

FIGURE 12.2
Stages for computing the AVR.

the artery and the vein widths are the inputs of the AVR function. In the following sections, we describe automatic procedures based on image-processing techniques to carry out these stages and develop a fully automatic AVR computation.

12.3 Optic Disc Location

The optic disc is a bright circular area formed by the optic nerve fibers. It has no photoreceptors so it causes a blind spot in the visual field. The importance of locating this structure lies in the fact that the vessel widths must be measured at equidistant points from the vessel tree center. Since the optic disc is the entrance point of the vessel tree in the retina, it can be considered that the center of this structure is within this region.

We can find several approaches to locate the optic disc in the literature. Some of the approaches are based on intensities since the optic disc is the brightest area in the retina [14–16]. Other approaches analyze the convergence of the vessel tree as well as the relations among the retinal structures [17,18]. Table 12.2 summarizes the success rates of several approaches found in the literature.

In this section, we describe a procedure that combines both approaches to deal with this problem in an efficient manner. This procedure has two main stages: the detection of the ROI where the optic disc is located and the precise adjustment to its boundaries.

12.3.1 Detection of ROI

The objective of this stage is the fast detection of all of the possible regions where the optic disc can be located. To this end, a fast blob detector, such as the difference of Gaussians (DoG), can be used.

The DoG operator is based on filtering the input image with two Gaussians at different scales, subtracting both filtered images, and looking for local maxima in the subtracted image. Since the Gaussian filters have a circular shape, they produce a high response in those image areas with a circular shape, such as the optic disc. In this problem, the scales of the Gaussians are adjusted to the approximate size of the optic disc.

Figure 12.3 shows the output of the DoG blob detector applied to a retinal image. Note that the optic disc area presents the highest filter responses. Once the ROI is located, the next step is to detect the optic disc boundaries and to select the optic disc center.

TABLE 12.2

Success Rates of Several Approaches for Locating the Optic Disc

	Based On	No. of Images	Correct Locations (%)
[17]	Vessel convergence	50 (healthy/pathological)	89
[18]	Vessel convergence	500 (healthy)	98.4
		100 (pathological)	94
[14]	Intensity	100 (healthy)	98
[16]	Intensity	233 (healthy)	100
		40 (healthy/pathological)	100

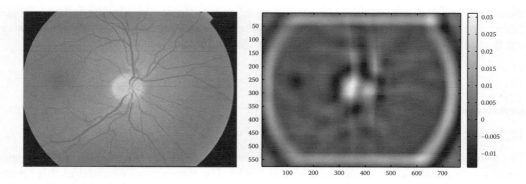

FIGURE 12.3
ROI detection by means of a DoG blob detector. (*left*) Input image; (*right*) output of the DoG operator. The brighter regions represent the higher filter responses.

12.3.2 Precise Segmentation

The standardized protocol to compute the AVR states that the vessel widths must be measured in several circumferences centered at the optic disc center. Moreover, their radii must be a multiple of the optic disc radius. For these reasons, a rough location of the optic disc is not enough and a precise segmentation is needed.

Since we are looking for the center and the radius of the optic disc, the circular Hough transform is one of the best choices for this stage [19]. The aim of this feature detector is the location of circles in the input image using a voting strategy.

The input of the Hough transform is usually the output of an edge detector such as a Sobel or a Canny detector. Each edge pixel votes for all the circles with a center (x, y) and a radius r, which passes through it. The votes are stored in an accumulator array indexed by the radius and the center coordinates. The elements with the highest values point out the circles in the image.

However, the application of the Hough transform to the segmentation of the optic disc is not straightforward. On the one hand, the presence of other structures in the ROI, in particular vessels, generates peaks in the accumulator array that do not correspond to circles. For this reason, it is necessary to remove all the edge pixels related to the vessel tree in the ROI. To this end, these structures must be detected in order to discard the corresponding edges from the output of the edge detector. This way, only the optic disc edges will vote for circles in the accumulator array.

On the other hand, the optic disc boundaries are not always well defined. Moreover, the background of the retina is not uniform so there could be spurious edges in areas where there are no structures. Therefore, the classic Hough transform could fail in some retinal images. The fuzzy Hough transform [20] is more robust so that it can deal with noise or irregular boundaries. In the fuzzy approach, the contribution of each edge pixel is weighted by some function, usually a Gaussian function.

Figure 12.4 shows an example of this segmentation approach [14]. The input of the fuzzy Hough transform is the output of a Canny edge detector (Figure 12.4a). The vessels are located by means of the multilocal creaseness technique (MLSEC-ST) operator [21]. The aim of this operator is the detection of tubular structures by means of analyzing the structure tensor of the input image. The output of this operator is the vessel centerlines, as shown in Figure 12.4b. This way, if an edge pixel is close to a vessel centerline, it is discarded for

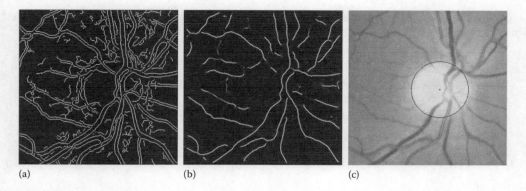

FIGURE 12.4
Segmentation of the optic disc using the fuzzy circular Hough transform. (a) Output of the Canny edge detector in the ROI. (b) Vessels detected by the MLSEC-ST operator in the ROI. (c) Final segmentation. These center coordinates and radius have obtained the largest number of votes in the accumulator array.

further computations. In order to speed up the voting process, the edge points only vote for radii in a range of typical optic disc sizes. Finally, the element in the accumulator array with the highest number of votes is selected. The radius and the center coordinates of this element represent the circle that segments the optic disc with the most accuracy, as shown in Figure 12.4c.

This procedure achieves a success rate of 90% in the DRIVE data set [22]. This approach is fast, efficient, and accurate in healthy retinal images. However, some pathologies, such as drusen, cause light circular spots in the retinal background that can affect the initial selection of the ROI. In these images, there will be several regions with a high blob detector response. In this case, an analysis of the vessel convergence (using, for example, the output of the MLSEC-ST operator) can be useful for discarding non-optic disc areas.

12.4 Vessel Width Measurement

Once the optic disc center (x_{od}, y_{od}) and the radius, r_{od}, are set, the vessels must be measured in several circumferences centered at (x_{od}, y_{od}). The radii of the circumferences are usually a multiple of the optic disc radius $(2r_{od}, 3r_{od}, \ldots)$.

The measurement of the vessel widths requires a precise segmentation of the retinal vessel tree. Over the last years, several approaches have been proposed in the literature to deal with this problem. For example, Gang et al. [23] used Gaussian filters to segment and measure the vessels; Al-Diri et al. [24] and Espona et al. [25] developed special active contour models; and Xu et al. [26] converted the vessel segmentation problem into a graph search problem. In these works, the whole vessel tree was segmented. However, a complete segmentation is not needed since the AVR only requires the widths at the intersection points between the vessel tree and the circumferences. Thus, in order to speed up this stage, we only need to segment the vessels in an area close to each circumference. Moreover, the branching and crossing points in the vessel tree should be avoided since their widths can produce incoherent AVR values.

Therefore, in an AVR computation framework, the measurement stage can be divided into three steps:

- Detect the intersection points between the vessel tree and each circumference
- Segment the vessels at those intersection points and measure their widths in the normal direction of the vessel centerline
- Discard conflicting measurements such as those obtained in branching or crossing points

In this section, we analyze in detail these steps and describe how they can be implemented.

12.4.1 Detection of Intersection Points

The first step of this stage is the detection of the intersection points between the vessel tree and the circumferences where the widths will be measured. To this end, we need an algorithm that identifies all the intersections. This algorithm should minimize the number of false negatives (vessels identified as background), whereas the false positives (background points labeled as vessels) are not important since they would be discarded in the segmentation step.

Since the vessels are darker than the retinal background, the simplest approach to detect the vessels is to analyze the values of the pixels located at each circumference, as shown in Figure 12.5. The lowest peaks correspond to vessels. However, this analysis is not straightforward due to the inter- and intraimage contrast variability. A more robust approach would require the segmentation of the vessel tree or the detection of the vessel centerlines in the vicinity of the circumference.

12.4.2 Vessel Segmentation and Measurement

In this step, the vessels are segmented and their widths are measured at the intersection points, which were computed in the previous step. On the one hand, we can apply any approach proposed in the literature to achieve precise vessel segmentation [23–26]. On the other hand, the widths must be measured in the normal direction of the vessel at the intersection point. Since the vessel is a thick line, its centerline should be computed in

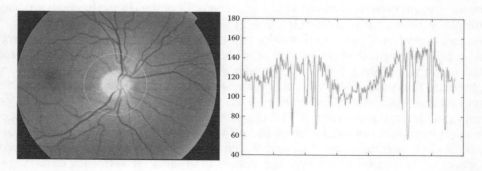

FIGURE 12.5
Detection of the intersection points. (*left*) Green channel of the input image; (*right*) the *y*-axis represents the gray levels of the pixels located at the circumference in the left image.

order to calculate its normal direction. To this end, we can use a specific operator [21,27] or transform the input image into a binary image with the aim of applying a thinning procedure [26].

Figure 12.6 shows an example of vessel segmentation using snakes [28]. In this approach, the vessel centerlines are obtained as a result of the MLSEC-ST operator (see Figure 12.6, top). These vessel centerlines are analyzed to compute the intersection points between each circumference and the vessel tree. However, the presence of noise in the retinal image can lead to the detection of lines that do not correspond to the vessels. Thus, the centerlines are checked in the radius $[r - n, r + n]$ of each vessel circumference with radius r in order to discard the lowest responses of the MLSEC-ST operator or discontinuous lines. Subsequently, a snake is initialized at each intersection in such a way that its number of nodes depends on the length of the centerline. The snake nodes are placed along the vessel centerline in the range $[r - n, r + n]$ (see Figure 12.7 left) and they evolve according to the external and internal energies of the snake. The internal energy ensures smoothness and continuity whereas the external energy moves the

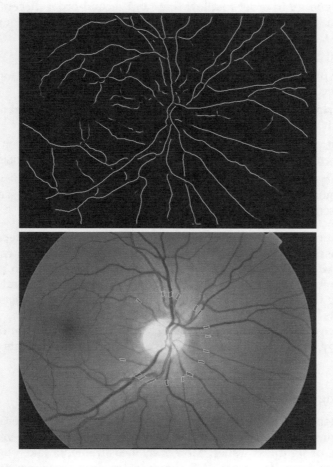

FIGURE 12.6
Vessel segmentation. (*top*) Output of the MLSEC-ST operator that represents the vessel centerlines; (*bottom*) segmentation of the vessels at the intersection points using active contours.

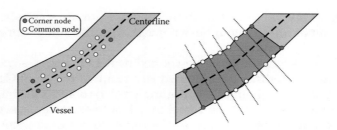

FIGURE 12.7

Snakes for vessel segmentation. (*left*) The nodes are initially located on both sides of the vessel centerline previously computed and they evolve in its normal direction. (*right*) Once the snake is adjusted to the vessel boundaries, the vessel width is measured several times along the snake in order to ensure a correct measurement.

nodes toward the vessel boundaries. This active model has been adapted to the vessel segmentation problem as follows:

- There are two kinds of nodes: common and corner nodes. The corner nodes have no internal energy in order to allow first- and second-order discontinuities. This way, the result of the segmentation is a parallelogram and not a smooth, rounded contour.
- The external energy has specific energy terms:
  - Dilation pressure, which moves the nodes in the normal direction of the vessel centerline.
  - Edge distance, which represents the distance between a pixel and its closest edge so it moves the nodes toward the vessel boundaries.
  - Gradient energy, which is computed as the difference between the previous and the current pixel. It is defined to allow movements only inside the vessel.
  - Stationary energy, which measures the adjustment among nodes and prevents uncommon node configurations. It solves the problems caused by noise or edge discontinuities.

Once the evolution stops, the final node locations are checked to detect possible deviations. In these cases, the position of the neighboring nodes is used to correct the wrong node positions. Afterward, the vessel width can be measured between both snake walls in the normal direction of the centerline. The vessel is measured several times along the snake, discarding the extrema and computing the final width as the average value of all the measurements (see Figure 12.7).

This step has two main outputs: the vessel width measurements and the vessel segments detected by the segmentation procedure. These vessel segments will be used in later stages.

12.4.3 Conflicting Measurements

In the previous step, all the detected intersections between the circumference and the vessel tree are measured. However, sometimes there are mistakes in the vessel widths due to noise, reflexes, or lightness issues. Moreover, measurements taken at bifurcations or crossing points are not valid for the AVR computation since these measurements involve two vessels. Therefore, it is necessary to use another step to discard outliers in the set of measurements.

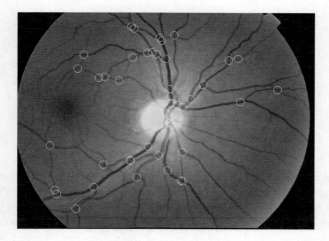

FIGURE 12.8
Detection of bifurcation and crossing points from the topological properties of both kinds of structures.

First, all of the bifurcations and crossings between vessels are detected. To this end, several algorithms have been proposed in the literature. Some approaches [29,30] use classifiers to detect these specific structures. Other approaches are based on analyzing the topological properties of both the bifurcations and the crossings [31,32]. The first step in this kind of algorithm is the segmentation of the vessel tree. Afterward, a thinning procedure is performed in order to obtain the skeleton of the vessels. Then, the 1 pixel-wide segments are joined in order to obtain the whole vessel tree structure. Finally, the crossing and bifurcation points are detected by means of checking the angles and distances between the segment junctions. Figure 12.8 shows the results of this procedure following the approach proposed by Calvo et al. [32].

Furthermore, we can define some rules in order to discard invalid or not useful measurements. On the one hand, experts do not select small vessels for the AVR computation since they are more difficult to measure and classify into an artery or a vein. On the other hand, outliers caused by wrong segmentations can be easily removed since they usually exceed typical vessel sizes.

12.5 Vessel Classification

One of the most difficult stages in the AVR computation is the classification of vessels into arteries or veins. According to the experts, the arteries are lighter than the veins so the color information of the vessels segmented in the previous stage can be used to separate both groups. However, the inter- and intraimage variability makes this distinction difficult. First, different retinal images have different lightness even though they are acquired with the same retinograph. Second, the lightness and contrast through the same image is not constant due to inhomogeneous light reflections. Third, biological features, such as skin pigmentation, produce different retinal color patterns. For these reasons, the vessel classification is a key issue in the development of an automatic procedure for the AVR computation.

TABLE 12.3

Success Rates of Several Vessel Classification Approaches
Found in the Literature

	Data Set	Correct Classifications (%)
[38]	505 segments	82.46 arteries, 89.03 veins
[36]	24 images	87.6
[37]	8 images	70
[39]	58 images	90.08

There are two main approaches in the literature to deal with this problem: tracking-based and color-based methods. The former methods are semiautomatic since they are based on tracking the vessel tree from several points manually labeled by the experts [33–35]. The latter methods are automatic and use classifiers to group both the artery and the vein color features [36–39]. Table 12.3 summarizes the success rates of the automatic approaches.

In this section, we describe the steps required for an automatic vessel classification procedure based on color information. This procedure has several steps. First, a lightness and contrast normalization algorithm is applied to the input image in order to minimize the interimage variability. Then, some feature vectors are computed from the vessel segments extracted in the previous stage. In the next step, these feature vectors are the input of a given classifier. Finally, the class of each vessel segment is ensured by linking the segments along the vessels.

12.5.1 Lightness and Contrast Normalization

Since vessel classification is based on color, the first step is to reduce the intraimage variability. Some approaches found in the literature are based on estimating the image variability and correcting it. For example, Figure 12.9b shows the output of the image normalization procedure proposed by Foracchia et al. [40]. This approach creates a model of the input image based on the fact that the intensity of the background pixels follows a normal distribution where the mean is the lightness and the standard deviation is the contrast of each pixel.

In this approach, a pixel is marked as background if its intensity value is close to the intensity mean in a local window. Then, the contrast and lightness are estimated from the set of background pixels by means of computing the mean value and standard deviation of the distribution in the neighborhood. Finally, the corrected image is computed by subtracting the estimated lightness of each pixel and dividing the result by the estimated contrast.

Figure 12.9c shows another procedure to enhance retinal images. It is based on the retinex theory that re-creates the model of the human visual system to obtain color constancy. In the image formation model, a color component of the image is the product of the illumination and the reflectance. The basis of the retinex methods is that the illumination varies slowly, so its frequency spectrum is assumed to be distributed at low frequencies. In this way, the illumination is approximated and the output image is obtained by subtracting this estimation from the original image. In the single-scale retinex (SSR), the illumination is estimated by means of a Gaussian, and it is then subtracted from the original image to obtain a description invariant to the illumination. The multiscale retinex (MSR) is simply a weighted sum of several SSR outputs at different scales.

In the approaches shown in Figure 12.9, note how the darker areas become lighter and the contrast between the vessels and the background is enhanced.

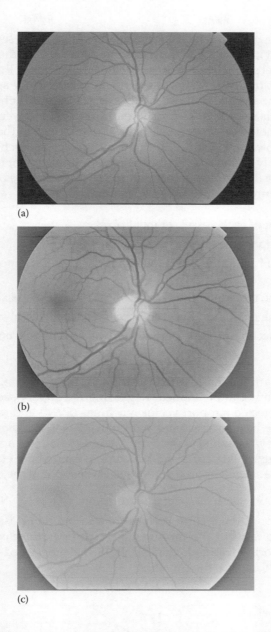

(a)

(b)

(c)

FIGURE 12.9
Lightness and contrast normalization. (a) Green channel of the input image. (b) Normalization of the green channel following the approach proposed by Foracchia et al. using a 201 × 201 neighborhood. (c) Normalization based on the multiscale retinex technique. ((b) From Foracchia, M., Grisan, E., and Ruggeri, A., *Medical Image Analysis*, 9, 179–190, 2005.)

12.5.2 Classification

Once the image lightness and contrast have been normalized, the next step is the classification of the vessel segments into arteries and veins using color information. This step requires making three important choices: an appropriate classifier, the most discriminant features to classify, and a procedure to perform the classification.

The inputs of this stage are the vessel segments obtained at the segmentation stage and normalized in the previous step. The inputs of the classifiers are the feature vectors computed from these vessel segments. A feature vector can be formed by one or more features that can be computed from the vessel segments in several color spaces (red-green-blue [RGB]; hue, saturation, and value [HSV]; hue, saturation, and light [HSL]; Commission Internationale de l'Éclairage Lab [CIE Lab]; etc.). Moreover, the feature vectors can be extracted from the whole vessel segment, from slices normal to the vessel centerline, or from each pixel, as shown in Figure 12.10. In the last two cases, each feature vector can be classified independently so that the final class of a vessel segment is set by analyzing all the outputs of the classifier in that vessel segment. Some examples of the feature vectors proposed in the literature are [36,41,42]:

- The R component of each vessel segment pixel
- The R and G components of each vessel segment pixel
- The mean of the H component and the variance of the R component in each vessel slice
- The mean and the median of the G component in each vessel slice
- The mean and the median of the G component in each vessel segment
- The value of a second-order Gaussian derivative centered on a vessel segment centerline pixel

The feature vectors are the input of the classifier. In this problem, both supervised and unsupervised algorithms can be applied. Regarding the supervised methods, Niemeijer et al. [41] trained and tested support vector machines (SVM) and k-NN, whereas Jelinek et al. [37] achieved the best success rates with naive-Bayes, decision table, and J48 algorithms. On the contrary, Grisan et al. [36] and Vázquez et al. [42] applied clustering techniques, in particular fuzzy clustering and k-means, to group both classes of vessels.

In addition, there are several approaches to select the input of the classifier and perform the classification:

- Global approach: All the feature vectors are selected and classified together [37]. This approach is fast but the intraimage variability can affect the results even when contrast normalization is applied. Both the supervised and unsupervised techniques can be used as the classifier.

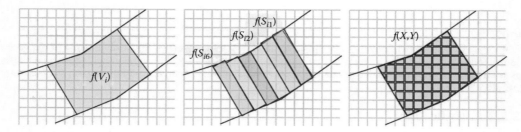

FIGURE 12.10
A feature vector can be computed as a function of all the pixels in the vessel segment (*left*), all the pixels in each slice (*center*), or as a function of each pixel (*right*). In the latter, the final class of a vessel segment is given by the combination of the classes of all its feature vectors. The grid represents the image pixels.

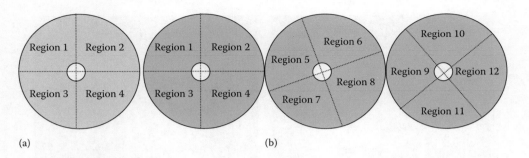

FIGURE 12.11
Local classification approaches. (a) Four local regions centered at the optic disc are defined and the classifier is applied in each region. (b) Several overlapped local regions are defined and the classifier is applied in all of these regions.

- Local approach: The image is divided into four regions centered at the optic disc and the feature vectors found in each region are classified together, independently of the feature vectors that belong to other regions [36], as shown in Figure 12.11a. In this case, a clustering algorithm is applied to each region to separate both groups of vessels. A supervised classifier cannot be used since it always gives the same result, independently of the vessel location, after the training stage. This approach reduces the effect of the intraimage variability so that it achieves better results than the global approach.

- Local overlapped approach: As in the previous approach, the image is divided into regions centered at the optic disc and the feature vectors found in each region are classified by means of a clustering algorithm. Subsequently, different regions, also centered at the optic disc, are defined and the feature vectors are classified again. These two steps are repeated several times, as shown in Figure 12.11b. As a consequence, the feature vectors of each vessel segment are classified in several regions with different neighboring vessel segments. The final class of the vessel segment is a combination of the outputs of the algorithm in all the regions where the feature vectors were classified [42]. This approach is the most robust and the least efficient since each feature vector is classified several times.

Figure 12.12a shows the result of the vessel classification using the approach proposed by Vázquez et al. [42] that combines a local overlapped classification with a k-means clustering technique. The feature vectors have only one component, the median of the G channel computed in each segment slice. Note that the output of the classifier is not always the same at different radii. Therefore, a new step is needed in order to unify the classifications along the vessel.

12.5.3 Vessel Tracking

The classifiers decide the kind of vessel segment but they only use the color information of each vessel segment for the classification. However, since the vessel segments are classified at several circumferences, they can be connected along the vessel tree in order to ensure the vessel type. To this end, we need an algorithm to track the retinal vessels.

Chrástek et al. proposed an approach for vessel tracking based on analyzing the vessel boundaries obtained with a Canny edge detector [34]. Martinez-Perez et al. [43] proposed

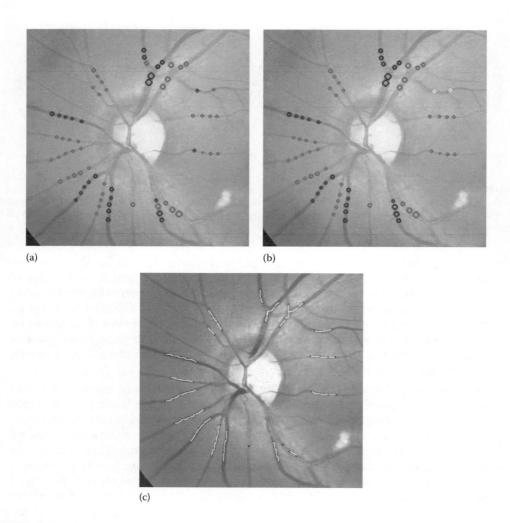

FIGURE 12.12
Classification of vessels into arteries and veins. (a) Output of the k-means classifier in local overlapped regions. (b) Output of the classifier including vessel tracking. Gray circles represent arteries, black circles represent veins, and white circles represent unclassified vessels. (c) Output of the vessel tracking procedure. The tracking procedure joins the vessel segments so that some misclassifications can be corrected.

a semiautomatic vessel tracking procedure. First, the vessel tree is segmented and its skeleton is extracted by thinning. Then, the user selects the initial point and its corresponding vessel tree is tracked along the skeleton. In the AVR computation, this algorithm can be fully automatic since the initial points lie on the vessel segments in the inner circumference.

Figure 12.12 shows the results of applying a tracking procedure to the vessel segments in several circumferences [39]. This procedure is based on the theory of minimal paths [44]. The aim of this theory is to find the path of minimal cost between two points in an efficient and consistent manner. A potential function is defined in such a way that it takes lower values near the desired features. A fast marching algorithm is used to compute the surface of minimal action using the potential function. The path of minimal cost is obtained by back propagation from the final point to the starting point in the surface of minimal action.

In the vessel tracking problem, the path of minimal cost must lie inside the vessels; therefore, the first step of this procedure involves the segmentation of the vessel tree. Subsequently, a surface of minimal action is computed by front propagation using a potential function that takes a low value inside the vessels and a high value in the retinal background. Some restrictions are included in order to set the direction of the propagation from the inner to the outer circumferences and to choose the correct path in case of crossings or bifurcations.

Once the vessel tracking procedure connects the segments along the vessel, a weight function is defined to give the vessel segments more weight or influence on the final classification. Thus, if the weight function is a constant, all the vessel segments will have the same influence on the result and the final vessel class will be the most repeated class along the vessel. Other weight functions can give more influence to the vessel segments located on particular circumferences, for example, the closest circumferences to the optic disc. In this way, the classification of three vessel segments was corrected, as shown in Figure 12.12b. Moreover, two segments that were detected along the same vessel were unclassified since they were labeled in different classes.

12.6 AVR Computation

The AVR is computed as the ratio between the artery and vein widths measured in several circumferences centered at the optic disc. In the literature, two main approaches have been proposed to calculate this value. The first approach computes the AVR as the ratio between the average artery and vein widths as follows [45,46]:

$$AVR = \frac{\sum_{i=0}^{n} W_{Ai}/n}{\sum_{j=0}^{m} W_{Vj}/m} \qquad (12.1)$$

where n and m represent the number of artery and vein segments, respectively. Usually, the number of artery and vein segments is the same, but this restriction is not necessary. Moreover, a minimum number of vessel segments is not required. In this way, it seems that the AVR values computed using this approach might depend on the subset of vessel segments that has been used.

In their work, Pose et al. [47] select a subset of vessel segments in circumferences from $2r$ to $4r$, where r is the optic disc radius. In their experiments, they have selected the same number of artery and vein segments. However, even though the experts select different sets of vessel segments, the correlation of their AVR values is high. This means that the experts actually follow some rules when they are computing the AVR.

Vázquez et al. analyzed the way that the experts selected the vessel segments in a set of 86 retinal images labeled by two experts [48]. They analyzed several hypotheses for selecting subsets of vessels, achieving the best correlation results with the following rules:

- Experts rule out vessels whose widths have been over- or underestimated.
- Experts do not take into account vessel segments found over branching or crossing points.
- Experts do not take into account thin vessels, either because it is more difficult to know their classes or because it is more probable to overestimate their width.

The first hypothesis can be implemented using the tracking procedure along the vessel and discarding the vessel segments whose widths are larger than double or smaller than one-half of the median width along the vessel. In addition, these extreme vessels can also be detected by means of percentiles, discarding the vessels whose widths are less than the p percentile or greater than the 100-p percentile. The second hypothesis needs an algorithm to detect the branching and crossing points in the vessel tree. In the case of the third hypothesis, the best results were obtained by discarding those arteries and veins whose widths were less than the 10 percentile computed for each class. Thus, because of these rules, it is possible to obtain an automatic and objective procedure to compute the AVR using the formula based on the ratio of average widths.

The second approach estimates the AVR as the ratio of two formulas derived empirically, the CRAE and the CRVE [49,8]:

$$AVR = \frac{CRAE}{CRVE} \tag{12.2}$$

The CRAE and CRVE are computed using Algorithm 12.6.1. The inputs of this algorithm are the arteriolar widths, when we compute the CRAE, or the venular widths, if we are computing the CRVE. In the inner loop, the largest and the smallest vessel widths are combined to obtain an equivalent width, whose value is stored in an array of equivalent widths. In the outer loop, this array of widths is processed until it has only one value, that is, the final CRAE or CRVE.

Algorithm 12.6.1: Central Retinal Vessel Equivalent (*Widths*, *Class*)

    while *size(Widths)* > 1
        Empty(Equivalent Widths)
        while *size(Widths)* > 1
            $W_a \leftarrow Max(Widths)$
            Remove(W_a, Widths)
            $W_b \leftarrow Min(Widths)$
            Remove(W_b, Widths)
    Do
        do
            if *Class* = Artery
            then $W_c \leftarrow$ *Artery Equivalent(W_a, W_b)*
            else $W_c \leftarrow$ *Vein Equivalent(W_a, W_b)*
            Insert (Equivalent Widths, W_c)
        Widths ← Equivalent Widths
    return *(Widths[0])*

Hubbard et al. [49] proposed the following equations for calculating the arteriolar and venular equivalents:

$$\text{Arteriolar } W_c = \sqrt{0.87W_a^2 + 1.01W_b^2 - 0.22W_aW_b - 10.76} \tag{12.3}$$

$$\text{Venular } W_c = \sqrt{0.72W_a^2 + 0.91W_b^2 + 450.05} \tag{12.4}$$

Knudston et al. [8] realized that this method was dependent on the number of selected vessels and they proposed a reformulation using only the six main arteries and veins. They also revised the equations for computing the arteriolar and venular equivalents as follows:

$$\text{Arteriolar } W_c = 0.88\sqrt{W_a^2 + W_b^2} \tag{12.5}$$

$$\text{Venular } W_c = 0.95\sqrt{W_a^2 + W_b^2} \tag{12.6}$$

In this approach, the vessels are measured in circumferences ranging from 1.5 to 2 times the optic disc radius. Moreover, since only the six main vessels are taken into account, the selection of vessel segments for performing the computations is not as subjective as the previous approach.

12.7 Conclusions

The AVR is an important variable to assess the condition of the patient regarding several relevant and critical pathologies such as hypertension, cerebrovascular diseases, or diabetes. Accordingly, there is a growing interest in the development of automatic image-processing tools to deal with the computation of the AVR from retinal images. However, the automatic computation of the AVR value is a challenging task due to the complexity of the retinal image domain and the stages involved in the calculus. In this chapter, we have analyzed in detail every stage of the AVR computation procedure, providing a brief review of the current state of the art and proposing a concrete implementation using well-known image-processing techniques.

The first stage in the AVR computation is the location of the ROI where the vessels will be measured, that is, some circumferences centered at the optic disc. We have described a methodology to locate the optic disc in the image based on a fast blob detector, which roughly locates the ROI, and the fuzzy circular Hough transform for fine adjustment. Nevertheless, since the manual location of the optic disc is fast and simple, the results of this stage are not critical in the development of the final methodology.

The second stage involves measuring the vessel widths at the ROIs defined previously. This stage is a crucial step in the methodology since the AVR is computed from the vessel widths. To this end, we have described an approach that is based on active contours to segment and measure the vessel widths. This technique presents several advantages over others since it is able to deal with noise or incomplete information. Moreover, we have presented a procedure to discard conflicting points, such as vessel crossings or bifurcations, because the widths at these points are not suitable for the computation since they involve two vessels.

In the third stage, the vessels are classified into arteries and veins using color information. This is a very difficult task due to the contrast and light variability of retinal images. In order to solve this problem, we have described a three-step procedure that starts with a contrast normalization stage. Subsequently, a classifier locally groups the vessel segments obtained in the previous stage into the artery and vein categories. This step is repeated several times in overlapping regions centered at the optic disc with the aim of overcoming the lightness issues. Finally, a vessel tracking procedure ensures the category of each segment along the vessel, allowing the correction of those segments that are incorrectly classified.

Finally, we have reviewed the approaches to compute the ratio of the vessel widths. The ratio of the mean vessel widths as well as the ratio of the central retinal artery and the vein equivalents are the two main algorithms found in the literature to compute the AVR. Both of these algorithms are based on the selection of a suitable set of vessel segments. The former approach has no explicit rules for performing the selection whereas the latter approach only takes into account the six main arteries and veins. Nevertheless, the best way to analyze the changes in the vascular tree with respect to some diseases is to always measure the same vessels at the same points. This method will guarantee a comparable measure over time that is not affected by outliers. To this end, we would require a two-stage methodology. In the first stage, the most suitable vessels are selected from a base image and the ROIs are defined. In the second stage, a registration procedure is performed between the base image and any other retinography of the same patient in order to align the vessel tree and find the measurement points in the same vessels. This way, the objectivity of the procedure is ensured since the AVR computation is always performed using the same subset of vessels.

The future work in this field includes not only the improvement of the current methodologies but also the development and validation of automatic tools for clinical practice. The wide use of these tools will allow the monitoring of several diseases as well as the screening of large populations. The early diagnosis of different pathologies has a double benefit. On the one hand, it can increase the life expectancy of the patient because the initial treatments are often more simple and more likely to be effective. On the other hand, an early disease diagnosis as well as fast and effective disease monitoring usually implies important savings for the health-care system.

References

1. C. Cuspidi, G. Macca, M. Salerno, L. Michev, V. Fusi, B. Severgnini, C. Corti, S. Meani, F. Magrini, and A. Zanchetti. Evaluation of target organ damage in arterial hypertension: Which role for qualitative funduscopic examination? *Italian Heart Journal*, 2(9):702–706, 2001.
2. T. Y. Wong, J. Coresh, R. Klein, P. Muntner, D. J. Couper, A. R. Sharrett, B. E. Klein, G. Heiss, L. D. Hubbard, and B. B. Duncan. Retinal microvascular abnormalities and renal dysfunction: The atherosclerosis risk in communities study. *Journal of the American Society of Nephrology: JASN*, 15(9):2469–2476, 2004.
3. T. Y. Wong, R. Klein, D. J. Couper, L. S. Cooper, E. Shahar, L. D. Hubbard, M. R. Wofford, and A. R. Sharrett. Retinal microvascular abnormalities and incident stroke: The atherosclerosis risk in communities study. *Lancet*, 358(9288):1134–1140, 2001.
4. T. T. Nguyen, J. J. Wang, and T. Y. Wong. Retinal vascular changes in pre-diabetes and prehypertension: New findings and their research and clinical implications. *Diabetes Care*, 30(10):2708–2715, 2007.
5. B. R. McClintic, J. I. McClintic, J. D. Bisognano, and R. C. Block. The relationship between retinal microvascular abnormalities and coronary heart disease: A review. *The American Journal of Medicine*, 123(4):374.e1–374.e7, 2010.
6. R. Kawasaki, N. Cheung, T. Mosley, A. F. M. Islam, A. R. Sharrett, R. Klein, L. H. Coker, et al. Retinal microvascular signs and 10-year risk of cerebral atrophy. *Stroke*, 41(8):1826–1828, 2010.

7. H. Yatsuya, A. R. Folsom, T. Y. Wong, R. Klein, B. E. Klein, A. R. Sharrett, and ARIC Study Investigators. Retinal microvascular abnormalities and risk of lacunar stroke: Atherosclerosis risk in communities study. *Stroke: A Journal of Cerebral Circulation*, 41(7):1349–1355, 2010.

8. M. D. Knudtson, K. E. Lee, L. D. Hubbard, T. Y. Wong, R. Klein, and B. E. Klein. Revised formulas for summarizing retinal vessel diameters. *Current Eye Research*, 27(3):143–149, 2003.

9. L. Tramontan, E. Grisan, and A. Ruggeri. An improved system for the automatic estimation of the arteriolar-to-venular diameter ratio (AVR) in retinal images. In *Conference Proceedings of 30th Annual International Conference of the IEEE Engineering in Medicine and Biology Society*, 20–25 August 2008, Vancouver, Canada, pp. 3550–3553.

10. M. Ortega, N. Barreira, J. Novo, M. G. Penedo, A. Pose-Reino, and F. Gómez-Ulla. Sirius: A web-based system for retinal image analysis. *International Journal of Medical Informatics*, 79(10):722–732, 2010.

11. M. Saez, S. G. Vázquez, M. G. Penedo, M. A. Barceló, M. Pena-Seijo, G. Coll de Tuero, and A. Pose-Reino. Development of an automated system to classify retinal vessels into arteries and veins. *Computer Methods and Programs in Biomedicine*, 108:367–376, 2012.

12. C. Muramatsu, Y. Hatanaka, T. Iwase, T. Hara, and H. Fujita. Automated selection of major arteries and veins for measurement of arteriolar-to-venular diameter ratio on retinal fundus images. *Computerized Medical Imaging and Graphics*, 35(6):472–480, 2011.

13. M. Niemeijer, X. Xu, A. V. Dumitrescu, P. Gupta, B. van Ginneken, J. C. Folk, and M. D. Abràmoff. Automated measurement of the arteriolar-to-venular width ratio in digital color fundus photographs. *IEEE Transactions of Medical Imaging*, 30(11):1941–1950, 2011.

14. M. Blanco, M. G. Penedo, N. Barreira, M. Penas, and M. J. Carreira. Localization and extraction of the optic disc using the fuzzy circular Hough transform. *Artificial Intelligence and Soft Computing—ICAISC: Proceedings of 8th International Conference*, Zakopane, Poland, 25–29 June 25–29, 2006. in: *Lecture Notes in Computer Science*, 4029:712–721, 2006.

15. R. Chrástek, M. Wolf, K. Donath, H. Niemann, D. Paulus, T. Hothorn, B. Lausen, R. Lämmer, C. Y. Mardin, and G. Michelson. Automated segmentation of the optic nerve head for diagnosis of glaucoma. *Medical Image Analysis*, 9(4):297–314, 2005.

16. J. Novo, M. G. Penedo, and J. Santos. Localisation of the optic disc by means of GA-optimised topological active nets. *Image Vision Computing*, 27(10):1572–1584, 2009.

17. A. Hoover and M. Goldbaum. Locating the optic nerve in a retinal image using the fuzzy convergence of the blood vessels. *IEEE Transactions on Biomedical Engineering*, 22:951–958, 2003.

18. M. Niemeijer, M. D. Abramoff, and B. van Ginneken. Segmentation of the optic disc, macula and vascular arch in fundus photographs. *IEEE Transactions on Medical Imaging*, 26(1):116–127, 2007.

19. D. H. Ballard. Generalizing the Hough transform to detect arbitrary shapes. *Pattern Recognition*, 13(2):111–122, 1981.

20. J. H. Han, L. T. Koczy, and T. Poston. Fuzzy Hough transform. *Pattern Recognition Letters*, 15(7):649–658, 1994.

21. C. Mariño, M. Penas, M. G. Penedo, J. M. Barja, V. Leborán, M. J. Carreira, and F. Gómez-Ulla. Methodology for the registration of whole SLO sequences. In *Proceedings of 16th International Conference on Pattern Recognition ICPR*, vol. 1, pp. 779–783. Spain, IEEE Computer Society 2002.

22. J. J. Staal, M. D. Abramoff, M. Niemeijer, M. A. Viergever, and B. van Ginneken. Ridge based vessel segmentation in color images of the retina. *IEEE Transactions on Medical Imaging*, 23(4):501–509, 2004.

23. L. Gang, O. Chutatape, and S. M. Krishnan. Detection and measurement of retinal vessels in fundus images using amplitude modified second-order Gaussian filter. *IEEE Transactions on Biomedical Engineering*, 49(2):168–172, 2002.

24. B. Al-Diri, A. Hunter, and D. Steel. An active contour model for segmenting and measuring retinal vessels. *IEEE Transactions on Medical Imaging*, 28(9):1488–1497, 2009.

25. L. Espona, M. J. Carreira, M. G. Penedo, and M. Ortega. Retinal vessel tree segmentation using a deformable contour model. In *Proceedings of the 19th International Conference on Pattern Recognition (ICPR '08)*, 8–11 December, Tampa, FL, IEEE Computer Society, pp. 1–4. December 2008.

26. X. Xu, M. Niemeijer, Q. Song, M. K. Garvin, J. M. Reinhardt, and M. D. Abramoff. Retinal vessel width measurements based on a graph-theoretic method. In *Proceedings of the IEEE International Symposium on Biomedical Imaging*: *From Nano to Macro* (ISBI), 30 March-2 April 2011, Chicago, IL, pp. 641–644, IEEE Signal Processing Society.

27. A. M. Mendonca and A. Campilho. Segmentation of retinal blood vessels by combining the detection of centerlines and morphological reconstruction. *IEEE Transactions on Medical Imaging*, 25(9):1200–1213, 2006.

28. N. Barreira, M. Ortega, J. Rouco, M. G. Penedo, A. Pose-Reino, and C. Mariño. Semi-automatic procedure for the computation of the arteriovenous ratio in retinal images. *International Journal for Computational Vision and Biomechanics*, 3(2):135–147, 2010.

29. V. Bevilacqua, L. Cariello, M. Giannini, G. Mastronardi, V. Santarcangelo, R. Scaramuzzi, and A. Troccoli. A comparison between a geometrical and an ANN based method for retinal bifurcation points extraction. *Journal of Universal Computer Science*, 15(13):2626–2639, 2009.

30. E. Grisan, A. Pesce, A. Giani, M. Foracchia, and A. Ruggeri. A new tracking system for the robust extraction of retinal vessel structure. In *Proceedings of the 26th Annual International Conference of the IEEE Engineering in Medicine and Biology Society* (IEMBS '04), 1–5 September 2004, San Francisco, CA, pp. 1620–1623. IEEE Engineering in Medicine and Biology Society.

31. A. Bhuiyan, B. Nath, J. Chua, and K. Ramamohanarao. Automatic detection of vascular bifurcations and crossovers from color retinal fundus images. In *Proceedings of the Third International IEEE Conference on Signal-Image Technologies and Internet-Based System* (SITIS'07), 16–18 December 2007, Shanghai, China, pp. 711–718. IEEE Computer Society.

32. D. Calvo, M. Ortega, M. G. Penedo, and J. Rouco. Automatic detection and characterisation of retinal vessel tree bifurcations and crossovers in eye fundus images. *Computer Methods and Programs in Biomedicine*, 103(1):28–38, 2011.

33. W. Aguilar, M. E. Martínez-Pérez, Y. Frauel, F. Escolano, M. A. Lozano, and A. Espinosa-Romero. Graph-based methods for retinal mosaicing and vascular characterization. In *Graph-Based Representations in Pattern Recognition: 6th IAPR-TC-15 International Workshop*, in *Lecture Notes in Computer Science*, 11–13 June 2007, Alicante, Spain. Springer, Berlin.

34. R. Chrástek, M. Wolf, K. Donath, H. Niemann, and G. Michelsont. Automated calculation of retinal arteriovenous ratio for detection and monitoring of cerebrovascular disease based on assessment of morphological changes of retinal vascular system. In *IAPR Workshop on Machine Vision Applications*, pp. 240–243. 11–13 December, Nara, Japan, 2002.

35. K. Rothaus, X. Jiang, and P. Rhiem. Separation of the retinal vascular graph in arteries and veins based upon structural knowledge. *Image and Vision Computing*, 27(7):864–875, 2009.

36. E. Grisan and A. Ruggeri. A divide et impera strategy for automatic classification of retinal vessels into arteries and veins. In *Proceedings of the 25th Annual International Conference of the IEEE Engineering in Medicine and Biology Society*, vol. 1, 17–21 September 2003, Cancún, Mexico, pp. 890–893. IEEE Engineering in Medicine and Biology Society.

37. H. F. Jelinek, C. Lucas, D. J. Cornforth, W. Huang, and M. J. Cree. Towards vessel characterization in the vicinity of the optic disc in digital retinal images. In *Proceedings of the Image and Vision Computing New Zealand*, 28–29 November 2005, Dunedin, New Zealand. Department of Computer Science, University of Otago.

38. H. Li, W. Hsu, M. L. Lee, and H. Wang. A piecewise Gaussian model for profiling and differentiating retinal vessels. In *Proceedings of the International Conference on Image Processing* (ICIP03), vol. 1, 14–17 September 2003, Barcelona, Spain, pp. 1069–1072. IEEE Signal Processing Society.

39. S. G. Vázquez, B. Cancela, N. Barreira, M. G. Penedo, and M. Saez. On the automatic computation of the arterio-venous ratio in retinal images: Using minimal paths for the artery/vein classification. In *Proceedings of the International Conference on Digital Image Computing*: *Techniques and Applications* (DICTA), 1–3 December 2010, Sydney, Australia, pp. 599–604. IEEE.

40. M. Foracchia, E. Grisan, and A. Ruggeri. Luminosity and contrast normalization in retinal images. *Medical Image Analysis*, 9(3):179–190, 2005.

41. M. Niemeijer, B. van Ginneken, and M. D. Abràmoff. Automatic classification of retinal vessels into arteries and veins. *Proceedings of the SPIE Medical Imaging 2009: Computer-Aided Diagnosis*, 7260:72601F–72601F–8, 2009.

42. S. G. Vázquez, N. Barreira, M. G. Penedo, M. Ortega, and A. Pose-Reino. Improvements in retinal vessel clustering techniques: Towards the automatic computation of the arterio venous ratio. *Computing*, 90(3–4):197–217, 2010.

43. M. E. Martinez-Perez, A. D. Highes, A. V. Stanton, S. A. Thorn, N. Chapman, A. A. Bharath, and K. H. Parker. Retinal vascular tree morphology: A semi-automatic quantification. *IEEE Transactions on Biomedical Engineering*, 49(8):912–917, 2002.

44. L. D. Cohen and R. Kimmel. Global minimum for active contour models: A minimal path approach. *International Journal of Computer Vision*, 24(1):57–78, 1997.

45. A. Pose-Reino, F. Gomez-Ulla, B. Hayik, M. Rodriguez-Fernández, M. J. Carreira-Nouche, A. Mosquera-González, M. González-Penedo, and F. Gude. Computerized measurement of retinal blood vessel calibre: Description, validation and use to determine the influence of ageing and hypertension. *Journal of Hypertension*, 23(4):843–850, 2005.

46. A. V. Stanton, B. Wasan, A. Cerutti, S. Ford, R. Marsh, P. P. Sever, S. A. Thom, and A. D. Hughes. Vascular network changes in the retina with age and hypertension. *Journal of Hypertension*, 13:1724–1728, 1995.

47. A. Pose-Reino, M. Pena Seijo, M. González Penedo, M. Ortega Hortas, M. Rodríguez Blanco, P. Vega, J. L. Díaz Díaz, N. Fernández, J. C. Estévez, and F. Gómez-Ulla Irazábal. Estimation of the retinal microvascular calibre in hypertensive patients with the snakes semiautomatic model. *Medical Clinic (Barc)*, 135(4):145–50, 2010.

48. S. G. Vázquez, N. Barreira, M. G. Penedo, M. Rodriguez-Blanco, F. Gómez-Ulla, A. González, and G. Coll de Tuero. Automatic arteriovenous ratio computation: Emulating the experts. In *Technological Innovation for Value Creation: Third IFIP WG 5.5/SOCOLNET Doctoral Conference on Computing, Electrical and Industrial Systems, DoCEIS*, 27–29 February 2012, Costa de Caparica, Portugal, pp. 563–570.

49. L. D. Hubbard, R. J. Brothers, W. N. King, L. X. Clegg, R. Klein, L. S. Cooper, A. R. Sharrett, M. D. Davis, and J. Cai. Methods for evaluation of retinal microvascular abnormalities associated with hypertension/sclerosis in the atherosclerosis risk in communities studies. *Ophthalmology*, 106:2269–2280, 1999.

13

Survey on Techniques Used in Iris Recognition Systems

Nagarajan Malmurugan, Shanmugam Selvamuthukumaran, and Sugadev Shanmugaprabha

CONTENTS

13.1 Introduction

Due to its high reliability for personal identification, the iris scores distinct merit and includes numerous irregular small blocks, similar to stripes, freckles, coronas, furrows, and other distinguishing features [1–3]. In addition, the divisions of these textures in the

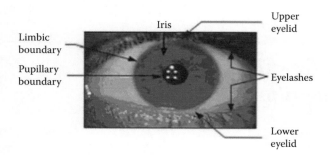

FIGURE 13.1
Structure of the eye.

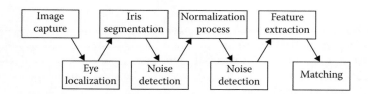

FIGURE 13.2
A typical iris recognition system.

iris are arbitrary. Hence, the technique of iris identification has become the focus of active research in recent years. A classic eye structure is shown in Figure 13.1, which illustrates the precise location of the iris and neighboring objects.

A typical iris recognition system which includes the above stages is shown in Figure 13.2.

We review existing techniques and limitations of iris segmentation, normalization, and matching phases.

13.2 Survey on Segmentation Phase

Typical iris segmentation steps focus the localization stage in the iris region of the object image. The segmentation process is the separation of a digital image into several regions (set of pixels), where the purpose of the segmentation is to simplify or change the representation of an image in one direction and facilitate the process of analysis. Image segmentation is normally used to locate objects and boundaries such as lines and curves in images [4–6].

The result of the segmentation of the image is either a set of regions which together cover the entire part of the image or a set of contours taken from the image. All pixels in an area are similar in respect of a quality or calculated property, such as color, intensity, or texture. Neighboring regions are significantly different with respect to that specific similarity. The eyelids and eyelashes generally seal the upper and lower portions of the iris region. In addition, specular reflections may occur within the iris region, corrupting the iris pattern [7,8]. Well-known methods such as the integro-differential Hough transform and active contour models have succeeded in detecting the iris boundaries [9,10]. These methods are described in subsequent sections and some of their weaknesses are emphasized.

13.2.1 Daugman's Integro-Differential Operator

For locating an iris, Daugman proposed the integro-differential operator [1,2,11], in which the operator assumes that the pupil and limbus are circular contours and operates as a circular edge detector. Detection of the upper and lower eyelids is also done using the integro-differential operator, adjusting the search from a circular contour with a precision designed [12,13]. The integro-differential is defined in Equation 13.1:

$$\left| G(r) \times \frac{\partial}{\partial_r} \oint_{x_0,y_0,r} \frac{I(x,y)}{2\pi r} \, ds \right| \tag{13.1}$$

where:
$I(x, y)$ is the eye image
r is the radius of search
$G(r)$ is a Gaussian smoothing function
s is the outline of the circle given by x_0, y_0, r

The operator searches for a circular path where there is a maximum change in the pixel values, by changing the radius and the center x and y position of the circular contour. The operator is applied iteratively to the amount of smoothing in order to achieve an exact localization. The eyelids are localized in a similar way, with the contour integration path modified from a circle to an arc.

Daugman achieved a false acceptance rate (FAR) of 1 in 4 million and a false rejection rate (FRR) of 0 [14,15]. Also, a series of experimental studies were carried out with several thousand images per eye, but these are not accessible to the public.

The algorithm does not give the desired precision if the noise level is high and works only locally.

13.2.2 Wilde's System

Wilde's system is also a patented system for iris recognition [9,16,17]. The iris is recognized based on a gradient-based Hough transform and its two circular boundaries are arrested. A binary edge map is generated using a Gaussian filter and three parameters of a circle (x_0, y_0, r) are estimated by a circular Hough space. A Hough space is defined in Equation 13.2:

$$H(x_0, y_0, r) = \sum_i h(x_i, y_i, x_0, y_0, r) \tag{13.2}$$

where (x_i, y_i) is an edge pixel and the location (x_0, y_0, r) with the maximum value of $H(x_0, y_0, r)$ is selected as the parameter vector for the largest circular boundary. Wilde's system models the eyelids as parabolic arcs. The upper and lower eyelids are detected using a linear Hough-based approach similar to that described above. The only difference is in voting for parabolic arcs instead of circles [9,16].

Wilde's system uses a Laplacian pyramid decomposition for encoding the iris texture pattern [18,19]. A normalized correlation technique is used for determining the similarity of iris codes. The final decision is obtained by Fisher's linear discriminant method with the strength of the correspondence of each frequency band. An accuracy of 100% verification was claimed during a test on 600 iris images. The test data set is not accessible to the public.

13.2.3 Active Contour Models

Ritter et al. [19,20] used active contour models to locate the pupil of the eye in images. Active contours meet preset internal and external forces and internal deformation, or move through an image until equilibrium is reached. Figure 13.2 contains a number of vertices whose positions are changed by two opposing forces: (i) an internal force, which depends on the desired characteristics, and (ii) an external force, which is a function of the image. Each vertex is moved between time t and $t + 1$, as in Equation 13.3:

$$v_i(t+1) = v_i(t) + F_i(t) + G_i(t) \tag{13.3}$$

where:
F_i is the internal force
G_i is the external force
v_i is the position of vertex i

For the location of the pupil region, the internal forces are calibrated such that the contour is a discretely expanding circle [20–22]. External forces are usually found using edge information. To improve accuracy, the use of the image of the variance instead of the image edge was attempted by Ritter et al. [23,24].

A point inside the pupil is a picture of the variance, and then a discrete circular active contour (DCAC) is created with this point as the center [25,26]. The DCAC is then moved under the influence of internal and external forces until it reaches equilibrium and the pupil is located.

13.2.4 Discrete Circular Active Contours

Ritter proposed an active contour model to locate the iris in an image [27,28]. The model detects the pupil and limbus by the activation and control of the active contour defined using two forces: internal and external. Internal forces are responsible for widening the ideal outline of a polygon with a radius larger than the average radius of the contour. This is shown in Figure 13.3.

The internal force $F_{\text{int}, i}$ is defined in Equation 13.4:

$$F_{\text{int}, i} = \bar{v}_i - v_i \tag{13.4}$$

where $\bar{v}_i$ is the expected position of the vertex in the perfect polygon.

The position of $\bar{v}_i$ can be obtained with respect to C, the average radius of the current contour, and the contour center is given by Equation 13.5:

$$C = (C_x, C_y) \tag{13.5}$$

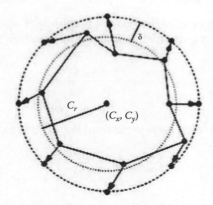

FIGURE 13.3
The internal forces of the discrete circular active contour.

The center of a contour is defined as in Equation 13.6:

$$C = (x_c, y_c) = \frac{1}{n} \sum_{i=1}^{n} v_i \qquad (13.6)$$

which is the average position of all contour vertices. The average radius of the edge is defined as in Equation 13.7:

$$C_r = \frac{1}{n} \sum_{i=1}^{n} \|v_i - c\| \qquad (13.7)$$

which is the average distance of all of the vertices of a defined center point. The position of the vertices of the polygon is then expected ideally as obtained in Equation 13.8

$$\bar{v}_i = \left(c_x + (c_r + \delta) \cos\left(\frac{2\pi i}{n} \right) c_y + (c_r + \delta) \sin\left(\frac{2\pi i}{n} \right) \right) \qquad (13.8)$$

where n is the total number of vertices.

Internal forces are designed to expand and maintain the circular contour. The model assumes that the strength of the pupil and limbus is generally circular, rather than local, to minimize undesirable deformations due to specular reflections and dark spots near the pupil boundary.

The method of detecting the contour of the model is based on the balance of domestic defined by external forces. The external forces are derived from the gray values of intensity at the image and are designed to push peaks inwardly. The magnitude of the external forces is defined in Equation 13.9:

$$\|F_{\text{ext}, i}\| = I(v_i) - I\left(v_i + \hat{F}_{\text{ext}, i} \right) \qquad (13.9)$$

where $I(v_i)$ is the value of the level of the nearest neighbor of V_i and $\hat{F}_{\text{ext},\,i}$ is the direction of the external force for each vertex, which is defined in Equation 13.10:

$$\hat{F}_{\text{ext},\,i} = \frac{C - v_i}{\|C - v_i\|} \tag{13.10}$$

Therefore, the external force on each vertex can be written as in Equation 13.11:

$$\hat{F}_{\text{ext},\,i} = \left\|\hat{F}_{\text{ext},\,i}\right\|\hat{F}_{\text{ext},\,i} \tag{13.11}$$

The displacement contour is based on the composition of the internal and external forces on the contour vertices. Each vertex is replaced by the iterative Equation 13.12:

$$v_i(t+1) = v_i(t) + \beta F_{\text{int},\,i} + (1-\beta)F_{\text{ext},\,i} \tag{13.12}$$

where β is a defined weight that controls the rate of flow and the contour defines the equilibrium condition of internal and external forces. The final equilibrium is reached when the average radius and the center of the outline are the same as in m iterations.

13.2.5 Masek Algorithm

In Masek's segmentation algorithm, both limits of the circular iris are localized [9,29]. A Canny detector is used to generate the edge map. It is based on the Hough transform, and is able to localize the iris region and circular pupil, eyelids and eyelashes occlusion, and reflections. Based on a survey of the presence of the recognition algorithm Masek confused with, it is clear that the performance of the iris segmentation step needs to be improved.

13.2.6 Graph Cut Method

Mehrabian and Hashemi-Tari [19,30] proposed a method for automatic segmentation of pupil detection limits for the purpose of accurate iris recognition using graph cuts. The theory uses a cut graph, which is used to minimize the energy function defined for segmenting the input image of the eye. During segmentation, terms such as vertex, the source is defined for the image. The pixels of the image are defined as the vertices. All pairs of adjacent pixels in the image are assumed to be interconnected by a link, and these links are called edges. The capacity of each link is defined in terms of the sharpness of the edge between the pixels. The sharpness of the edge is defined by the difference between their intensity values. The "object" can be attributed to a set of pixels to specify the source or object terminal and "white" can be assigned to another set representing the background pixels or sink. The objective is to find a cut or a set of edges that separate the object and the background in a way that sets the cup has a minimum cost. To perform the minimization process, the cost of energy and the function are defined.

The 2D graph of the iris shows two terminals designated as "source" and "sink", and the cut between the regions. Thick lines connect the terminal to the pixels in the same region, while the thin lines show its relationship with the pixels of the other region (Figure 13.4).

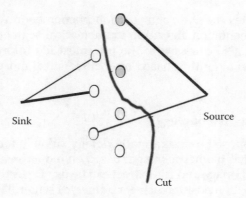

FIGURE 13.4
Graph cut method.

This method can be used to detect the limit regardless of the shape of the pupil, which allows us to avoid considering some parts of the pupil as a diaphragm or removal of parts of the iris with the non-circular shape of the pupil. Most segmentation algorithms of pupils take the pupil as a circular object and try to fit a circle to its edge. The algorithm has been tested on all 756 images of the CASIA eye image database. All images have been successfully segmented with high accuracy, which proves the effectiveness of the method.

13.2.7 Fuzzy Mathematical Morphology

Yucheng and Yubin [21,31] proposed a new image segmentation algorithm based on fuzzy mathematical morphology to noise and the small size of the watershed resulting image oversegmentation phenomenon when adopting traditional algorithm basin segmenting an image. The approach first employed an opening–closing algorithm based on fuzzy mathematical morphology to soften the image and then calculate its gradient operators based on the basic morphology. This operation is shown in Figure 13.5.

In addition, the method of image segmentation was based on gradient fuzzy mathematical morphology in order to obtain the result. The simulation experiment results showed

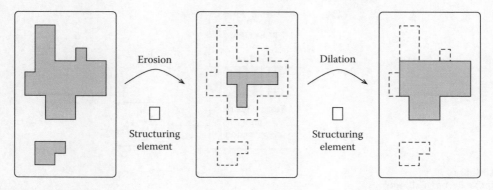

FIGURE 13.5
Fuzzy operation.

that it not only eliminates the oversegmentation phenomenon resulting from the traditional morphology segmentation algorithm mathematical segmentation achieve the goal of full background, but also can save to the uttermost file information when using the new image segmentation algorithm based on mathematical morphology blurred picture segment.

13.2.8 Adaptive Design Methodology

Scotti and Piuri [32] proposed a design methodology suitable for the detection of reflection and the location of iris biometric images based on inductive classifiers such as neural networks. The measured image and iris extract can be used effectively to achieve a precise identification of the reflection position using a trained classifier. The schematic representation is given in Figure 13.6.

In addition, the use of radial symmetry transformation (RST) is presented to identify reflections in iris images.

13.2.9 Hugo Proenca Method

Proenca [8,33] proposed a segmentation method for the treatment of degraded iris images taking into account the sclera, which is the most easily distinguishable in degraded images of the eye; measuring the proportion of sclera in each direction is fundamental in the segmentation of the iris, the execution of the whole procedure deterministic time linear in the size of the image, which makes the method suitable for real-time applications. Close-up iris images acquired at a distance, with movement between 4 and 8 m, and under dynamic lighting conditions are shown in Figure 13.7.

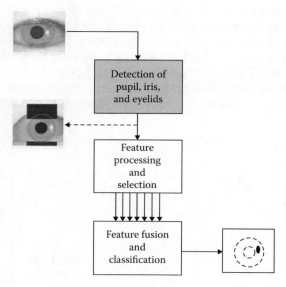

FIGURE 13.6
Adaptive design methodology.

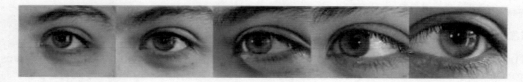

FIGURE 13.7
Close-up iris images.

13.2.10 Optimized Iris Segmentation Using Sobel Edge Detection

Malmurugan and Selvamuthukumaran [32,34,35] proposed segmentation-optimized iris detection using a Sobel edge for improvement in the segmentation phase. The process begins with the application of the Sobel edge detector to the acquired image to generate an edge map, which is the key to accurately detecting the boundaries of the iris. As local thresholding, morphology blurred applied for further improvements. The resulting edge map contains the exact limit of both the inner and outer boundaries of the iris.

Subsequently, a circular Hough transform is applied to obtain the exact iris. It identifies the pupillary and limbic boundaries of the iris and the segments of the iris from the eye image. To remove the eyelashes and eyelids from the region of the iris, a linear Hough transform is applied. The result of this process leads to a segmented image consisting of the exact boundaries of the iris. The complete process is illustrated in Figure 13.8.

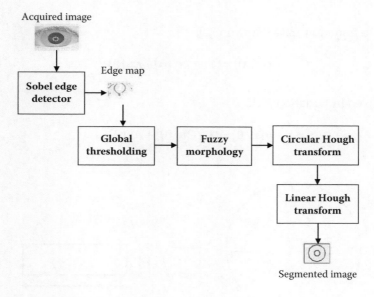

FIGURE 13.8
Block diagram of optimized iris segmentation using Sobel edge detection.

13.3 Survey on Normalization Phase

The next goal of this work is the normalization of the iris. Most normalization techniques are based on the transformation of the iris into polar coordinates, known as the process of unpacking. The pupil boundary and limbus boundary are generally two nonconcentric contours. The condition of nonconcentricity led to different choices of reference points for the transformation of the iris into polar coordinates. The appropriate choice of reference point is very important because the radial and angular information is defined with respect to this point [18,36].

Inconsistencies between the sizes of ocular images are mainly due to stretching of the iris caused by pupil dilation as a result of different lighting levels. Other sources of inconsistency include variable distance imaging, camera rotation, head tilt, and rotation of the eye in the eye socket. The standardization process occurs in the iris regions, which have the same constant dimensions, so that two images of the same iris under different conditions have the same spatial location [24].

13.3.1 Daugman's Rubber Sheet Model

The homogeneous rubber sheet model developed by Daugman [2,16] remaps each point in the iris region with a pair of polar coordinates (r, θ), where r is present in the range of $[0, 1]$ and θ is the angle $[0, 2\pi]$.

Reconfiguration of the iris region from (x, y) Cartesian coordinates to the normalized nonconcentric polar representation is modeled in Equation 13.13:

$$I\big(x(r, \theta), y(r, \theta)\big) \rightarrow I(r, \theta) \tag{13.13}$$

with $x(r, \theta)$ as in Equation 13.14 (Figure 13.9):

$$x(r, \theta) = (1-r)x_p(\theta) + rx_i(\theta) \tag{13.14}$$

and $y(r, \theta)$ is given in Equation 13.15:

$$y(r, \theta) = (1-r)y_p(\theta) + ry_i(\theta) \tag{13.15}$$

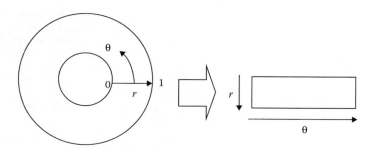

FIGURE 13.9
Daugman's rubber sheet model.

where:

$I(x, y)$ is the image of iris region

(x, y) are the Cartesian coordinates of origin

(r, θ) are the polar coordinates corresponding to standardized x_p, y_p

x_1, y_1 are the coordinates of the pupil and iris boundaries along the θ direction

The rubber sheet model takes account of pupil dilation and inconsistencies in size to produce a normalized representation with constant dimensions.

In this way, the iris region is modeled by a flexible rubber sheet anchored at the iris boundary with the pupil center as the reference point. The normalized iris is shown in Figure 13.10.

Although the rubber sheet model has uniform dilation of pupils, the imaging distance and moving pupils are not concentric, and it does not compensate for inconsistencies in rotation. In Daugman's system, rotation is recorded in correspondence shifting patterns in the iris in the θ direction, until the two iris patterns are aligned [71,80].

13.3.2 Image Registration

Wilde has proposed a technique for recording an image [77] for the normalization of iris textures. In this method, a newly acquired image I_a $(u; v)$ is aligned with an image in the database I_d $(u; v)$ so that a comparison can be performed. The alignment process is a transformation with the aid of a selection of the mapping function $(U(x; y); V(x; y))$ to minimize the function, as in Equation 13.16:

$$\iint_{x\ y} I_d\left(x,\ y\right) - I_a\left(x - u,\ y - v\right)^2 \mathrm{d}x\mathrm{d}y \tag{13.16}$$

The alignment process compensates for changes in rotation and scale. The mapping function is forced to take a similarity transformation of the image coordinates $(x; y)$ to $(x'; y')$, given by Equation 13.17:

$$\begin{pmatrix} x' \\ y' \end{pmatrix} = \begin{pmatrix} x \\ y \end{pmatrix} - sR(A') \begin{pmatrix} x \\ y \end{pmatrix} \tag{13.17}$$

with s as the factor of scaling and $R(A')$ a matrix representing the rotation A'. The parameters s and A' are recovered by an iterative minimization.

The Wilde standardization process is based on a different approach to the Daugman method. In this process, the normalization is performed corresponding time.

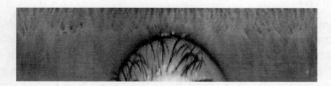

FIGURE 13.10
Normalized iris after conversion.

Compared with the standard method, Daugman's approach is very time consuming regarding identification applications. However, verification of the method compensates for undesirable factors such as changes in rotation and scale.

13.3.3 Nonlinear Normalization Model

The unwrapping method proposed by Daugman [2,3] assumes that iris patterns are distributed linearly in the radial direction which allows the mapping procedure in the range. The technique is based on two main factors:

1. The image acquisition process adjusts the size of the pupil in a large radius with appropriate control of lighting.
2. The feature extraction process is applied locally to different positions of the texture of the iris, which compensates for variations in local nonlinear.

The nonlinear normalization method proposed by Yuan and Shi considers nonlinear behavior of iris patterns due to changes in pupil size [37,38]. To place an iris region correctly, a nonlinear model and a linear normalization model are combined. The nonlinear method, which is firstly applied to an image of the iris, is based on three assumptions:

1. The edge of the pupil and the iris root (which correspond to the inner and outer boundaries of the iris) are concentric circles.
2. The margin of the pupil does not rotate significantly during changes in the size of the pupils.
3. The shape of the pupil does not change and remains circular when resizing pupils.

The nonlinear model is defined by virtual arcs, which are called "fiber" Wyatt after work [39,40], which connect a point on the boundary equaling to a point on the blade. The polar angle traversed by the arc between the two points is $\pi/2$. Virtual arcs are defined on the basis of a pupil normalized to a fixed value by using a predefined λ_{ref} which is obtained by averaging all λ, values defined as $\lambda = r/R$ in the iris database. r and R represent the radius of the pupil and limbus, respectively. The reference annular zone with λ_{ref} is then linearly mapped into a fixed-size rectangle zone of $m \times n$ by equal sampling points in each concentric circle m virtual sampling with a fixed radial resolution.

It is concluded by the authors that the approach presented by the nonlinear model further simplifies the actual physiological mechanism of deformation of the iris, and further assumptions and approximations are needed to support the model. The model is also believed to explicitly show the nonlinear behavior of iris textures due to improvements in the experiments.

13.3.4 Virtual Circles

In the Boles system [27,41], iris images are first scaled for a constant diameter so that when comparing two images a reference image is considered. It works differently to other techniques because standardization is not performed until trying to match two iris regions, rather than proceeding with the standardization and recording the results of subsequent comparisons. Once the two irises have the same dimensions, the characteristics are extracted from the iris region by storing the intensity values along concentric virtual circles, with the origin at the center of the pupil.

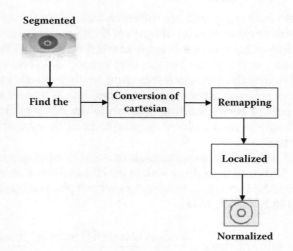

FIGURE 13.11
Optimized rubber sheet model.

Standardization is a resolution selected so that the number of data points extracted from each iris is the same. This is essentially the same as the Daugman rubber sheet model, but scaling is fixed at one game rather than setting some dimensions in a constant. In addition, Boles does not mention how rotational invariance is obtained.

13.3.5 Optimized Rubber Sheet Model for Iris Normalization

Malmurugan and Selvamuthukumaran [35,42] proposed a rubber sheet model optimized for the normalization of the iris to further improve the standardization phase. In this method, the segmented image is taken as input for the standardization process. First, the coordinate system of the iris region is converted from the Cartesian spherical. Then, the mapping process is obtained for normalization. Histogram equalization is applied to the localized region of the iris for greater standardization. The complete methodology is given in Figure 13.11.

13.4 Survey on Matching Phase

With different systems feature extraction, one iris image is transformed into a single representation in the feature space. To make the decision of acceptance or rejection, a distance is calculated to measure the closeness of the match [5]. Systems in iris recognition, such as distance measures, include the Hamming distance (HD), the normalized correlation (NC), and the weighted Euclidean distance (WED) [8,56].

13.4.1 Hamming Distance Method

The key to iris recognition is the failure of a test of statistical independence, which involves many degrees of freedom that this test is almost guaranteed to be transmitted whenever the iris codes for both eyes compared are different, but uniquely has failed in any eye iris code is compared with another version of himself [10,16].

The test of statistical independence is implemented by a simple Boolean Exclusive OR operator (XOR) applied to the phase vectors that encode 2048 bits for both iris patterns, masked (associated with) the two corresponding to their mask bit vectors to prevent objects from nonirises influencing comparison irises. The XOR operator detects disagreement between any pair of corresponding bits, while the AND operator ensures that the compared bits are both deemed to have been corrupted by eyelashes, eyelids, specular reflections, or other noises.

The norms ($\|\ \|$) of the said bit vectors result in an XOR'ed phase mask and the vectors are then associated with measures to calculate an HD as a fraction of the measure of the dissimilarity between the two irises, two vectors whose phase of code bits are designated {mask A, mask B} as in Equation 13.18:

$$\text{hamming distance} = \frac{\|\text{code A} \otimes \text{code B} \cap \text{mask A} \cap \text{mask B}\|}{\|\text{mask A} \cap \text{mask B}\|} \tag{13.18}$$

The denominator counts the total number of relevant phase bits in iris comparisons after artifacts such as eyelashes and specular reflections have been updated so that the HD that results is a dissimilarity measure; fractional "0" represents a perfect match. Boolean operators AND and XOR are applied as a vector of binary strings of length to the word length of the CPU as a single machine instruction. Thus, for example, on a single 32-bit machine, the two integers between 0 and 4 billion can be XOR'ed in a single machine instruction for generating a third integer such that each of the bits of a binary development is the XOR of the corresponding bits of the combination of two original integers. The implementation of the HD calculation in parallel 32-bit chunks enables extremely rapid comparisons of iris codes when searching through a large database to find a match. On a single processor of 300 MHz, these exhaustive searches are performed at a speed of about 100,000 irises per second.

Search speed scales linearly with the clock frequency, except I/O overhead, and of course the search process is inherently parallelizable. And databases that can contain millions of iris codes can be grown in parallel pieces, each managed by a single processor adapted to maintain the desired speed of response.

It is clear that two individuals are distinct, and the resulting binary matrices encoding functionality are essentially random matrices. Therefore, an elementary statistical analysis will suffice to make the decision as to whether the subjects are the same person or are different individuals. Further improvements can be made in which the individual noise masks are used to eliminate the possibility of including the eyelashes, eyelids, and specular reflections factoring in the decision-making process. In addition, an image of the eye obtained at different angles of head movement can be used to reduce the FRR.

13.4.2 Normalized Correlation

Wilde's system uses the NC between two iris images coded to measure the closeness of their match [13,29]. The NC is defined in Equation 13.19:

$$\text{NC} = \sum_{i=1}^{n}\sum_{j=1}^{m}\left(p_1[i, j] - u_1\right)\left(p_2[i, j] - u_2\right)\big/nm\sigma_1\sigma_2 \tag{13.19}$$

where:

p_1 and p_2 are the two encoded iris templates of size $n \times m$

u_1 and u_2 are averages of images

σ_1 and σ_2 are the standard deviations of the images p_1 and p_2

13.4.3 Weighted Euclidean Distance

Euclidean distance is a way of defining the proximity of the correspondence between two models of iris [13,27]. It is calculated by measuring the norm between two vectors. For the WED, another factor is taken into consideration because the percentage of decision-making varies in different dimensions.

Zhu et al. [23,47] tried to use the WED to measure the proximity of an unknown iris for a model in the existing database [26,33], as defined in Equation 13.20:

$$WED = \sum_{i=1}^{N} \frac{(f-g)^2}{\delta^2} \tag{13.20}$$

where:

f is the unknown model to be adapted

g is the matrix of the iris in an existing database to compare therewith

i is used to denote the index of features in the models

δ is the standard deviation of the ith feature in template g

Similar to the HD, the WED is a distance measure in another biometric system. In a complete system, the designer must interpret the metric for identification or verification. In the Wilde algorithm, the iris template g with a minimum WED to the template f is identified as being from the same subject.

13.4.4 Matching Pursuit

Lee et al. [21,36] proposed a new adaptive dynamic programming pursuit (DPMP) algorithm for iris recognition. This method modifies the matching pursuit (MP) algorithm to select the most representative atoms for the iris rec power. The experiments show that our system has (1) better performance for both personal identification and verification, and (2) a better ROC curve, with less computation than the conventional MP-based iris recognition.

13.4.5 Optimized Iris Matching Using Cyclic Redundancy Check

Malmurugan and Selvamuthukumaran [43] proposed an optimized adaptation using iris CRC for an exact match of the iris. In this method, CRC-32 is used to generate the CRC code and then the codes are processed to match the iris images. The CRC is used to detect changes in the code of an image of the iris at its comparison with a further image of the iris. It is used to perform matching between the iris codes of the acquired iris and irises in the database. To determine whether two irises are of the same class, this method compares the similarity between the codes. The two irises can be accepted or rejected based on the similarity found in the iris code by using the cyclic redundancy check. A diagram of this method is given in Figure 13.12.

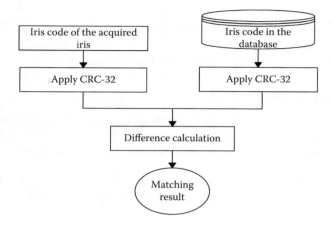

FIGURE 13.12
Optimized iris matching using CRC.

13.4.6 Other Algorithms

Bolle et al. [21,44] addressed the problem of the analytical modeling of the "personality" of the texture of the iris as a biometric. Building on concepts developed by Daugman, they considered the probability of binary values in an iris code and the HD between the iris codes to develop an analytical model of FRR and FAR as probability functions p if a bit in the iris code is "flipped" due to noise. The model predicts that the iris FAR performance is relatively stable and is not affected by p, and that the performance of the FRR theoretical accuracy degrades rapidly when the bit flip p increases. They also indicate that the performance predicted by the model FAR above analytic is in excellent agreement with the empirical data reported by Daugman.

Kong et al. [13,33] presented an analysis to show that "the iris code is a clustering algorithm," in the sense of using a "cosine measure to assign an image patch to one of the prototypes." They proposed the use of cream texture coding and gave a brief discussion on the basis of the impostor distribution being shown in tandem. There are no experimental results for image segmentation and iris matching.

13.5 Summary

In this chapter, research efforts on segmentation, normalization, and the corresponding phases of iris recognition and their limitations have been discussed. The chapter reviews the existing techniques and their limitations. This further motivates engineers to undertake additional research into developing new algorithms in the segmentation, normalization, and matching phases of iris recognition.

References

1. J.G. Daugman, High confidence visual recognition of persons by a test of statistical independence, *IEEE Transactions on Pattern Analysis and Machine Intelligence*, 15(11): 1148–1161, 1993.

2. J. Daugman, Biometric personal identification system based on iris analysis, U.S. Patent No. 5, 291, 560, 1994.
3. J. Daugman, Demodulation by complex-valued wavelets for stochastic pattern recognition, *International Journal of Wavelets, Multi-resolution and Information Processing*, 1(1): 1–17, 2003.
4. J. Daugman, The importance of being random: Statistical principles of iris recognition, *Pattern Recognition*, 36(2): 279–291, 2003.
5. J. Daugman, Statistical richness of visual phase information: Update on recognizing persons by iris patterns, *International Journal of Computer Vision*, 45(1): 25–38, 2001.
6. J.G. Daugman, How iris recognition works, *IEEE Transactions on Circuits and Systems for Video Technology*, 14(1): 21–30, 2004.
7. J.G. Daugman, New methods in iris recognition, *IEEE Transactions on Systems, Man and Cybernetics*, 37(5): 1167–1175, 2007.
8. J.R. Matey, O. Naroditsky, K. Hanna, R. Kolczynski, D. LoIacono, S. Mangru, M. Tinker, T. Zappia, and W.Y. Zhao, Iris on the move: Acquisition of images for iris recognition in less constrained environments, *Proceedings of the IEEE*, 94(11): 1936–1946, 2006.
9. H. Proenca and L.A. Alexandre, Iris segmentation methodology for non-cooperative recognition, *IEEE Proceedings: Vision, Image and Signal Processing*, 153(2): 199–205, 2006.
10. X. Li, Modeling intra-class variation for non-ideal iris recognition. In Springer LNCS 3832: International Conference on Biometrics, pp. 419–427. Hong Kong, China, 2006.
11. X. Liu, K.W. Bowyer, and P.J. Flynn, Experiments with an improved iris segmentation algorithm. In *Proceedings of the Fourth IEEE Workshop on Automatic Identification Advanced Technologies*, pp. 118–123. AUTO ID 2005, Buffalo, NY, October, 2005.
12. K. Chang, K.W. Bowyer, and P.J. Flynn, An evaluation of multi-modal 2d+3d face biometrics, *IEEE Transactions on Pattern Analysis and Machine Intelligence*, 27(4): 619–624, 2005.
13. L. Ma, T. Tan, Y. Wang, and D. Zhang, Personal identification based on iris texture analysis, *IEEE Transactions on Pattern Analysis and Machine Intelligence*, 25(12): 1519–1533, 2003.
14. V. Dorairaj, N. Schmid, and G. Fahmy, Performance evaluation of non-ideal iris based recognition system implementing global ICA encoding, *Proceedings of IEEE International Conference on Image Processing*, 3: 285–288, 2005.
15. L. Yucheng and L. Yubin, An algorithm of image segmentation based on fuzzy mathematical morphology. In *Proceedings of the IEEE International Conference on Information Technology and Applications, International Forum on Information Technology and Applications*, 2009.
16. N. Schmid, M. Ketkar, H. Singh, and B. Cukic, Performance analysis of iris based identification system at the matching score level, *IEEE Transactions on Information Forensics and Security*, 1(2): 154–168, 2006.
17. F. Scotti and V. Piuri, Adaptive reflection detection and location in iris biometric images by using computational intelligence techniques, *IEEE Transactions on Instrumentation and Measurement*, 59(7): 1825–1833, 2010.
18. H. Proenca, Iris recognition: On the segmentation of degraded images acquired in the visible wavelength, *IEEE Transactions on Pattern Analysis and Machine Intelligence*, 32(8): 831–846, 2010.
19. C. Xu and J. Prince, Gradient vector flow: A new external force for snakes. In *Proceedings of IEEE Conference on Computer Vision and Pattern Recognition*, pp. 66–71. San Juan, Puerto Rico, 1997.
20. N. Malmurugan and S. Selvamuthukumaran, Investigation on optimization in iris segmentation phase of iris recognition, *Journal of Applied Computer Science & Mathematics*, 8(4): 41–44, 2010.
21. C. Xu and J. Prince, Snakes, shapes, and gradient vector flow. *IEEE Transactions on Image Processing*, 7(3): 359–369, 1998.
22. J. Zuo, N.K. Ratha, and J.H. Connel, A new approach for iris segmentation. In *Proceedings of the IEEE Computer Society Conference on Computer Vision and Pattern Recognition Workshops*, pp. 1–6. San Francisco, California, 2008.
23. A. Zaim, M. Quweider, J. Scargle, J. Iglesias, and R. Tang, A robust and accurate segmentation of iris images using optimal partitioning. In *Proceedings of the International Conference on Pattern Recognition*, pp. 578–581. IEEE, Piscataway, 2006.

24. N. Malmurugan and S. Selvamuthukumaran, Optimization in iris recognition, *Journal of Computer Applications*, II(I): 41–42, 2009.
25. W. Boles and B. Boashash, A human identification technique using images of the iris and wavelet transform, *IEEE Transactions on Signal Processing*, 46(4): 1185–1188, 1998.
26. N. Malmurugan and S. Selvamuthukumaran, Optimization in iris recognition. In *Proceedings of the International Conference on Information and Advanced Computing*, pp. 23–25. Bharat University, Chennai, July 2008.
27. N.B. Puhan, N. Sudha, and X. Jiang, Robust eyeball segmentation in noisy iris images using Fourier spectral density. In *Proceedings of the 6th International Conference on Information, Communications and Signal Processing*, pp. 1–5. Singapore, 2007.
28. J. Thornton, M. Savvides, and B.V.K. Vijaya Kumar, An evaluation of iris pattern representations. In *Proceedings of the First IEEE International Conference on Biometrics: Theory, Applications, and Systems*, pp. 1–6. Washington, DC, 2007.
29. H. Mehrabian and P. Hashemi-Tari, Pupil boundary detection for iris recognition using graph cuts. In *Proceedings of Image and Vision Computing New Zealand* 2007, pp. 77–82. Hamilton, New Zealand, December 2007.
30. Institute of Automation, Chinese Academy of Sciences, Database of eye images. http://biometrics.idealtest.org/dbDetailForUser.do?id=1.
31. G. Castagnoli, S. Brauer, and M. Herrmann, Optimization of cyclic redundancy-check codes with 24 and 32 parity bits, *IEEE Transactions on Communications*, 41(6): 883–892, 1993.
32. G.-D. Guo and C.R. Dyer, Learning from examples in the small sample case: Face expression recognition, *IEEE Transaction System, Man and Cybernetics—Part B*, 35(3): 477–488, 2005.
33. J. Canny, A computational approach to edge detection, *IEEE Transaction on Pattern Analysis and Machine Intelligence*, 8(6): 679–698, 1986.
34. S.J. Pundlik, D.L. Woodard, and S.T. Birchfield, Non-ideal iris segmentation using graph cuts. In *Proceedings of the IEEE Computer Society Conference on Computer Vision and Pattern Recognition Workshops*, pp. 1–6, 2008.
35. R.P. Wildes, Iris recognition. In *Biometric Systems: Technology, Design and Performance Evaluation*. Springer-Verlag, pp. 63–95, 2005.
36. N.D. Kalka, J. Zuo, N.A. Schmid, and B. Cukic, Image quality assessment for iris biometric. In *Proceedings of 2006 SPIE Conference on Biometric Technology for Human Identification III*, Vol. 6202, pp. 6202:D1–6202:D11, 2006.
37. J. Thornton, M. Savvides, and B.V.K. Vijaya Kumar, A Bayesian approach to deformed pattern matching of images, *IEEE Transactions on Pattern Analysis and Machine Intelligence*, 29(4): 596–606, 2007.
38. N.D. Kalka, Image quality assessment for iris biometric, Master's Thesis, the Lane Department of Computer Science and Electrical Engineering, West Virginia University, 2005.
39. Y. Chen, S. Dass, and A. Jain, Localized iris quality using 2-D wavelets. In *Proceedings of the International Conferences on Advances in Biometrics*, pp. 373–381. Hong Kong, China, 2006.
40. L. Masek, Recognition of human iris patterns for biometric Identification, PhD Thesis, The University of Western Australia, 2003. http://www.csse.uwa.edu.au/~pk/studentprojects/libor/LiborMasekThesis.pdf.
41. ISO/IEC Standard 19794–6. Information technology—Biometric data interchange formats, part 6: Iris image data. Technical report, International Standards Organization, 2005.
42. Case study of International Biometrics Group page on Independent Testing of Iris Recognition Technology (ITIRT). https://ibgweb.com/about/case-studies/independent-testing-iris-recognition-technology-itir.
43. N. Malmurugan and S. Selvamuthukumaran, Optimization in iris segmentation phase, *International Journal of Emerging Technologies and Applications in Engineering, Technology and Science*, 2(2): 302–304, 2009.
44. N. Malmurugan and S. Selvamuthukumaran, Optimization in iris recognition. In *Proceedings of the Second National Conference on New Frontiers in Computing*. K.S. Rangasamy College of Technology, Tiruchengode, 2008.

14

Formal Design and Development of an Anterior Segment Eye Disease Classification System

Oliver Faust, Chan Wei Yan, Muthu Rama Krishnan Mookiah,
U. Rajendra Acharya, Eddie Y. K. Ng, and Wenwei Yu

CONTENTS

14.1 Introduction

The majority of visual impairments are caused by disease and malnutrition. Studies from the World Health Organization (WHO) indicate that more than 42 million people worldwide are currently blind [1]. In 2002, the most common causes of blindness were cataract (47.8%), glaucoma (12.3%), age-related macular degeneration (AMD) (8.7%), trachoma (3.6%), corneal opacity (5.1%), and diabetic retinopathy (4.8%) [2]. These figures indicate that cataract, which is an anterior segment eye disease, is the leading cause of blindness in the world. Currently, approximately 1 million free cataract operations are performed every year, but there are 1.5 million new cases of blindness worldwide per year that are directly linked to cataract. In other words, cataract-related eye disorders cause the world population to gradually become blinder. This increase in blindness causes lots of suffering; even more worrying is the fact that this suffering is unnecessary, because early diagnosis and correct treatment greatly reduce the probability of cataract-related vision loss [3].

Early diagnosis is especially important, because cataracts develop slowly and many patients are not aware of their gradual loss of sight until very late in the disease when vision is irreversibly affected. Therefore, improving methods for cataract screening is an important field of research. This research involves the combination of engineering and medical methods in order to create physical solutions which eliminate suffering caused by cataract-related blindness. These methods must address cost effectiveness and reliability issues [4]. One way to address these issues is to use inexpensive computer technology to design and develop automated cataract classification systems for diagnosis support. Computer-based systems come with their own set of challenges, which result from the immense flexibility of modern processing machines [5]. One of these shortcomings is state space explosion and nondeterminism of large-scale systems. To overcome, or at least manage, these challenges, this type of medical support system must be designed with a formal and model-driven design methodology [6,7].

This chapter shows the models which were used during design and development of an automated eye disease classification system. The classification system was able to discriminate optical eye images that show signs of anterior segment eye diseases from those of healthy eyes with an accuracy of 90%. This result instills trust into the design, because we have established that it is possible to diagnose anterior segment eye diseases based on optical images. Furthermore, with these performance figures we are able to set a benchmark for the implemented system. This benchmark is used to construct the so-called *use cases* with which the implemented system is tested. This use case testing will instill trust in the implemented anterior segment eye abnormalities classification system.

The content of this chapter follows the formal and model driver design approach, which we have adopted to create a physical solution for the problem of an anterior segment eye disease diagnosis. The literature review introduces the medical background which is necessary to understand the materials and methods. Section 14.3 introduces data-processing methods necessary to model the proposed diagnosis system. Section 14.4 states the results that were obtained by testing the model. These results, and indeed the merits of the model itself, are discussed in Section 14.5. Section 14.6 concludes the chapter.

14.2 Literature Review

The literature review describes the working of the normal eye before the different anterior segment eye diseases are introduced. We show sample pictures for each of these diseases.

14.2.1 Working of Normal Eye

Understanding the working of the normal human eye is a prerequisite for modeling an anterior segment eye abnormalities classification system. The working of a normal eye is based on the principle that light rays, reflected from physical objects, are detected by the eye and interpreted by the brain [8,9]. Once these rays have entered the eye, they have to pass the iris, which controls the quantity of light entering the eye by either increasing or decreasing the pupil size. The remaining light travels through a lens which focuses a picture of the physical objects on the retina in the back of the eye. The retina converts the picture to electrical impulses which are transmitted to the brain through the optic nerve. Once the signals are received by the brain, it interprets them as images of physical objects. Figure 14.1 shows a cross section of the human eye and Figure 14.2(a) shows an optical image of the anterior segment of a normal eye.

14.2.2 Cataract Eye

Cataract refers to the clouding of the eye's natural lens [10,11]. This lens consists mainly of water and protein. The protein is arranged in a precise way that keeps the lens clear and allows light to pass through. But, with age or disease, some protein molecules may clump together and start to cloud a small area of the lens, forming the cataract. The initial cataracts may grow larger over time and cloud more of the lens, blocking more light, and hence vision deteriorates. Figure 14.2b shows the anterior segment of a typical cataract eye. Cataracts are categorized into four main types: (i) age-related cataract, (ii) congenital cataract, (iii) secondary cataract, and (iv) traumatic cataract.

Research on cataract has focused on the effect of pupil size [12]. The researchers determined that the pupillary dilation that improved the image quality in most of the subjects was small. Subjects with small undilated pupils and/or cataracts, however, may benefit most from pupillary dilation.

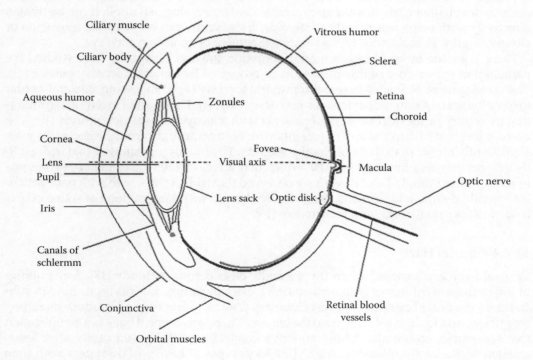

FIGURE 14.1
Cross section of human eye with major parts labeled.

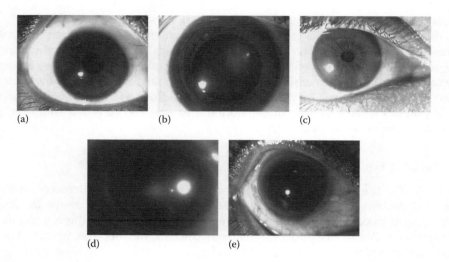

FIGURE 14.2
Typical optical images: (a) normal, (b) cataract, (c) iridocyclitis, (d) corneal haze, and (e) postcataract.

14.2.3 Iridocyclitis (Iritis)

Iridocyclitis is a condition where both iris and ciliary body show signs of inflammation. Symptoms of iridocyclitis may include eye pain, redness, blurred vision and light sensitivity. Acute or chronic inflammation of iris and ciliary body is characterized by exudates in the anterior chamber, iris discoloration, and a constricted, sluggish pupil. It can be treated effectively with tropane alkaloids or steroids. Iridocyclitis can be classified into acute or chronic. Figure 14.2c shows a typical anterior segment of an iridocyclitis eye.

There is a wide range of research on iridocyclitis. Job and Thompson have studied the pathological appearance of this disease in an advanced lepromatous leprosy patient [13]. The development of Fuchs' heterochromic iridocyclitis (FHI) following bilateral ocular toxoplasmosis in Asian Indian females was described [14]. The effect of macrophage migration inhibitory factor (MIF) in sera of patients with iridocyclitis was determined [15]. The average levels of MIF in the sera of patients with both acute and chronic iridocyclitis were significantly higher than those of healthy subjects. The researchers showed that iridocyclitis induces the elevation of serum MIF, which may affect various inflammatory symptoms in iridocyclitis. Prahalad and Passo have observed that iridocyclitis, seen with pauciarticular juvenile rheumatoid arthritis, was usually chronic with long periods of active ocular inflammation, remissions, and recurrences [16].

14.2.4 Corneal Haze

Corneal haze is diagnosed when the normally clear cornea is cloudy [17]. Any buildup of inflammatory infiltrates (white blood cells), extra moisture, scar tissue, or foreign substances (like drugs) can cause cornea clouding. Cataract surgery can introduce moisture, scar tissue, and foreign substances to the cornea. Therefore, corneal haze is a complication that sometimes occurs after photorefractive keratectomy (PRK), and rarely after laser-assisted *in situ* keratomileusis (LASIK) [18]. Most types of haze will disappear with time or drug treatment, but sometimes it can be permanent. Figure 14.2d shows a picture of the anterior segment of a typical corneal haze eye.

14.2.5 Postcataract

The term postcataract refers to a condition which occurs after a cloudy lens has been surgically replaced by an artificial one. Currently, there are two surgical procedures for removing cataracts: (i) extracapsular and (ii) intracapsular surgery. Extracapsular surgery is a technique where the surgeon removes the lens while keeping most of the lens capsule intact. Sometimes, a process called *phacoemulsification* is used, where high-frequency sound waves break up the lens before extraction [19]. During intracapsular surgery, the entire lens, together with the lens capsule, is removed. Figure 14.2e shows an optical image of a postcataract eye.

14.3 Materials and Methods

Figure 14.3 shows a block diagram of the proposed anterior segment eye disease classification system. The data flow from left to right though a two-step processing structure. The first step is nonlinear feature extraction. We have used nine different algorithms to extract significant features from the optical eye image data. The second step is classification. This step uses the support vector machine (SVM) algorithm to discriminate between optical eye images which show signs of eye disease and normal optical eye images. The optical eye image data and all the individual processing algorithms are discussed in the following sections.

14.3.1 Data

The optical eye images were obtained from the Department of Ophthalmology at Kasturba Medical College Hospital, Manipal, India. The hospital ethics committee has approved the use of these optical eye images for research. The images were grouped into four sets, the details of which are shown in Table 14.1. The images are in 24-bit TIFF format with an image size of 128×128 pixels.

14.3.2 Radon Transform

The Radon transform is widely used in computed tomography to create images from scattering data, which are associated with cross-sectional scans of an object [20]. It transforms

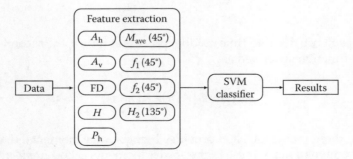

FIGURE 14.3
Block diagram of the proposed feature extraction and classification system.

TABLE 14.1

Details of Age, Gender, and Number of Subjects Used in Each Class

	Cataract	Postcataract	Iridocyclitis	Normal	Corneal Haze
Age (years)	68 ± 13	68 ± 13	56 ± 12	42 ± 8	62 ± 10
Males	25	22	25	35	24
Females	15	15	15	25	24

two-dimensional images into a line parameter domain. Each line in the original image will yield a peak in the transform domain; the position of this peak indicates the corresponding line parameters [21]. Hence, lines within images are transformed into points in the Radon domain.

Mathematically, a line can be expressed as: $\rho = x \times \cos\theta + y \times \sin\theta$, where θ is a line angle and ρ is the offset from the origin of the coordinate system.

Given a continuous function $g(x, y)$, the Radon transform is defined as:

$$Rg(\rho, \theta) = \int_{-\alpha}^{+\alpha} g\left[\rho\cos\theta - s\sin\theta, \rho\sin\theta + s\cos\theta\right]ds \tag{14.1}$$

Equation 14.1 describes an integral from $-\alpha$ to $+\alpha$ along a line s through the image. So, the Radon transform converts two-dimensional (2-D) signals into 1-D parallel beam projections, at various angles θ. In this work, we have used $\theta = 5°$.

14.3.3 Higher-Order Spectra (HOS)-Based Features

Higher-order spectra (HOS) techniques were first applied to signal processing problems in 1970, and subsequently these techniques were applied to economics, speech, seismic data processing, plasma physics, optics, and biomedical applications [21]. We start the discussion of HOS by introducing second-order statistics which evaluate both the mean value (m) and variance (σ^2) of input data. These statistical measures are based on the expectation operation $\mathbb{E}(\ldots)$ which operates on a random process A:

$$m_A = \mathbb{E}\{A\}$$

$$\sigma_A^2 = \mathbb{E}\left\{\left(A - m_A\right)^2\right\} \tag{14.2}$$

If $A(n)$ is the result of a discrete-time random process at time n, the second-order moment autocorrelation function is defined as:

$$m_A^2(i) = \mathbb{E}\left\{A(n) \times A(n+i)\right\} \tag{14.3}$$

In addition to these moments, HOS provides higher-order moments, that is, m^3, m^4, $\ldots$, and nonlinear combinations of these higher-order moments called *cumulants*, that is, c_1, c_2, c_3, $\ldots$ [22]. Thus, HOS consists of both moment and cumulant spectra. It can be used for both deterministic signals and random processes [23].

Third-order statistics of the signal *bispectrum* were used in this work. The bispectrum is defined as the Fourier transform of the third-order correlation of the data, and is given by:

$$B(f_1, f_2) = \mathbb{E}\{A(f_1)A(f_2)A^*(f_1 + f_2)\} \tag{14.4}$$

where $A(f)$ is the discrete-time Fourier transform of the $A(n)$, which is usually computed using the fast Fourier transform (FFT) algorithm. The expectation operation is not necessary for deterministic signals, because the third-order correlation is a time-averaging operation.

The features used in our work are based on phases of the integrated bispectrum and they are described briefly below: Assuming that there is no bispectral aliasing, the bispectrum of a real signal is uniquely defined with a triangle which is formed by $0 \le f_2 \le f_1 \le f_1 + f_2 \le 1$. Parameters are obtained by integrating along straight lines which pass through the origin in bifrequency space. Figure 14.4 shows both the region of computation and the line of integration. $P(a)$ is the bispectral invariant, which is defined as the phase of the integrated bispectrum along the radial line with slope equal to a. Mathematically, this is expressed as:

$$P(a) = \arctan\left(\frac{I_i(a)}{I_r(a)}\right) \tag{14.5}$$

where:

$$I(a) = I_r(a) + jI_i(a)$$

$$= \int_{f_1=0}^{\frac{1}{1+a}} B(f_1, af_1) df_1 \tag{14.6}$$

for $0 < a \le 1$ and $j = \sqrt{-1}$. The variables I_r and I_i refer to real and imaginary parts of the integrated bispectrum, respectively.

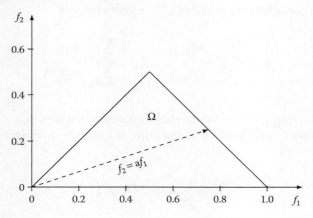

FIGURE 14.4
Ω is the nonredundant region that results from computing the bispectrum for real signals. Integrating along the dashed line with slope a yields the bispectrum features. The frequencies on the axes are normalized with the Nyquist frequency.

Chua et al. have shown that $P(a)$ contains information about the waveform shape within the window, that the information is robust against shift as well as amplification, and that it is invariant to timescale changes [24]. They are particularly sensitive to changes in the left–right waveform asymmetry. For windowed segments of a white Gaussian random process, these features will tend to be distributed symmetrically and uniformly about zero in the interval from $-\pi$ to $+\pi$. When a process is both chaotic and exhibits a colored spectrum with third-order time correlations or phase coupling between Fourier components, it is found that the mean value and distribution of the invariant feature may be used for process identification. Changing the slope value (a) yields different sets of $P(a)$.

The equations for determining the mean magnitude of both bispectrum and phase entropy for HOS are given below [21]:

$$M_{ave} = \frac{1}{L} \sum_{\langle \Omega \rangle} \left| B(f_1, f_2) \right| \tag{14.7}$$

$$P_h = \sum_{\langle n \rangle} p(\Psi_n) \log \left[p(\Psi_n) \right] \tag{14.8}$$

where:

$$p(\Psi_n) = \frac{1}{L} \sum_{\langle \Omega \rangle} l\{\phi[B(f_1, f_2)]\} \in \Psi_n$$

$$\Psi_n = \{\phi \mid -\pi + 2\pi n / N \le \phi < -\pi + \pi(n+1)/N \mid\}, n = 0, 1, \ldots, N-1$$

L is the number of points within the region Ω
ϕ is the phase angle of the bispectrum
$l(\cdot)$ is an indicator function that gives a value of 1 when the phase angle is within the range of Ψ_n

The weighted center of bispectrum (WCOB) is given by [25]:

$$f_{1m} = \frac{\sum_{\langle \Omega \rangle} iB(i,j)}{\sum_{\langle \Omega \rangle} B(i,j)}, \quad f_{2m} = \frac{\sum_{\langle \Omega \rangle} jB(i,j)}{\sum_{\langle \Omega \rangle} B(i,j)} \tag{14.9}$$

where i and j are the frequency indices in the nonredundant region.

The following equation defines H_2 as the sum of logarithmic diagonal element amplitudes in the bispectrum:

$$H_2 = \sum_{\langle \Omega \rangle} \log \left[\left| B(f_k, f_k) \right| \right] \tag{14.10}$$

In this work, we derived bispectral phase entropy (P_h), mean magnitude of the bispectrum (M_{ave}), WCOB, and logarithmic amplitudes of diagonal elements in the bispectrum (H_2) for each Radon-transformed normal and abnormal eye image.

14.3.4 DWT-Based Features

Wavelets are mathematical functions that decompose data into different frequency components. This technique allows us to study each component with a resolution that is matched to its scale [26]. This property, of representing an image at various resolutions, is the reason why the wavelet transform is a better tool for extracting features from images than the widely used Fourier transform. Wavelet analysis can be done using continuous wavelet transforms (CWT) and discrete wavelet transforms (DWT). In our work, we have used DWT for feature extraction, which is explained below.

The DWT transforms a 2-D signal $x(n)$ by sending it through a sequence of down-sampling low- and high-pass filters [27]. The low-pass filter is defined by the transfer function $L(n)$ and the high-pass filter is defined by the transfer function $H(n)$. The output of the low-pass filter is known as the approximation coefficients. Equation 14.11 provides a mathematical formulation which describes how these coefficients are obtained.

$$A(n) = \sum_{k=-\infty}^{\infty} x(k)L(2n-k)$$

(14.11)

The high-pass filter output, $D(n)$, is referred to as the detailed coefficients. Equation 14.12 describes the process of obtaining these coefficients.

$$D(n) = \sum_{k=-\infty}^{\infty} x(k)H(2n-k)$$

(14.12)

Cascading two or more basic filter operations increases the frequency resolution. The cascading is done by feeding the output of the first-level low-pass filter to the same high- and low-pass filter combination. In other words, the detailed coefficients from a lower level form the coefficients for the next higher level. Therefore, each level doubles the frequency resolution and halves the number of samples. In the final level, both detailed and approximation coefficients constitute the level coefficients.

In this work, images are represented as an $m \times n$ grayscale matrix $I(i, j)$. Each matrix element represents the intensity of one pixel. All nonborder pixels in $I(i, j)$, where $i \notin \{0, m\}$ and $j \notin \{0, n\}$, have eight immediate neighboring pixels. These eight neighbors can be used to traverse through the matrix [28]. However, the 2-D DWT coefficients are the same when the direction in which the matrix is traversed is changed by 180°, because the sequence of pixels is just reversed. Hence, there are four possible decomposition directions: 0° (horizontal, D_h), 90° (vertical, D_v), and 45° or 135° (diagonal, D_d). For this work, we found that significant features could be obtained from Level 1 decomposition results.

We have evaluated 54 wavelet functions, each of which has a unique high-pass filter transfer function $H(n)$ and a unique low-pass filter transfer function $L(n)$ [27]. Our results show that Biorthogonal 3.1 (*bior3.1*) yields the most significant features. The name Biorthogonal indicates that the wavelet transform is invertible, but it is not necessarily orthogonal. In general, Biorthogonal wavelets can cope with signals that have more degrees of freedom.

The first-level 2-D DWT decomposition results in four matrices: D_{h1}, D_{v1}, D_{d1}, and A_1. The matrix elements are intensity values. In this work, we have computed a range of average and mean values. The following equations show the mathematical procedures which yield the features:

$$\text{Average } D_{h1}\,(A_h) = \frac{1}{N \times M} \sum_{x=\langle N \rangle} \sum_{y=\langle M \rangle} |D_{h1}\,(x,\,y)|$$

$$\text{Average } D_{v1}\,(A_v) = \frac{1}{N \times M} \sum_{x=\langle N \rangle} \sum_{y=\langle M \rangle} |D_{v1}\,(x,\,y)|$$

$$\text{Average } D_{d1}\,(A_d) = \frac{1}{N \times M} \sum_{x=\langle N \rangle} \sum_{y=\langle M \rangle} |D_{d1}\,(x,\,y)|$$

$$\text{Energy }(E_d) = \frac{1}{N^2 \times M^2} \sum_{x=\langle N \rangle} \sum_{y=\langle M \rangle} \left(D_{d1}\,(x,\,y)\right)^2$$

$$\text{Energy }(E_v) = \frac{1}{N^2 \times M^2} \sum_{x=\langle N \rangle} \sum_{y=\langle M \rangle} \left(D_{v1}\,(x,\,y)\right)^2$$

(14.13)

14.3.5 Hurst Exponent (*H*)

The texture of an abnormal eye can be analyzed based on the ideas of Brownian motion [29–31]. One way to describe an image with Brownian motion is in terms of an intensity and distance map. It can be defined as the expected value of this intensity difference, which is proportional to $\left|\sqrt{(x_2 - x_1)^2 + (y_1 - y_2)^2}\right|^H$, where the Hurst exponent H indicates the Hurst coefficient, $0 < H < 1$.

$$\mathbb{E}\left(|I(x_2,\,y_2) - I(x_1,\,y_1)|\right) = C\left(\left|\sqrt{(x_2 - x_1)^2 + (y_1 - y_2)^2}\right|^H\right)$$

$$\therefore \log\left(\mathbb{E}\left(|(x_2,\,y_2) - I(x_1,\,y_1)|\right)\right) = H\log\left(\left|\sqrt{(x_2 - x_1)^2 + (y_1 - y_2)^2}\right|\right) + \log(C)$$

(14.14)

To satisfy this equation across all types of images, H must vary from zero to one. This variation represents the image texture. This textural analysis method has a high computational complexity, because it involves distance calculations which require many multiplication operations. We overcame this problem by using Chebyshev's distance with some degree of approximation. Under the assumption that we have an $M \times N$ image, the intensity difference vector for that image can be calculated as:

$$\text{IDV} = \left[ID(1),\, ID(2),\, \dots,\, ID(k),\, \dots,\, ID(s)\right]$$

(14.15)

where s indicates the maximum possible scale and $ID(k)$ is defined as follows:

$$Id_1(k) = \frac{\sum_{x=1}^{M} \sum_{y=1}^{N-k} |I(x,\,y) - I(x,\,y+k)|}{M(N-k) - (\text{count of } I(x,\,y) = 0)}, \quad \forall I(x,\,y) \neq 0$$

$$Id_2(k) = \frac{\sum_{x=1}^{M-k}\sum_{y=1}^{N}\left|I(x,y)-I(x+k,y)\right|}{N(M-k)-\left(\text{count of } I(x,y)=0\right)}, \quad \forall I(x,y) \neq 0$$

$$Id_3(k) = \frac{\sum_{x=1}^{M-k}\sum_{y=1}^{N-k}\left|I(x,y)-I(x+k,y+k)\right|}{(M-k)(N-k)-\left(\text{count of } I(x,y)=0\right)}, \quad \forall I(x,y) \neq 0$$

(14.16)

$$Id_4(k) = \frac{\sum_{x=1}^{M-k}\sum_{y=1}^{N-k}\left|I(x,n-y+1)-I(x+k,n+1-(y+k))\right|}{(M-k)(N-k)-\left(\text{count of } I(x,y)=0\right)}, \quad \forall I(x,y) \neq 0$$

$$ID(k) = \frac{\sum_{j=1}^{4} Id_j(k)}{4}, \quad \forall k = 0, 1, \ldots, (m \times n)-1$$

where all pixel pairs calculated in the absolute difference ($Id_i(k)$ with $i \in \{1, 2, 3, 4\}$) are along horizontal, vertical, diagonal, and asymmetric-diagonal directions, respectively. A function $f(k)$ is defined, which describes normalized intensity difference vectors. These vectors are normalized to the neighbor of each pixel, in order to compensate for staining variation. Mathematically, we have:

$$f(k) = \log\left[\left|ID(k)\right| - \log\left|ID(1)\right|\right], \ k > 1$$

(14.17)

Thus, from Equation 14.14:

$$f(k) = H\log(k), \quad \text{where } k = 1, 2, \ldots, \min(M, N)$$

(14.18)

The value of H can be estimated using least squares estimation [31] from the Brownian motion curve ($f(k)$ versus $\log(k)$).

14.3.6 Fractal Dimension

Fractal dimension (FD) is another texture analysis method. Optical images of abnormal eyes can be viewed as 3-D objects which have an intensity variation as covering surface on the 2-D spatial plane. Any surface S in a Euclidean n-dimensional space is self-similar if S is the union of N_r distinct (nonoverlapping) copies of itself scaled up or down by a factor of r. Mathematically, FD is computed using the following formula [32,33]:

$$D = \frac{\log(N_r)}{\log\left(\dfrac{1}{r}\right)}$$

(14.19)

where D is the fractal dimension. In this work, we have used modified differential box counting together with a sequential algorithm. The input to the sequential algorithm was a grayscale image where the grid size is a power of two for efficient computation. Maximum and minimum intensities for each box (2 × 2) were obtained to sum their difference, which gives the N and r as:

$$r = \frac{s}{M}$$

$$M = \min(R \vee C)$$

(14.20)

where s denotes a scale factor, and R and C denote the number of rows and the number of columns, respectively. When the grid size doubles, R and C are reduced to half of their original value and the above procedure is repeated iteratively until max($R \vee C$) is not greater than 2. A linear regression model was used to fit a line to plots of $\log(N)$ versus $\log(1/r)$. The slope of this line is used to calculate the FD:

$$\log(N_r) = D \log(1/r)$$

(14.21)

14.3.7 Feature Selection Test: Student's *t*-Test

Student's *t*-test is a method for assessing whether or not the means of two groups are statistically different from each other. The result of this test is called the *p*-value [34,35]. A low *p*-value indicates that the two groups are statistically different. The ability to determine the difference between data groups is important for this study, because we want to assess the capability of the extracted features to discriminate between images which show signs of anterior segment eye disease and normal eye images. The feature significance is inversely proportional to the *p*-value. Typically, features with *p*-values below 0.05 are regarded as clinically significant. The *p*-value was calculated for each of the nine features.

14.3.8 Support Vector Machine (SVM)

The SVM classification algorithm was initially designed for two-class problems. However, shortly after the invention of this algorithm it was extended to multi-class problems [36]. The following paragraph introduces a two-class SVM algorithm.

The SVM algorithm establishes a hyperplane which forms as a decision surface [37,38]. This surface separates the two classes from each other with a maximum margin. This involves orienting the separating hyperplane perpendicular to the shortest line separating the convex hulls of the training data for every class, and locating it midway along this line. The separating hyperplane is modeled as $x \cdot w + b = 0$, where w is its normal. For linearly separable data $\{x_i, y_i\}$ where $x_i \in \mathbb{R}^n$ and $y_i = \{-1, 1\}$ for $i = 1, \ldots, N$, the optimum boundary, chosen with the maximal margin criterion, is found by minimizing the objective function:

$$O = \|w\|^2$$

(14.22)

subject to $(x_i \cdot w + b) y_i \geq 1 \quad \forall i.$

The solution for the optimum boundary w_0 is a linear combination of a subset of the training data, $s \in \{1, ..., N\}$, known as the *support vectors*.

Kernel functions can be used to extend the solution to nonlinear boundary problems. To be specific, the dot product ($\cdot$) in the feature space is expressed by some functions (i.e., kernels) of two vectors from the input space. Commonly used kernels are radial basis function (RBF) and polynomial. With these kernels, it is not necessary to transform the data to a feature space.

14.4 Results

Table 14.2 shows the *t*-test results (mean $\pm$ standard deviation) of the features extracted for classification. It can be seen from the table that phase entropy is more for "normal" because of higher variation in the pixel values. For biomedical engineering and medicine, sensitivity is defined as the proportion of people with a specific disease who are tested positive for this disease. In general, a higher sensitivity indicates a higher detection rate as well as a lower false negative (FN) rate. Specificity indicates the proportion of people who are disease free and who have negative test results. A higher specificity implies a lower false positive (FP) rate. High levels of specificity are important, because a high specificity ensures that only a small proportion of people without the disease will be unnecessarily worried or exposed to unnecessary treatment. Accuracy measures the probability of a patient with a positive test having the disease. The classification model shows a sensitivity of 93.8%, a specificity of 100%, and an accuracy of 90%. Therefore, the results are clinically significant.

Table 14.3 shows the classification results for the SVM classifier.

TABLE 14.2

Results (Mean $\pm$ Standard Deviation) of the Features Extracted for Classification

Features	Normal	Abnormal	*p*-Value
A_h	0.975 ± 1.06	3.18 ± 2.96	$<.0001$
A_v	0.760 ± 2.53	7.42 ± 9.76	$<.0001$
FD	$2.12 \pm 3.933 \times 10^{-2}$	$2.18 \pm 3.945 \times 10^{-2}$	$<.0001$
H	$0.355 \pm 4.817 \times 10^{-2}$	$0.456 \pm 5.695 \times 10^{-2}$	$<.0001$
P_h	3.01 ± 0.301	2.76 ± 0.375	$.0008$
$M_{ave}(45°)$	2.35 ± 0.781	2.99 ± 0.755	$<.0001$
$f_1(45°)$	6.99 ± 3.80	4.27 ± 2.43	$<.0001$
$f_2(45°)$	2.77 ± 0.829	2.27 ± 0.340	$<.0001$
$H_2(135°)$	2.35 ± 0.790	2.98 ± 0.792	$.0002$

TABLE 14.3

True Negative, False Positive, True Positive, False Negative, Sensitivity, Specificity, and Accuracy of the SVM Classifier

Classifier	TN	TP	FP	FN	Sensitivity	Specificity	Accuracy
SVM	12	2	18	0	93.8%	100%	90%

14.5 Discussion

As humans get older, they are more likely to depend on biomedical support systems for their well-being. Hence, over recent years, we have seen the rapid development and widespread deployment of biomedical systems. Gains in both pervasiveness and complexity have transformed single-purpose island systems into massively networked health-care systems which hold millions of personal health records [39,40]. The success of biomedical systems is also documented by the ever-increasing amount of biomedical data that is distributed by health-care networks [41,42]. From these facts we draw the conclusion that our civilization is increasingly dependent on biomedical systems which get more and more complex. In particular, physicians who base their diagnosis on biomedical data suffer from the almost limitless availability of physiological information. However, this is not a problem of too much technology; on the contrary, we need more technology to cope with the impending information overload. To be specific, computer-aided diagnosis (CAD) technology can be used to support physicians during their data analysis tasks by providing them with an automated quantitative analysis of biomedical data [43–45]. As a consequence, CAD is a major research topic, especially for medical imaging and diagnostic radiology [7,46,47].

In general, high-reliability systems, such as anterior segment eye disease CAD systems, need extensive modeling during the design phase [48]. Modeling is widely used in biomedical engineering; despite this fact, Kent et al. argue that designers in this field assign a low priority to the modeling tasks [49]. In practice, designers hasten to design and implement software and hardware solutions after only a little time spent on understanding the domain requirements. This design approach results in a rapid development cycle, but unfortunately the resulting systems usually do not, or do not completely, satisfy the user requirements and the developers are forced to re-design or re-program certain aspects of the system. Furthermore, projects with this type of rapid development cycle result in an evolutionary design methodology [50,51]. Moreover, this approach makes it difficult for the designer to cope with steep increases in the requirements complexity. This slow progress results from the evolutionary approach, which relies on progress that is made in distinct steps from one system generation to another. However, even with the fast turnover cycles of rapid development, the product or system lifecycle is still counted in years instead of months or weeks, and therefore evolutionary progress takes time. However, given the anticipated exponential rise in difficulty for biomedical systems, the requirements (or demand) surpass the rate of progress possible with standard evolutionary system design methodologies [6,52].

14.5.1 Treatment

Wound-healing processes are known to be more rapid in young subjects. Hence, the effect of patient age on refractive outcome of PRK was investigated [53]. Results from Hefetz et al. show that patient age had no statistical significance on refraction and corneal haze 1 year after PRK [53]. The effect of intact corneal epithelium on stromal haze and myofibroblast cell formation after excimer laser surgery was studied [54]. The researchers determined that the intact corneal epithelium may play an important part in curbing subepithelial haze and differentiation of myofibroblasts in corneal wound healing.

14.5.2 Cataract Classification

Both the volume and complexity of data produced during videokeratography examinations make interpretation a challenge. As a consequence, results are often analyzed qualitatively by subjective pattern recognition or reduced to comparisons of summary indices [55]. Twa et al. have applied the objective methods of decision tree induction and automated machine learning to discriminate between normal and keratoconic corneal shapes [55]. Their classification method was interpretable and it can be sourced from any instrumentation platform which is capable of raw elevation data output.

Field tests have been done with slit lamp-based classification systems [56,57]. Both cataract type and disease severity were assessed after dilating the pupil. The tested methods required an ophthalmologist who assessed and graded patient lenses against a collection of pictorial standards. Slit lens approaches show good intraobserver agreement for nuclear cataract grading in these studies [57,58]. Furthermore, the scale coarseness was used to evaluate nuclear cataract, that is, the methods may not be sensitive to small (but clinically or biologically significant) differences in nuclear cataract severity. Hockwin has classified different cataract types by measuring lens transparency or lens opacity based on slit image documentation which follows the Scheimpflug principle, combined with the retroillumination technique [59]. Photo-documented measurements of lens thickness were performed on cataract eyes and compared with the same measurements carried out on normal eyes. The experimenters found that the lens thickness in normal eyes usually increased with age (0.015 mm per year).

Carvalho has used the combination of Zernike coefficients and an artificial neural network (NN) to classify specific types of corneal shapes with an accuracy of more than 80% [60]. Automated machine classifiers based on optical coherence tomography (OCT) data are useful for enhancing both the specificity and sensitivity of this glaucoma detection technology [61].

Grabner et al. have found that dynamic corneal imaging yields a reproducible and reversible change in the corneal topography corresponding to different indentation depths [62]. Another set of results points toward the fact that several clinical parameters were correlated with corneal elastic behavior *in vivo* and that the technology could increase the predictability of refractive corneal surgery as well as help in the early diagnosis of corneal diseases. The Age-Related Eye Disease Study Research Group has built a system which has the ability to classify different types of cataracts from photographic images [63].

In this study, we have extracted nine features: A_h, A_v, FD, H, P_h, $M_{ave}(45°)$, $f_1(45°)$, $f_2(45°)$, and $H_2(135°)$. We feel that quality, that is, the practical relevance, of the system can further be increased by increasing the size (training data more than 200) and quality of the training set. The classification results can be enhanced by extracting features which are even more discriminative from the optical images. Environmental conditions such as reflection of light influence the quality of the optical images and hence the percentage of classification efficiency. MATLAB® 7.0.4 was used to create the software for both feature extraction and classification of eye images.

14.6 Conclusion

In this chapter, we have used a formal and model-driven design methodology to specify an anterior segment eye disease classification system. The classification system was based on optical eye images. These images were subjected to feature extraction using HOS, DWT, and texture methods. The significance of these features was established using Student's *t*-test before they were used as input to the SVM classification algorithm. The resulting system could detect whether or not a particular optical eye image is normal or abnormal with an accuracy of 90%. This result supports the premise that it is possible to build automated disease detection systems based on optical eye images. This support is necessary in order to proceed to the implementation phase, which aims to create a physical solution for the disease diagnosis problem. Furthermore, the results were obtained in a best-case scenario, where the system was fed with well-defined input in a system state where this input is legal.* The implemented system must show the same level of accuracy when tested with the same input. This use case testing instills trust in the implemented system.

Biomedical systems design is a great deal about trust, and modeling is one way to earn this trust. Formalizing a design methodology means to use modeling very early in the design process. An important aspect of the design methodology is that the project is steered by the modeling results; that is, if the results support a specific underlying premise, like our assumption that it is possible to do automated disease detection based on optical eye images, the project goes ahead. In all other cases, either more modeling is needed or the initial assumption is not supportable and hence the project must be stopped in the design phase. Once modeling results have been obtained, they can be used for testing in a later stage of the project. Modeling and testing are a necessary part of the design methodology which aims to support the creation of reliable and trustworthy biomedical processing systems.

14.7 Acronyms

AMD	Age-related macular degeneration
CAD	Computer-aided diagnosis
CWT	Continuous wavelet transform
DWT	Discrete wavelet transform
FHI	Fuchs' heterochromic iridocyclitis
FD	Fractal dimension
FFT	Fast Fourier transform
FN	False negative
FP	False positive
H_2	Logarithmic amplitudes of diagonal elements in the bispectrum
H	Hurst exponent
HOS	Higher-order spectra
LASIK	Laser-assisted *in situ* keratomileusis
M_{ave}	Mean magnitude of the bispectrum
MIF	Migration inhibitory factor
NN	Neural network
OCT	Optical coherence tomography
P_h	Bispectral phase entropy
PRK	Photorefractive keratectomy

---

* Where the system expects this input.

RBF   Radial basis function
SVM   Support vector machine
TN   True negative
TP   True positive
WCOB   Weighted center of bispectrum
WHO   World Health Organization

References

1. S. Resnikoff, D. Pascolini, S. P. Mariotti, and G. P. Pokharel. Global magnitude of visual impairment caused by uncorrected refractive errors in 2004. *Bulletin of the World Health Organization* 86.1 (2004), pp. 1–80.
2. S. Resnikoff, D. Pascolini, D. Etya'ale, I. Kocur, R. Pararajasegaram, G. P. Pokharel, and S. P. Mariotti. Policy and Practice: Global data on visual impairment in the year 2002. *Bulletin of the World Health Organization* 82 (2004), pp. 844–851.
3. A. Foster. Vision 2020: The cataract challenge. *Community Eye Health* 13(34) (2000), 17–19.
4. O. Faust, U. R. Acharya, and T. Tamura. Formal design methods for reliable computer aided diagnosis: A review. *IEEE Review in Biomedical Engineering* 5 (2012), 15–28.
5. A. M. Turing. On computable numbers, with an application to the entscheidungsproblem. *Proceedings of the London Mathematical Society.* 42 (1936), 230–265.
6. O. Faust, U. Acharya, B. Sputh, and T. Tamura. Design of a fault-tolerant decision-making system for biomedical applications. *Computational Methods Biomechanics and Biomedical Engineering* 16(7) (2013), 725–735.
7. O. Faust, R. Shetty, V. S. Sree, S. Acharya, U. R. Acharya, E. Ng, C. Poo, and J. S. Suri. Towards the systematic development of medical networking technology. *Journal of Medical Systems* 35(6) (2010), 1431–1445.
8. R. Fletcher, D. Still, and R. J. Allen. *Eye Examination and Refraction.* Wiley, New York, 1998.
9. C. R. S. Jackson and R. D. Finlay. *The Eye in General Practice.* Churchill Livingstone, London, 1991.
10. L. A. Remington. *Clinical Anatomy of the Visual System.* Elsevier, St. Louis; MO, 2005.
11. R. S. Snell and M. A. Lemp. *Clinical Anatomy of the Eye.* Blackwell Science, Malden, MA, 1998.
12. L. Zangwill, I. Irak, C. C. Berry, V. Garden, M. S. Lima, and R. N. Weinreb. Effect of cataract and pupil size on image quality with confocal scanning laser ophthalmoscopy. *Archives of Ophthalmology* 115(8) (1997), 983–990.
13. C. K. Job and K. Thompson. Histopathological features of lepromatous iridocyclitis: A case report. *International Journal of Leprosy and Other Mycobacterial Diseases* 66(1) (1998), 29–33.
14. S. K. Ganesh, S. Sharma, K. M. Narayana, and J. Biswas. Fuchs' heterochromic iridocyclitis following bilateral ocular toxoplasmosis. *Ocular Immunology and Inflammation* 12(1) (2004), 75–77.
15. N. Kitaichi, S. Kotake, Y. Mizue, H. Matsuda, K. Onoé, and J. Nishihira. Increase of macrophage migration inhibitory factor in sera of patients with iridocyclitis. *British Journal of Ophthalmology* 84(12) (2000), 1423–1425.
16. S. Prahalad and M. H. Passo. Long-term outcome among patients with juvenile rheumatoid arthritis. *Frontiers in Bioscience* 3 (1998), e13–e22.
17. S. A. Greenstein, K. L. Fry, J. Bhatt, and P. S. Hersh. Natural history of corneal haze after collagen crosslinking for keratoconus and corneal ectasia: Scheimpflug and biomicroscopic analysis. *Journal of Cataract & Refractive Surgery* 36(12) (2010), 2105–2114.
18. R. Ambrósio and S. E. Wilson. LASIK vs LASEK vs PRK: Advantages and indications. *Seminars in Ophthalmology* 18(1) (2003), 2–10.
19. J. M. Emery and J. H. Little. *Phacoemulsification and Aspiration of Cataracts: Surgical Techniques, Complications, and Results.* Mosby, St. Louis, MO, 1979.

20. S. Helgason. *The Radon Transform: Progress in Mathematics*. Birkhäuser, Boston, MA, 1999.
21. U. R. Acharya, C. K. Chua, E. Y. Ng, W. Yu, and C. Chee. Application of higher order spectra for the identification of diabetes retinopathy stages. *Journal of Medical Systems* 32(6) (2008), 481–488.
22. K. C. Chua, V. Chandran, U. R. Acharya, and C. M. Lim. Application of higher order statistics/spectra in biomedical signals—A review. *Medical Engineering & Physics* 32(7) (2010), 679–689.
23. C. L. Nikias and A. P. Petropulu. *Higher-Order Spectra Analysis: A Nonlinear Signal Processing Framework*. Prentice Hall signal processing series. PTR Prentice Hall, Englewood Cliffs, NJ, 1993.
24. K. C. Chua, V. Chandran, U. R. Acharya, and C. M. Lim. Cardiac state diagnosis using higher order spectra of heart rate variability. *Journal of Medical Engineering & Technology* 32(2) (2008), 145–155.
25. K. C. Chua, V. Chandran, U. Rajendra Acharya, and C. M. Lim. Analysis of epileptic EEG signals using higher order spectra. *Journal of Medical Engineering & Technology* 33(1) (2009), 42–50.
26. M. Vetterli and C. Herley. Wavelets and filter banks: Theory and design. *IEEE Transactions on Signal Processing* 40(9) (1992), 2207–2232.
27. S. Dua, U. R. Acharya, P. Chowriappa, and S. V. Sree. Wavelet-based energy features for glaucomatous image classification. *IEEE Transactions on Information Technology in Biomedicine* 16(1) (2012), 80–87.
28. H. Yuan, J. Gao, H. Z. Guo, and C. Lu. An efficient method to process the quantized acoustoelectric current: Wavelet transform. *IEEE Transactions on Instrumentation and Measurement* 60(3) (2011), 696–702.
29. E.-L. Chen, P.-C. Chung, C.-L. Chen, H.-M. Tsai, and C.-I. Chang. An automatic diagnostic system for CT liver image classification. *IEEE Transactions on Biomedical Engineering* 45(6) (1998), 783–794.
30. C. S. Fortin, R. Kumaresan, W. J. Ohley, and S. Hoefer. Fractal dimension in the analysis of medical images. *Engineering in Medicine and Biology Magazine, IEEE* 11(2) (1992), pp. 65–71.
31. T. Lundahl, W. J. Ohley, S. M. Kay, and R. Siffert. Fractional Brownian motion: A maximum likelihood estimator and its application to image texture. *IEEE Transactions on Medical Imaging* 5(3) (1986), 152–161.
32. B. B. Mandelbrot. *The Fractal Geometry of Nature*. W. H. Freeman, New York, 1983.
33. M. K. Biswas, T. Ghose, S. Guha, and P. K. Biswas. Fractal dimension estimation for texture images: A parallel approach. *Pattern Recognition Letters* 19(3–4) (1998), 309–313.
34. J. F. Box. Guinness, Gosset, Fisher, and small samples. *Statistical Science* 2(1) (1987), 45–52.
35. C. A. Boneau. The effects of violations of assumptions underlying the *t* test. *Psychological Bulletin* 57(1) (1960), 49–64.
36. I. Steinwart and A. Christmann. *Support Vector Machines. Information Science and Statistics*. Springer, New York, 2008.
37. V. N. Vapnik. *The Nature of Statistical Learning Theory*. Springer-Verlag, New York, 1995.
38. V. N. Vapnik. *Estimation of Dependences Based on Empirical Data (Springer Series in Statistics)*. Springer-Verlag, Secaucus, NJ, 1982.
39. N. Archer, U. Fevrier-Thomas, C. Lokker, K. A. McKibbon, and S. E. Straus. Personal health records: A scoping review. *Journal of the American Medical Informatics Association* 18(4) (2011), 515–522.
40. D. Detmer, M. Bloomrosen, B. Raymond, and P. Tang. Integrated personal health records: Transformative tools for consumer-centric care. *BMC Medical Informatics and Decision Making* 8(1) (2008), 1–45.
41. J. S. Duncan and N. Ayache. Medical image analysis: Progress over two decades and the challenges ahead. *IEEE Transactions on Pattern Analysis and Machine Intelligence* 22(1) (2000), 85–106.
42. A. Burgun and O. Bodenreider. Accessing and integrating data and knowledge for biomedical research. *Yearbook of Medical Informatics* (2008), 91–101.

43. K. Doi. Computer-aided diagnosis in medical imaging: Historical review, current status and future potential. *Computerized Medical Imaging and Graphics* 31(4–5) (2007), 198–211.

44. U. R. Acharya, O. Faust, V. S. Sree, F. Molinari, and J. S. Suri. ThyroScreen system: High resolution ultrasound thyroid image characterization into benign and malignant classes using novel combination of texture and discrete wavelet transform. *Computer Methods and Programs in Biomedicine* 107(2) (2012), 233–241.

45. K. Doi. Current status and future potential of computer-aided diagnosis in medical imaging. *British Journal of Radiology* 78(Suppl. 1) (2005), S3–S19.

46. K. Doi, M. Giger, R. Nishikawa, K. Hoffmann, H. MacMahon, and R. Schmidt. Potential usefulness of digital imaging in clinical diagnostic radiology: Computer-aided diagnosis. *Journal of Digital Imaging* 8 (1995), 2–7.

47. H. P. Chan, K. Doi, S. Galhotra, C. J. Vyborny, H. MacMahon, and P. M. Jokich. Image feature analysis and computer-aided diagnosis in digital radiography. I: Automated detection of microcalcifications in mammography. *Journal of Medical Physics* 14(4) (1987), 538–548.

48. Z. Song, Z. Ji, J.-G. Ma, B. H. C. Sputh, U. R. Acharya, and O. Faust. A systematic approach to embedded biomedical decision making. *Computer Methods and Programs in Biomedicine* 108(2) (2012), 656–664.

49. J. Kent S. Hoo and S. T. C. Wong. Information system modeling for biomedical imaging applications. In: *Medical Imaging 1999: PACS Design and Evaluation: Engineering and Clinical Issues*, Eds G. J. Blaine and S. C. Horii, Vol. 3662, pp. 202–208. SPIE, San Diego, CA, 1999.

50. K.-S. Lee and K. Lee. Framework of an evolutionary design system incorporating design information and history. *Computers in Industry* 44(3) (2001), 205–227.

51. C. Haubelt, J. Falk, J. Keinert, T. Schlichter, M. Streubühr, A. Deyhle, A. Hadert, and J. Teich. A systemC-based design methodology for digital signal processing systems. *EURASIP Journal on Embedded Systems* 2007(1) (2007), 15–15.

52. O. Faust, U. R. Acharya, B. H. C. Sputh, and L. C. Min. Systems engineering principles for the design of biomedical signal processing systems. *Computer Methods and Programs in Biomedicine* 102(3) (2011), 267–276.

53. L. Hefetz, Y. Domnitz, D. Haviv, D. Krakowsky, Y. Kibarsky, S. Abrahami, and P. Nemet. Influence of patient age on refraction and corneal haze after photorefractive keratectomy. *British Journal of Ophthalmology* 81(8) (1997), 637–638.

54. K. Nakamura, D. Kurosaka, H. Bissen-Miyajima, and K. Tsubota. Intact corneal epithelium is essential for the prevention of stromal haze after laser assisted in situ keratomileusis. *British Journal of Ophthalmology* 85(2) (2001), 209–213.

55. M. D. Twa, S. Parthasarathy, C. Roberts, A. M. Mahmoud, T. W. Raasch, and M. A. Bullimore. Automated decision tree classification of corneal shape. *Optometry & Vision Science* 82(12) (2005), 1038–1046.

56. A. Laties, E. Keates, E. Lippa, C. Shear, D. Snavely, M. Tupy-Visich, and A. N. Chremos. Field test reliability of a new lens opacity rating system utilizing slit-lamp examination. *Lens and Eye Toxicity Research* 6(3) (1989), 443–464.

57. J. M. Sparrow, W. Ayliffe, A. J. Bron, N. P. Brown, and A. R. Hill. Inter-observer and intra-observer variability of the oxford clinical cataract classification and grading system. *International Ophthalmology* 11(3) (1988), 151–157.

58. A. Laties, E. Keates, E. Lippa, C. Shear, D. Snavely, M. Tupy-Visich, and A. N. Chremos. The age-related eye disease study (AREDS) system for classifying cataracts from photographs: AREDS report no. 4. *Lens and Eye Toxicity Research* 6(3) (1989), 443–464.

59. O. Hockwin. Cataract classification. *Documenta Ophthalmologica* 88(3) (1995), 263–275.

60. L. A. Carvalho. Preliminary results of neural networks and zernike polynomials for classification of videokeratography maps. *Optometry & Vision Science* 82(2) (2005), 151–158.

61. Z. Burgansky-Eliash, G. Wollstein, T. Chu, J. D. Ramsey, C. Glymour, R. J. Noecker, H. Ishikawa, and J. S. Schuman. Optical coherence tomography machine learning classifiers for glaucoma detection: A preliminary study. *Investigative Ophthalmology & Visual Science* 46(11) (2005), 4147–4152.

62. G. Grabner, R. Eilmsteiner, C. Steindl, J. Ruckhofer, R. Mattioli, and W. Husinsky. Dynamic corneal imaging. *Journal of Cataract & Refractive Surgery* 31(1) (2005), 163–174.
63. Age-Related Eye Disease Study Research Group. The age-related eye disease study (AREDS) system for classifying cataracts from photographs: AREDS report no. 4. *American Journal of Ophthalmology* 131(2) (2001), 167–175.

15

Modeling of Laser-Induced Thermal Damage to the Retina and the Cornea

Mathieu Jean and Karl Schulmeister

CONTENTS

15.1 Introduction

The very properties that make laser radiation a valuable tool in many fields—namely its high intensity and collimation—are also the critical reasons for potential eye and skin hazards (Sliney and Freasier 1973; Henderson and Schulmeister 2001). In general, optical radiation—be it ultraviolet, visible light, or infrared—is absorbed in the superficial layers of the body due to its high water content (mostly relevant for infrared) and the various pigments and chromophores it contains (mostly relevant in the ultraviolet and visible ranges). The absorbed energy can then be converted into a thermoelastic pressure wave and heat, and can even trigger chemical reactions. All these interactions can ultimately lead to tissue damage if injury thresholds are exceeded. Among all organs, the eye is by far the most sensitive as it combines several critical factors: (i) pigments and water-based constituents provide high absorption capacity, (ii) irradiance can be greatly increased as optical radiation is focused onto the retina, and (iii) a lesion is rarely reversible and can be severely impairing.

Exposure limits for laser-based applications are first set in guidelines by expert committees such as the International Commission on Non-Ionizing Radiation Protection (ICNIRP), then adopted by IEC 60825-1 on an international level or ANSI Z136 in the United States. These guidelines are based on experimentally determined levels of minimal injuries that—combined with an appropriate safety factor—correspond conceptually to an acceptable hazard level (known as maximum permissible exposure or exposure limit). The experimental basis consists of identifying just-discernible lesions ophthalmoscopically assessed in the hours following exposure under laboratory conditions (typically 1–48 h). The so-called minimum visible lesion (MVL) is the standard threshold in the field of laser safety. Rabbits and macaque monkeys usually serve as experimental models to provide threshold data for the human cornea and retina, respectively. However, given the time-consuming nature of the experiments as well as ethical and economical considerations, the experimental approach cannot solely provide all necessary information or encompass all potential exposures. Computer modeling therefore is an appealing complementary support for safety questions and for improving scientific knowledge of laser–tissue interactions.

In this chapter, we concentrate on the investigation of thermally induced threshold damage to the cornea and retina (discussion on photochemical and mechanical interactions can be found in, for instance, Glickman 2002). We describe the fundamns of physics-based models intended for this specific laser–tissue interaction and for reproducing experimental threshold values. We briefly review the optics of the eye and the optics of layered tissues and discuss setting up the bioheat equation and modeling the occurrence of macroscopic damage.

15.2 Beam Propagation in the Eye

In principle, laser-induced threshold damage levels depend on three parameters: exposure duration, wavelength, and—as long as the damage mechanism is thermal in nature—the size of the irradiated area (or spot size). In the case of retinal exposure, exposure duration and intraocular power are known but the retinal spot size cannot be directly measured. Only the beam divergence and source size are systematically measured while the irradiance profile at the retina has to be predicted mathematically.

The optics of the eye has been extensively studied in recent decades and precise data on various ocular properties are available. However, a simple and accurate representation of the retinal image is not straightforward and is complicated by the fact that it depends on many anatomical factors specific to the involved subject: instantaneous refractive state, local ocular aberrations, eccentricity, intraocular inhomogeneities, pupil size, and more (Milsom et al. 2006). Moreover, dynamic effects may play a crucial role: residual eye movements for long exposures or thermal lensing in the case of strongly attenuated infrared-A (IR-A) wavelengths (780–1400 nm, due to high irradiance levels within the lens in Maxwellian view for instance; Vincelette et al. 2008). Nevertheless, all these phenomena tend to increase the power level required to induce a lesion, which implies that— when addressing the question of safety limits—only the worst cases must be predicted accurately.

15.3 Minimum Spot Size

Investigators in the field of laser-induced damage to the retina designate the radial extent of light absorption within the retina—and the following source term in the heat equation—as spot size. A major challenge lies in the determination of the *minimum* spot size. The determination of a characteristic lower limit to the focus of a collimated laser beam is crucial for setting safety guidelines (see discussion in Sliney 2005) since the threshold level varies with the square of the spot size for short exposures and linearly for longer ones. Yet, recent experimental results show strong evidence that thresholds do not further decrease for spot sizes below 70–100 μm (i.e., beam divergence ~5 mrad; Lund et al. 2007; Zuclich et al. 2008).

Attempts to achieve best-focused retinal spots show that the spot size can be reduced further on purpose in specific conditions; for example, by optimizing the beam positioning in order to avoid ocular inhomogeneities (Birngruber et al. 1979) or by using wavefront correction (Lund et al. 2008b). In an idealized aberration-free rhesus monkey eye, with a beam diameter at the cornea of, say 4 mm, and a laser wavelength of 590 nm, the diffraction-limited beam waist diameter approaches 3–4 μm. Investigators have traditionally assumed that retinal diameters smaller than 20–30 μm are not achievable in the typical conditions of laser-induced threshold lesion experiments (guidelines assume 25.5 μm for the human eye), but for the purpose of modeling, this consensus is questioned and assumptions such as 60–70 μm (Connolly et al. 1978) are more common (Welch et al.1979; Lund et al. 2008a).

Only intraocular scattering is unlikely to enlarge the retinal spot size to such an extent since the postulated retinal image is approximately one order of magnitude above the limit of diffraction and smaller spots have been measured *in vivo* (Birngruber et al. 1979). However, scattering does reduce the part of energy contained in the central portion of the spot. For instance, if only 40% of the energy reaching the retina is efficiently focused (Birngruber et al. 1983), then additional input power is required in order to compensate for this loss. But in modeling, such widening of the retinal irradiance distribution is usually not directly modeled, but can be accounted for by defining an enlarged *effective* spot. As an attempt to account for the relative impact of scattering, an alternative can consist of considering a reduced spot-size-dependent ocular transmission (Jean and Schulmeister 2013).

Intraretinal scattering has also been suggested as a reason for augmenting the radial extent of light distribution at the retinal pigment epithelium (RPE) in the extrafoveal region (Welch et al. 1979; Schulmeister et al. 2006). Another possible explanation for the discrepancy between observed thresholds and model predictions in the minimal spot size regime involves limitations in the experimental detection techniques. According to this hypothesis, the absolute minimum lesions are not detectable by ophthalmoscopy and the ophthalmoscopically observed lesions are actually above threshold (Davis and Mautner 1969). Meanwhile, awaiting strong evidence of a reliable minimum spot size, the current uncertainty necessitates safety factors between experimentally found thresholds and exposure limits to be of about 10 for collimated laser beams (Schulmeister et al. 2011).

15.4 Optical Models

15.4.1 Single Lens Approximation

Several investigators have shown that the retinal spot size can be measured *in vivo* using invasive techniques (Sanders 1974; Birngruber et al. 1979). In the case of extended sources, the following linear relationship between source size θ and retinal spot size d, $d = \theta f$, yields acceptable results (assuming a relaxed eye; θ in milliradians, d and the focal length f in millimeters; see Figure 15.1a). Here the eye is considered as a single thin lens in air and in the paraxial approximation, source size and image size are linearly related. However, this does not hold for collimated beams. Moreover, it has to be considered that the focal length of an optical system depends on the wavelength of radiation, implying that chromatic dispersion can increase the spot size beyond its reference value. In the relaxed eye, a collimated beam reaches focus at the retinal plane for 590 nm (Atchison and Smith 2002; the helium d line at 587.6 nm is often used as a reference for estimating chromatic dispersion of materials such as in the Abbe value). A first refinement is thus to account for chromatic dispersion such as $d(\lambda) = \theta f(\lambda)$ (Figure 15.1c). The wavelength-dependent focal

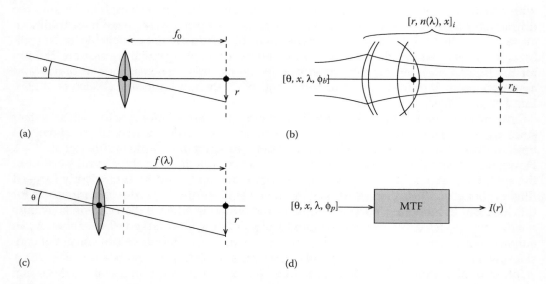

FIGURE 15.1
Review of optical models used in modeling of threshold damage to the retina (θ, subtense angle; f, focal length; λ, wavelength; rb, spot radius; x, position; ϕ_b, beam diameter; ϕ_p, pupil diameter; r, radius of curvature; n, index of refraction; I, intensity). (From (a) Henderson, R. and Schulmeister, K., *Laser Safety*, Taylor & Francis, New York, 2004. (b) Birngruber, R., Gabel, V.-P., and Hillenkamp, F., *Health Phys*, 44, 519–531, 1983. (c) Vincelette, R.L., Rockwell, B.A., Oliver, J.W., et al., *Laser Surg Med*, 41, 382–390, 2009. (d) Takata, A.N., Kuan, L.P., Goldfinch, L., Thomopoulis, N., Hinds, J.K., and Weigandt, A., Thermal model of laser-induced eye damage, USAF School of Aerospace Medicine, Brooks City-Base, TX, 1974.)

length is obtained from refractive error measurements and a wavelength of reference. The refractive error or chromatic difference of refraction can be expressed as:

$$R(\lambda) = \frac{1}{f_0} - \frac{1}{f(\lambda)}$$

The chromatic difference of refraction (in diopters) can be fitted by polynomials (Atchison and Smith 2005), thus obtaining a first estimate of the wavelength-dependent image size. This approach has been used, for instance, to extrapolate damage thresholds from one wavelength to others (this procedure is sometimes referred to as action spectrum, Lund et al. 2008a). The proposed dispersion equations slightly overestimate dispersion in the IR-A range (Vincelette et al. 2008). However, this representation still cannot provide a reliable measure of the retinal image in the case of either a collimated beam near best focus or varying iris apertures.

15.4.2 Ray Tracing

Since the single thin lens approach is too coarse for representing the complexity of the eye, ray-tracing methods provide a finer view of more complex optical systems such as thick lenses. Basically, each ocular tissue—that is, cornea, aqueous chamber, lens, and vitreous—can be treated as a homogeneous medium delimited by two refractive surfaces, each having a given curvature. Their combination forms the schematic eye, whose primary task is to reproduce the optical properties of a system (see cardinal points) by adequately designing geometrical and optical properties: radii of curvature and spacing between surfaces, and indices of refraction, respectively (Figure 15.1b; more details in Atchison and Smith 2002).

Since chromatic aberration is the most dominant source of spot size variation—besides beam divergence—and because interindividual variations are minimized by the averaging effect of using several animals, a schematic eye is a convenient approach for including wavelength-dependent refractive indices. Formulae such as Cornu and Herzberger equations provide reasonable fitting of refractive error (the Herzberger equation is more appropriate in the IR-A range; Atchison and Smith 2005). Schematic eyes can also include complex properties such as asphericity, gradient refractive index, and eccentricity (e.g., tilt for modeling astigmatism).

A schematic eye is a useful basis for the application of ray transfer matrix analysis—also known as ABCD matrix analysis—where each component of the system is represented in a second-order matrix. In the paraxial approximation, both phenomena—propagation and refraction—are linear transformations of the input ray with respect to its angle:

$$\text{Propagation:} \begin{bmatrix} 1 & d \\ 0 & 1 \end{bmatrix} \quad \text{Refraction:} \begin{bmatrix} 1 & 0 \\ \dfrac{n_{in} - n_{out}}{R\,n_{out}} & \dfrac{n_{in}}{n_{out}} \end{bmatrix}$$

where d, n, and R stand for distance, index of refraction, and radius of curvature, respectively. Consequently, the combination of all optical elements is achieved by matrix multiplications.

$$M_{\text{eye}} = M_n \cdot M_{n-1} \cdot \ldots \cdot M_0$$

For Gaussian beams, input and output rays are computed in the form of a basis vector incorporating the complex beam parameter. The image size can thus be calculated at any axial position. In ocular lesion experiments, lasers are often operated in the fundamental transversal mode in which the laser beam exhibits axial symmetry and its profile is described by a Gaussian function. This property is very convenient since a Gaussian profile remains Gaussian after transformation by an optical system. An in-depth discussion on ray transfer matrix analysis can be found in Gerrard and Burch (1994). Schematic eyes downscaled from human to monkey and ray-tracing methods have already been applied in laser-induced retinal damage modeling (e.g., Rockwell et al. 1997; Birngruber et al. 1983).

15.4.3 Modulation Transfer Function

The eye can be conceived as a linear and time-invariant system described by its modulation transfer function, that is, the Fourier transform of the point spread function (Figure 15.1d). This analytic method exhibits peculiar advantages, namely its validity for any source profile and the consideration of any kind of linear transformation, scattering, and attenuation (attenuation must be considered separately in geometrical optics). However, this method is not easily applicable in practice since the function needs to be measured at every single wavelength of the spectrum and requires a large number of subjects for averaging purposes. Consequently, this approach has not yet been used for retinal injury threshold modeling, but it is worth consideration for future efforts. An interesting way of formulating wavelength and eccentricity components is proposed by Hodgkinson et al. (1994).

From scalar diffraction theory, especially in the Fresnel approximation, that is, near field, a formulation of the Fourier transform of the pupil can be obtained as a combination of aberration and defocusing phase functions. The near-field approximation is valid for all relevant values of pupil size and wavelength. Formulation and appropriate parameters have been developed by Takata et al. (1974).

15.4.4 Practical Aspects

A comparison of the results obtained by ray transfer matrix analysis and diffraction theory is shown in Figure 15.2 (applied by Jean and Schulmeister (2013) and Takata et al. (1974), respectively). As in laser-induced damage experiments, we consider the rhesus monkey eye in a relaxed state (after anesthetization) and fully dilated (pupil diameter 7 mm).

Aberrations of high order and diffraction by the pupil have a limited impact on spot size but they do modify the wide-angle irradiance profile on the retina. The one obtained from the diffraction theory has more pronounced tails than the Gaussian function assumed in ray tracing. This effect is also observed in the study of intraocular forward scattering, where energy is spread over a few degrees while the spot itself contains only 40%–50% of the transmitted intraocular energy (Birngruber et al. 1979). Even though there are some discrepancies, both models show to what extent the retinal spot size is affected by chromatic aberrations.

It should be mentioned that small-scale variations of the spot size—in the order of micrometers—have no direct effect on retinal damage levels for various reasons: (i) inter-individual and interlocation variations are randomly distributed, (ii) heat diffusion overcomes these irregularities within a few microseconds, that is, shorter than the thermal

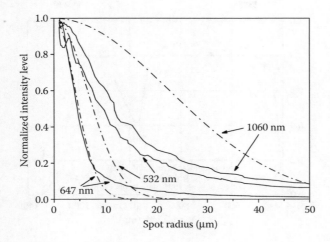

FIGURE 15.2
Retinal intensity distribution at three wavelengths from two models: modulation transfer function (solid line) and ray tracing (dashed line).

damage regime, and (iii) damage is detected at a larger scale, that is, at least over a few tenths of micrometers (see Section 15.8). Consequently, light distribution at the retinal plane is commonly treated as a simple mathematical function (such as Gauss) and parameterized only by its diameter. Further refinements are thought not to be critical for the purpose of modeling retinal injury, except if minimum retinal spot sizes can be proven to be of the order of 10 μm or smaller.

15.5 Ocular Transmission

A critical aspect is the degree of ocular transmission, which, in the range of 400–1400 nm, varies between practically 0% and 80%. This optical property is commonly obtained from *ex vivo* measurements (e.g., Boettner and Dankovic 1974). Two types of measurements are available, referred to as direct and total transmission. Transmitted light is distinguished into the part of collimated light (typically within 1°) associated with direct transmission and the part of both collimated and diffuse light (i.e., within almost 180°) associated with total transmission. We use these two types of characterization for representing ocular transmission for collimated beams and extended sources, respectively. However, no data are available for in-between cases. Attenuation is assumed to follow the Beer–Lambert law.

Above approximately 1150 nm, the eye filters optical radiation similarly to pure water (van den Berg and Spekreijse 1997) and transmission can be modeled well by considering a 19 mm equivalent path length of water for the young rhesus monkey eye (Bradley et al. 1999). At shorter wavelengths, the transmission spectra of water and those of all ocular tissues diverge significantly from each other. In the visible spectrum, the cornea exhibits the highest optical density while the lens and the cornea steeply cut off transmission below approximately 400 nm. Figure 15.3 shows the spectral optical density of the young rhesus monkey eye for both transmission types (direct and total) along with the pure water model. Attenuation is assumed to follow the Beer–Lambert law in both cases.

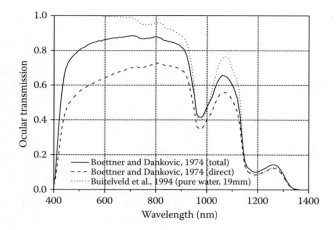

FIGURE 15.3
Transmission of the rhesus monkey eye (solid and dashed lines) and of pure water (dotted line).

15.6 Optical Properties of Ocular Tissues

15.6.1 Retina

The sketch in Figure 15.4 schematically depicts a section of the retina. In principle, optical radiation strikes the back of the eye at the neural retina and to a large degree passes through the photoreceptors. The underlying layers—RPE, choriocapillaris, and choroid—are primarily devoted to anatomically and physiologically supporting the sensory organ, but they also play a determinant role in light absorption. A reasonable physiological

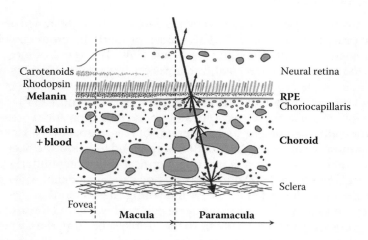

FIGURE 15.4
Section of the primate retina with emphasis on pigments (labeled on the left) and the most relevant layers (labeled on the right). Idealized light paths are indicated (arrows). Retinal areas of importance are labeled at the bottom.

explanation is that the highly absorbing RPE layer eliminates backscattering, thereby improving image contrast. Furthermore, pigmentation of the RPE shields the cell nucleus from phototoxic UV radiation. A pernicious effect of the highly absorbing layer is that the retina becomes more vulnerable regarding thermal injury from exposure to intense light.

In terms of light absorption, the retina can be reduced to two relevant layers, namely RPE and choroid. They both contain melanosomes, the primary retinal absorber in the wavelength range from approximately 300 to 1200 nm. Additionally, there are many other relatively minor absorbers: oxyhemoglobin and melanocytes in the choroid, lipofuscin and derivates in the RPE, carotenoids (yellow pigments) in Henle's fiber layer (Borland et al. 1992), and rhodopsin contained in the photoreceptors (Figure 15.5).

In the RPE (a single-cell layer), the melanosomes—approximately 1 μm large spheroids—are densely packed in the apical half of the cuboidal cells. Locally, the spacing between granules varies between 0 and 2 μm. Since we are investigating thermally induced damage, the exposure duration of interest starts in the order of 10–50 μs (concerning shorter pulses, the mechanism of damage is microbubble formation; Lee and Alt 2007; Schüle et al. 2005). As a consequence, local variations shorter than the thermal diffusion length can be neglected. Assuming that the surrounding medium has thermal properties similar to water, the diffusion length already reaches 2.5 μm at 10 μs. It is therefore justified to consider bulk absorption in the apical portion of the RPE, which moreover simplifies both the treatment of light distribution and solving of the heat equation (see further discussion in Section 15.7.1).

The measurement of absorption properties in solutions of extracted melanosomes is very sensitive to the experimental approach (Stolarski et al. 2002) and it cannot be directly applied to the RPE since the concentration *in situ* is not identical. Furthermore, data over the whole spectral range of interest are—to the knowledge of the authors—not available. The optical density of the RPE as a whole has been measured *in vitro* for the wavelength range of 400–1100 nm (Gabel et al. 1976), 1200 nm (Coogan et al. 1974), and 1500 nm (Geeraets et al. 1962). The data from Gabel are commonly used in a mathematical description of RPE bulk absorption. A fitting equation was first proposed by Jacques et al. (1996).

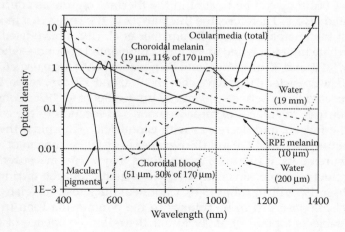

FIGURE 15.5
Optical density of various ocular absorbers. (Thicknesses taken from Jean, M. and Schulmeister, K., Validation of a computer model to predict laser-induced thermal injury thresholds to the retina. In: *ILSC 2013 Conference Proceedings*, Laser Insitute of America 1002:229–238, 2013.)

Similar expressions in exponential or power functions are found in Vincelette et al. (2008) and Jean and Schulmeister (2013).

In the choroid, the distribution of melanosomes is much sparser as well as inhomogeneous (i.e., there is significant clustering). However, again, the assumption of a homogeneous distribution can be argued to be valid for pulse durations that are relevant for thermal injury. Indeed, since damage is mainly located at the RPE level (see Section 15.8), local variations of several tenths of micrometers in the choroid do not affect temperature diffusion as seen from the RPE. It is, however, critical to define both an appropriate equivalent layer thickness and its separation distance to the RPE, considering the observation that the outer choroid can appear under the light microscope more than two times darker than its inner part (Weiter et al. 1986).

The choroid is densely perfused by vessels of various sizes and bordered by a dense network of capillaries (Spraul et al. 1996) in which blood is highly oxygenated (~95%, commonly assimilated to pure oxyhemoglobin; Berendschot et al. 2003). With a concentration of 30%–50% in blood (e.g., Hammer et al. 1995), the red pigment found in red blood cells is a relevant absorber for wavelengths shorter than approximately 590 nm (Figure 15.5). Similarly to melanin, heterogeneous blood distribution is not critical and the choriocapillaris can also be modeled as a homogeneous blood layer with a representative absorption coefficient.

In the central region of the retina (Hammond et al. 1997), Henle's fiber layer (see Figure 15.4) possesses distinctive pigments that selectively absorb blue light (thus called yellow pigment). They are carotenoids such as xanthophylls and zeaxanthins whose function is to shield the photoreceptors from phototoxicity (Snodderly et al. 1991) induced by high-energy photons (sometimes referred to as actinic radiation). A formula in the form of exponential functions has been derived by Zagers and van Norren (2004) for their absorption spectrum (Figure 15.5).

15.6.1.1 Distribution of Absorbers and Layer Geometry

As seen previously, the various layers are heterogeneously pigmented from an anatomical point of view, but they can be treated in the thermal regime as equivalent homogeneously pigmented layers. Therefore, the thicknesses of the layers in a model may not be representative of the anatomical ones. Birngruber et al. (1985) have used three layers—RPE, an intermediate nonpigmented layer, and a pigmented choroid—whose thicknesses are, respectively, 5, 25, and 80 µm; Vogel and Birngruber (1992) have used 6, 4, and 400 µm, while Jean and Schulmeister (2013) have chosen 10, 4, and 170 µm, respectively. The RPE cell height is expected to lie between 10 and 12 µm (Gabel et al. 1976; Coogan et al. 1974), depending on sources, references of measurement, and location in the retinal map. It is the thickest at the foveola and decreases with eccentricity. Choroidal thickness is often reported to be between 80 and 170 µm (Birngruber et al. 1985; Coogan et al. 1974) following *in vitro* measurements. It has to be emphasized that *in vivo* measurements can yield up to a twofold thicker tissue, since large vessels usually collapse during manipulation (Delori and Pflibsen 1989; Birngruber 1991). Choroidal thickness, correlated with size and density of vessels, is observed to be thinner in the paramacula than in the macula of elderly human subjects (Spraul et al. 1996) but there is no evidence of any significant change over the region of interest for laser-induced damage studies in young monkey subjects (typically the central 30°).

Between the pigmented layers, the pigment-free volume consists of the basal part of RPE cells (~3–5 µm) and Bruch's membrane (3 µm in elderly human subjects; Spraul et al. 1996), and the innermost layer of the choroid is sometimes also included (about 20 μm, Birngruber et al. 1985). Such a separation distance between the RPE and pigmented choroid has an effect of several tenths of a microsecond in delaying the heat wave traveling from the choroid toward the RPE (the RPE is the critical layer for thermal injury at threshold level). Therefore, it has a minor effect, only impacting very short pulses or exposures at the long wavelength end of IR-A where the choroid plays an important role.

15.6.1.2 Regional Variations

Also of importance is the variation of morphology throughout the retinal surface. Photoreceptor distribution, vessel density, layer thickness, cell dimensions, and pigment concentration are more or less concentric functions centered about the foveal pit. Concentric regions of importance in laser-induced damage experiments are marked in Figure 15.4.

The RPE cell diameter increases with distance from the foveola: the diameter reaches 13.5 μm on average at the foveola and 18 μm at 2–4 mm from the center (Snodderly et al. 2002). It follows that RPE cell density is twice as large in the foveal region as in the outer regions of the retina. Even if the melanosome concentration (per cell) is slightly lower in the macula than in the peripheral region (Feeney-Burns et al. 1984), pigment concentration per surface area, and consequently local optical density, is higher within the central portion (Weiter et al. 1986). Since RPE melanin also plays a role in protecting the retina from oxidative stress (Sarna 1992; Wang et al. 2006), this change in pigment concentration is consistent with the increased density of photoreceptors and subsequent metabolic activity in the central retina (Wikler and Rakic 1990). In the same fashion, fluorescence, which is correlated with the amount of RPE melanin and its derivates, reveals a Gaussian-shaped distribution almost centered about the fovea in human subjects (Keilhauer and Delori 2006). Finally, RPE light transmission measurement allows quantification of this variation: the central region absorbs about 75% more energy than the paramacula (at approximately 3 mm away from the foveola; Gabel et al. 1978). These variations are large enough to necessitate differentiating model parameters for central or peripheral exposures. Threshold lesions require between 25% and 100% more energy in the paramacula than in the macula (for instance, see Cain et al. 2000; Lappin 1971). Variable regional sensitivities can be simulated by modifying pigment concentration or layer thickness. In the latter approach, the difference vanishes if diffusion is negligible or if the absorption depth is shorter than the layer thickness, that is, short pulse duration and short wavelength, respectively.

15.6.1.3 Fundus Reflectance

Due to the presence of scatterers and layers of varying refractive indices, diffuse and specular reflections occur in the retina. Backscattered light from the back of the eye (fundus) is used to examine the retina noninvasively. Since the spectral distribution of reflected light depends on the optical density of the various retinal layers, it can also be used to infer retinal pigmentation quantitatively (see review by Berendschot et al. 2003).

The sclera is a strong reflector (Delori and Pflibsen 1989), as light is both backscattered by collagen fibrils and reflected at its surface because of its relatively high refractive index (Fine et al. 1985). Other important sources of reflection are identified at the RPE level, at the inner limiting membrane as well as in the choroid (Berendschot et al.

2003). Additionally, blood, photoreceptors, and macular pigments play a substantial role in interpreting reflectance in the visible spectrum (Hammer and Schweitzer 2002). Melanin concentration, in both the RPE and the choroid, is the predominant signature of reflectance from about 600 nm to the end of the IR-A range (Hammer and Schweitzer 2002), which can reach up to 15% in lightly pigmented human individuals (Delori and Pflibsen 1989).

Quantitatively, the main part of the reflectance can therefore be approximated with a basic model consisting of two reflectors on both sides of the pigmented region. This model uses a wavelength-dependent reflection at the sclera and an eccentricity-dependent reflectance at the RPE (proposed by van Norren and Tiemeijer 1986). This basic model is satisfactory for approximating the amount of light measured out of the eye but suffers from strong simplifications such as the absence of diffusion, thus leading to an overestimation of the pigmentation (Delori and Pflibsen 1989).

A similar model has already been used in combination with a thermal model for controlling the size of photocoagulation (Pflibsen et al. 1989). It appears that the change in choroidal pigmentation is the main factor for suprathreshold lesion size variation. Therefore, reliable fundus reflectance data can effectively provide additional information on both absolute and relative pigmentation. Other approaches for the modeling of light propagation in attenuating media are discussed in Welch and van Gemert (1995).

15.6.2 Cornea

The cornea is the outermost transparent part of the eye, with a diameter of about 11 mm in humans. The space between the cornea and the lens of the eye is filled with the aqueous humor. The cornea acts as the primary diffractive element of the eye, while the lens serves mostly for accommodation.

In nonhuman primates from the genus *Macaca*, the central cornea is in the order of 500–550 μm thick (Boettner and Dankovic 1974 and Maher 1978, respectively), while corneal thickness is only 300 μm in common rabbits (Zhang et al., 2009). In general, corneal thickness is also subject to variation of ocular pressure, thickening with increasing eccentricity and interindividual variability.

Due to the high water content of the cornea (80%) and of the aqueous humor (99%), optical radiation of wavelengths longer than approximately 1.2 μm is predominantly absorbed by these anterior media, reaching the retina or even the lens only weakly. Above a wavelength of 2.5 μm, absorption of optical radiation is entirely concentrated in the first few hundreds of micrometers (Figure 15.6). Noticeably, for an absorption coefficient larger than 1000 cm^{-1}, the penetration depth—shorter than 10 μm—is even reduced to the tear film.

The estimation of normal tear film thickness is subject to controversy, with values ranging between 3 and 40 μm (King-Smith et al. 2000). Differences between species are large as well (Prydal and Campbell 1992) and, depending on the environment and the application of saline (or lack thereof), evaporation plays a critical role in the evolution of the precorneal tear film thickness in the time course of minutes (Iwata et al. 1969). Thus, the method used for preventing corneal dryness during *in vivo* corneal exposures must be considered for the sake of consistency when comparing corneal lesions (Fine et al. 1968).

Scattering and refraction in the cornea are negligible for modeling corneal injury, since we are only interested in light distribution within the cornea, not behind it. It is commonly accepted that the cornea is homogeneously absorbent because it does not contain pigments and its water content is homogeneous throughout the various sublayers.

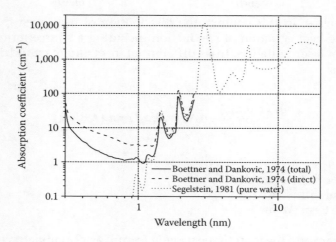

FIGURE 15.6
Absorption coefficient of the rhesus monkey cornea (sampled up to 2.5 μm) and of pure water.

The Beer–Lambert law, which describes the exponential decay of local irradiance with distance, is used to calculate optical attenuation within the cornea (thus referring to absorption coefficient). Specular reflection at the front surface can be taken into account by the Fresnel equations. The assumption that the corneal refractive index is similar to that of water for all wavelengths of relevance is thought to be acceptable (e.g., data from Segelstein 1981). At the interface between cornea and aqueous, reflection (corresponding to the second Purkinje image) is assumed to be negligible given the small difference between refractive indices.

From a thermal point of view, we believe that the curvature of the cornea does not play a substantial role for modeling. Simple geometrical optics allows confirmation that optical power does not constitute a primary variable. By applying Snell's law of refraction, it can be shown that the largest angle of refraction reaches only 11° (worst case obtained with a centered and collimated 8 mm beam). The larger the beam, the less important local variations at the edges become. Thus it can be assumed that the beam diameter remains constant throughout the corneal depth, unless the laser beam is strongly focused to a tiny spot at the corneal surface.

15.7 Heat Transfer

15.7.1 Heat Equation

When addressing the issue of thermal interaction in the modeling of laser-induced thermal injury at threshold level, only heat generation and conduction are critical. Convection and evaporation are secondary, while metabolism—through the rate of work performed continuously within the tissue—and radiation from the cornea are comparatively negligible (Chen et al. 2006; McCally et al. 1992). Consideration of vascular convection in the case of the retina and free air convection on the corneal surface are discussed below. In this context, the distribution of heat over space and time is described by the heat equation of conduction including a source term resulting from the absorption of laser radiation. In its differential form and in cylindrical coordinates, this is written as:

$$\frac{\partial T(r,\theta,z,t)}{\partial t} - \alpha \Delta T(r,\theta,z,t) = q_s(r,\theta,z,t)$$

where:

   T is the increase in temperature (K)
   α is the thermal diffusivity (m^2 s^{-1})
   q_s is the source term (W m^{-3})

As the laser beam and the local tissue usually feature axial symmetry, the angular component θ vanishes and the problem can be reduced to two dimensions (r for radius and z for depth). The symmetry is lost in cases of complex beam profiles and scanning.

The equation is linear with respect to laser power, provided that thermal properties are constant (i.e., are assumed not to depend on temperature). Variation in thermal diffusivity of water does not exceed 7% between 40°C and 80°C, thus having a very limited impact on damage levels. Within the retina, melanosomes exhibit a significantly higher mass density (~1400 kg m^{-3}) and lower specific heat capacity (~2700 J kg^{-1} K^{-1}) than water (Neumann et al. 2005). Nevertheless, only the product of these two properties is relevant and it remains similar to that of water. This approximation is convenient since it greatly simplifies the problem geometry and the solving process. In general, biological tissues are 10%–20% less thermally conductive than water (e.g., 0.58 W m^{-1} K^{-1} in Ooi et al. 2008; nonlinear relation as a function of water content in Chen et al. 2006). In addition to conduction, heat convection can take place in vascular layers (e.g., choroid) or on both sides of the cornea (due to temperature gradient at the air/cornea interface and aqueous flow; Ooi and Ng 2008). A convenient approach is to consider convection as simple heat dissipation or, in other words, as removal of heat from the system. The concept of heat sink represents losses without transfer from one location to another and is mathematically formulated in the heat equation as an additional and negative source term on its right-hand side (see derivation in Roider and Birngruber 1995):

$$q_b(T) = \rho_b c_b w_b (T_b - T)$$

where the terms on the right-hand side are, from left to right, mass density, specific heat capacity, perfusion rate, and incoming blood temperature (SI units). The perfusion rate is expressed in sec^{-1} (e.g., 1 sec^{-1} means 100% of the perfused tissue is renewed within 1 sec by tissue at body temperature). Perfusion rates in the range of 0.15–0.35 sec^{-1} have been estimated in the rabbit retina (Kandulla et al. 2006; Herrmann et al. 2007). The assumption of global perfusion underestimates real flow rates but at the same time it overestimates heat losses since heat vanishes instead of being actually displaced. In general, modeling of blood flow is relevant only for exposure durations longer than several seconds (Welch et al. 1980; Birngruber et al. 1985). A different approach for heat convection is addressed in the next section.

15.7.2 Initial and Boundary Conditions

In association with the heat equation, it is necessary to define initial and boundary conditions. Initially, the temperature distribution is at equilibrium—that is, body temperature—and constant throughout the retina:

$$T(t=0) = T_{body}$$

In the case of tissues at the body surface, three approaches are discussed. First, a constant temperature can be assumed because, as the temperature gradient is close to 0.3 K mm⁻¹ (Ng and Ooi 2007), the much larger local temperature increase required to induce damage makes such variation secondary.

This can, however, be refined by imposing heat transfer at the corneal surface. Scott (1988a) proposed a model and numerical values for taking into account evaporation, free air convection, and radiation:

$$-k \cdot \frac{\partial T(z=0)}{\partial z} = q_e + h(T - T_\infty) + \sigma \varepsilon (T^4 - T_\infty^4)$$

In the field of laser-induced damage, this boundary model—neglecting emissivity—has been applied to the skin by Chen et al. (2006). It includes a temperature-dependent outward flux for modeling vaporization. It is expected to underestimate heat loss at the corneal surface since—although lipid components slow down evaporation—the tear film remains subject to loss of water to a greater extent than the comparatively drier epidermis.

In normal conditions, say at an ambient temperature of 22°C, evaporation accounts for 40–100 W m⁻², free convection for 120 W m⁻², and radiation for 30 W m⁻² (data from Scott 1988a). The steady-state temperature can be obtained by solving the time-independent heat equation or it can be approximated by a linear equation (the gradient being approximately 0.38 K mm⁻¹ in Scott's data):

$$T(t=0) = T_{surface} + z \cdot \frac{dT}{dz}$$

Alternatively, when using numerical methods, it is possible to take into account a volume of air in front of the cornea, in which case outward conduction and convection can be included directly in the heat equation. Calculations by the authors show that the two approaches give almost identical results (within 10% for typical spot sizes and absorption coefficients). Explanations for this similitude are (i) the investigated pulse durations are too short for observing a significant difference, (ii) the differences are insignificant regarding the relatively large temperature increase within the cornea, and (iii) the model and values proposed by Chen et al. (2006) for the skin may underestimate heat losses at the cornea.

Due to the transient nature and the extent of the temperature rise, parameterizing the boundary conditions does not impact threshold levels much. It follows that the initial surface temperature is actually of greater importance than the aforementioned assumptions on boundary conditions. The normal corneal surface temperature fluctuates by about 1°C around 34°C (e.g., Mapstone 1968; Scott 1988a) depending on several factors such as ambient temperature, humidity, circadian phase, anesthesia, and blink rate.

Using numerical methods, boundary conditions are usually of the Neumann type due to the limited volume being modeled. That is, the normal component of the temperature derivative is set to zero. In a two-dimensional problem with axial symmetry, it writes:

$$\vec{r} \cdot \frac{\partial T(r,\vartheta,z,t)}{\partial r}\bigg|_{r=0,r=R} = \vec{z} \cdot \frac{\partial T(r,\vartheta,z,t)}{\partial z}\bigg|_{z=0,z=Z} = 0$$

15.7.3 Solving the Bioheat Equation

Under certain circumstances (symmetry, homogeneity, etc.), analytical solutions of the bioheat equation can be found. A review of the solutions in the field of laser–tissue interactions was published by Roider and Birngruber (1995). Noticeably, a semianalytical solution to the specific problem of laser-heated retina using a Gaussian laser beam profile and exponentially decaying absorption has been developed by Birngruber et al. (1978) but its formulation in the form of error functions impedes numerical evaluation for high levels of absorption (e.g., those relevant in the short-wavelength range). An unconditional stable analytical solution exists, however, for a sphere. Its application to the problem of retinal laser irradiation consists of considering each melanin granule as a spherical absorber embedded in an infinite homogeneous medium. The linearity of temperature with respect to laser power makes it possible to superimpose the solutions obtained for a set of spheres (typically a few thousand) at any time and at any location in space. The approach developed by Thompson et al. (1996) (referred to as the Thompson Gerstman model) takes intergranule shading into account and serves as a valuable basis for modeling short-term variations in temperature at the micrometer scale, that is, within and between melanosomes. Phenomena relevant to short pulse exposures are mainly hot spots and microbubble formation. A drawback is that this approach is inherently associated with homogeneous properties and infinite volumes. Consequently, significant limitations of analytical solutions and today's powerful computational methods give growing support for the use of numerical solutions. They simplify the treatment of nonlinearity, allow for the introduction of inhomogeneities and handling of complex geometries. These potentials, although still not fully capitalized in current models, may prove beneficial in the future.

Among numerical methods, the finite element method (FEM) appears to be the most enticing, as user-friendly and powerful commercial software is available. As with other methods, such as finite differences, the fundamental concept relies on discretization. The mathematical and computational procedures are beyond the scope of this chapter but they are widely discussed in the literature (e.g., Reddy and Gartling 2001). The FEM has already been applied for the modeling of ocular temperature (Ng and Ooi 2007), ocular hyperthermia, (e.g., Scott 1988b) and retinal coagulation (Glenn et al. 1996).

15.7.4 Characteristic Results

In this section, absolute threshold levels are not discussed because they depend on various model parameters, the type of tissue studied, the species involved, and so on, but it is worth highlighting the fundamental characteristics shared by all models. Retinal and corneal models typically exhibit the same trends when results are observed as a function of exposure duration, spot size, or absorption coefficient (i.e., wavelength).

As the damage mechanism is purely thermal, three regimes can be distinguished: (i) thermal confinement, where heat diffusion does not apply, (ii) transient phase where heat diffusion is under progress, and (iii) steady state where conduction of heat away from the source has reached equilibrium.

Two interesting asymptotic behaviors are mathematically described by the definition of internal energy and Fourier's law, respectively:

$$\begin{cases} \text{thermal confinement: } \dfrac{\Delta T}{Q} = \dfrac{1}{\rho c V} \\ \text{steady state: } \dfrac{\Delta T}{Q} = \dfrac{l}{S \kappa t} \end{cases}$$

where:
Q is the absorbed energy
ΔT is the increase in temperature
ρ is the mass density
c is the specific heat capacity
V is the volume
S is the surface of conduction
κ is the conductivity
t is the time
l is a characteristic length (all in SI units)

Regarding the spatial variables, one can consider an idealized heated volume that is radially delineated by the spot radius and by the penetration depth in the depth dimension, conceptually representative of a thin cylinder, whose total surface area is assumed to be representative of the exchange surface of conduction. Finally, the characteristic length is set to the spot radius since it has been shown to be a good measure of thermal diffusion (Schulmeister et al. 2006).

These basic regimes are compared with model simulations in Figure 15.7a (run with arbitrary parameters; typical for the macula at 530 nm). The ordinate (in kelvin per joule) is representative of the heat capacity of the system. Besides the fact that the two aforementioned limiting cases are time independent and inversely proportional to time, respectively, we observe a breakpoint whose position varies with spot size in a following a power law with respect to time (Figure 15.7b). This relationship becomes inexact for very small spots because the definitions of volume and surface are inappropriate.

The theoretical breakpoint can be simply calculated by resolving the system of equations mentioned before. It is worth mentioning that damage thresholds (expressed as energy) do not exactly vary linearly with respect to time in the long exposure regime because the damage model is nonlinear (purposely neglected in this study in order to characterize the purely thermal behavior of the laser/tissue system).

A similar analysis of the thermal interaction in our laser/tissue system can be performed over the dependence of thresholds on spot size. Three regimes are clearly identified (see Schulmeister et al. 2006): (1) a constant threshold level below a certain spot size, referred to as minimum angular subtense, (2) a variation proportional to the square of the spot size (i.e., to the surface area) above a certain spot size, referred to as maximum angular subtense, and (3) a transition phase that can be approximated (for instance in laser safety guidelines) to vary linearly with spot size.

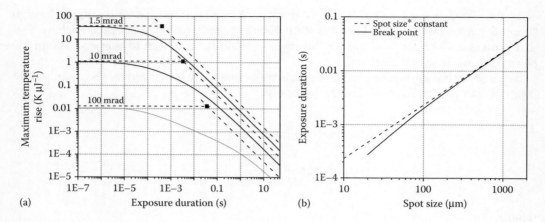

(a)   (b)

FIGURE 15.7
(a) Representation of the thermal capacity of the retina by asymptotic analysis. (b) Variation of the breakpoint in time with retinal spot size.

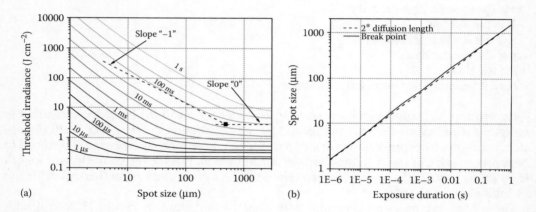

(a)   (b)

FIGURE 15.8
Threshold irradiance as function of spot size for various exposure durations; at each exposure duration, the cross-point between asymptotes representative of slope 0 and −1 yields a spot size, which can be directly compared with twice the diffusion length.

When irradiance thresholds are plotted as a function of spot size, a breakpoint is also identified by examining the asymptotic behavior (Figure 15.8a). For each exposure duration, this breakpoint is compared with the theoretical diffusion length that applies to this duration (Figure 15.8b). A good agreement is therefore indicative of a direct correlation between the spot size and the effect of radial diffusion with respect to time.

15.8 Modeling of Damage

15.8.1 Lesion Definition

The definition of a lesion is dependent on the observation method and the scale as well as the investigated tissue reaction (referred to as end point). For safety reasons, a threshold injury is roughly defined as the smallest lesion that can be reasonably detected with a given method, usually under ophthalmoscopic examination. In laser safety, what is referred to as "threshold" is the statistical product of results from several exposures at various energy levels (doses), and it represents the dose at which 50% of exposures lead to an observable injury (known as ED_{50}; its relevancy is discussed in Sliney et al. 2002). This experimentally determined value is commonly taken as a reference for the validation of a threshold injury computer model.

The damage mechanism discussed here is purely thermal in nature. At the subcellular level and at threshold level, elevated temperatures lead to denaturation of proteins, which leads to cascading processes that ultimately kill the cell if a sufficient fraction of critical proteins have been affected. Proteins are plausible targets as they are basic cellular components. Proteins can undergo unfolding—a potentially reversible process—above melting temperature. This transition occurs above 42°C–47°C (Deaton et al. 1990; Lepock 2003; Dewirsht et al. 2003). Accumulation of denatured proteins within a cell impedes vital functions and if repair mechanisms are insufficient, the cell ultimately dies. Several observations tend to confirm that a single mechanism, namely protein denaturation, is the basis of thermally induced injuries across a wide variety of tissues and over a wide range of temperatures (Lepock 2003). In the case of retinal damage, preferred targets might be the melanosome coat or cellular membranes (Wright 2003). At the cellular level, thermally induced injury is associated with cell death. A severe insult involves necrosis, characterized by swelling followed by removal of cell debris through phagocytosis (Verheyen 1996). Histopathological studies suggest that this process is dominant following intense increase in temperature (i.e., short exposure, Zuclich et al. 1998; Marshall et al. 1975). Apoptosis occurs mostly after moderate thermal insult and this process lasts longer (Matylevitch et al. 1998) since the cell can be only partially damaged without its integrity being compromised, that is, the cell can still fight to recover homeostasis (Verheyen 1996). This may explain the observation of increasing delay in the appearance of threshold lesions following long exposures (i.e., up to 48 h after second-long exposures).

When the temperature rise exceeds approximately 20°C for a very short period, there is strong evidence that thermotolerance does not play any role during the heating time (Dewirsht et al. 2003), although the synthesis of protective products (heat shock proteins) is already triggered (Desmettre et al. 2001). The effect of long exposures involving relatively low temperature increases (i.e., 10–15°C) may however be impacted by thermotolerance at threshold level (Deaton et al. 1990). A schematic representation in Figure 15.9 gives a simplified review of the damaging process.

15.8.2 Mathematical Description

The effect of temperature on organic components has been widely studied in biochemistry and the rate of chemical reactions can be described mathematically by the Arrhenius equations. In the so-called Arrhenius model, a rise in temperature defines the rate at which a given reaction occurs, assuming that the pathway remains identical. The temperature-dependent reaction rate is given by:

$$k(t) = A \cdot e^{\frac{-E}{T(t)}}$$

where:
  T is the absolute temperature (K)

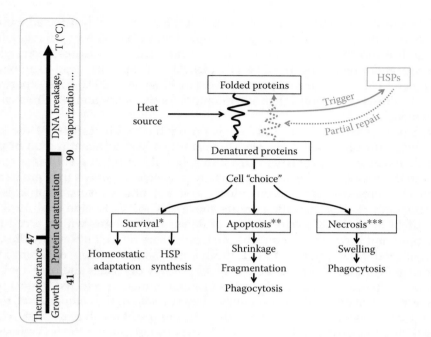

FIGURE 15.9
Schematic of simplified processes and scenarios of cellular response to acute heat stress (responses to * light, ** moderate, and *** severe heating).

A is a frequency factor (sec^{-1})
E is an inactivation energy divided by the gas constant (K)

The factor *A* is assumed to be temperature independent (Jacques 2006; Criado 2005; a temperature-dependent formulation is provided by the Eyring equation). Subdamage accumulation Ω is then described by its integration over time, which leads to:

$$\Omega = \int_0^t k(t)\,dt$$

This measure of damage also has a statistical interpretation. The cell or tissue is conceived as a system containing billions of targets that are, independently from each other, transformed to a degenerative state of lower energy (e.g., protein unfolding). A macroscopic observation of this phenomenon leads to an overall single process, represented by a concentration of affected targets:

$$c_{\text{denatured}} = 1 - e^{-\Omega}$$

Setting $\Omega = 1$ corresponds therefore to 63% of damaged targets (commonly accepted for representing threshold damage). It has also been suggested that 5% is enough to achieve cell death (Lepock 2003) but these numerical values and their importance must be put into perspective because they are directly dependent on the choice of the preexponential factor.

For instance, different degrees of skin burns (redness, edema, thrombosis) can be modeled with a single set of Arrhenius parameters simply by associating the different degrees of lesion with appropriate values of Ω (Henriques 1947).

It appears that this first-order model is appropriate in the range of time and temperatures under investigation. It is worth mentioning that the timescale at which protein dynamics occurs is much shorter than the laser exposure in the thermal regime (Day et al. 2002). It follows that the dynamics of each molecular reaction can be neglected. Furthermore, we are only interested in quantifying the first step of the cellular damage process or, in other words, only the component that is the most sensitive to a temperature rise (known as the limiting step). Subsequent reactions are triggered in cascade. In the case of very long exposures (several minutes to hours), a model of higher order might be necessary (Jacques 2006) since long-term processes such as thermotolerance or refolding come into play and can partly counterbalance the destructive action of temperature increase.

As shown by Wright (2003) and Jacques (2006), the two coefficients of the Arrhenius integral can be mathematically linked (see Gibbs free energy and Van't Hoff equation) so that only one independent coefficient is representative of the chosen end point. The inactivation energy commonly used for cutaneous, corneal, and retinal injuries is consistent with the order of magnitude characteristic of protein denaturation (100–200 kcal mol^{-1} or 50,000–100,000 K; Deaton et al. 1990; Lepock 2003). It has been inferred that all corneal layers—epithelium, stroma, and endothelium—have similar sensitivity to elevated temperature, thus allowing the use of a unique set of damage parameters for the whole tissue (Farrell et al. 1985). Some values found in the literature are plotted in Figure 15.10a. These curves show the temperature jump required for achieving an isoeffect (in this case for modeling minimum injury). The approximate intersection—suggestive of a typical transition temperature—is believed to be representative of the general form of thermal damage. The discrepancies between sets of parameters may not be of physical meaning but, instead, may be attributed to possible inconsistencies between end points, possible inconsistencies between model parameters, or the fact that the various models have not been validated against the same set of experimental results.

To our knowledge, there are few alternatives to the Arrhenius approach. An empirical time-dependent critical temperature has been applied to both minimal damage

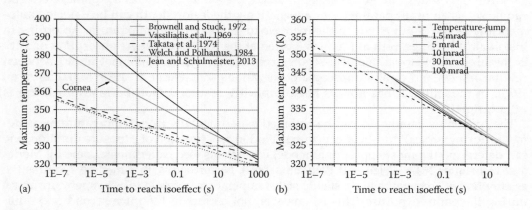

FIGURE 15.10
(a) Isoeffect curves for various Arrhenius sets applied in models of retinal and corneal damage. (b) Comparison between temperature-jump assumption and simulated time-temperature histories.

and vaporization (Bargeron et al. 1989) but doubt remains regarding its applicability to exposures shorter than about 10 ms (McCally et al. 1992).

15.8.3 Lesion Size and Computation

The Arrhenius model must be solved iteratively (e.g., up–down method) by scaling the increase in temperature in order to find the unique exposure level that leads to $\Omega = 1$. One can take advantage of the linearity of the heat equation with regards to power by solving it once for an arbitrary exposure level and subsequently scaling the temperature to reach threshold. When computation time is of importance, this is a reason for assuming model properties that retain linearity (such as constant and homogeneous thermal properties).

Several investigators have examined the size of ophthalmoscopic minimum visible lesions (MVL) by means of histological sections or flat preparations (e.g., Welch and Polhamus 1984; Bresnick et al. 1970). It appears that thermally induced lesions are detectable down to a size of 30–50 µm although variability increases under approximately 80 µm (Vincelette et al. 2008). It is known that the MVL is at least as large as one epithelial cell in *in vitro* conditions, that is, 10–20 µm in diameter (Milsom et al. 2006). The assessment of an MVL is also impacted by several parameters not related to its actual size: optical quality, contrast and dynamic range of the ophthalmoscopic apparatus, delay after exposure, damage depth (i.e., wavelength), pigmentation, local molting, and changes in contrast over the retinal map, among others. In the cornea, lesions investigated with a slit lamp are detectable between 80 µm (Stuck et al. 1981) and 200 µm (Byer et al. 1972).

Since MVL are finite in size, damage must be numerically evaluated also over a certain tissue volume. Given the fact that the beam profile for threshold experiments is either top hat or Gaussian and exhibits axial symmetry, it follows that the temperature will always decrease monotonically with increasing distance from the spot center. As a consequence, if damage is detected at a distance r_0, the domain that satisfies $r \leq r_0$ is *de facto* damaged. The increase in temperature must be monitored at the edge of the MVL domain only. Most thermal models have been developed with MVL diameter between 20 and 50 µm (Takata et al. 1974; Birngruber et al. 1985).

Within the tissue of interest, the depth where the model calculates the damage integral can be set as an input parameter or alternatively the lesion depth can be detected automatically as the depth at which the increase in temperature is maximum. According to histological findings, retinal lesion is located at the RPE level, where absorption density is the highest. Histopathological studies confirm the good agreement found between cellular effects and ophthalmoscopic observations (Zuclich et al. 1998; Marshall et al. 1975). In modeling, it has always been implicitly assumed that the MVL thickness is infinitesimal.

The Arrhenius parameters can be obtained experimentally from temperature measurements during typical threshold exposures. Plotted as a function of exposure duration, one can determine the most appropriate model coefficients (see experimental data by Moritz and Henriques 1947; Welch and Polhamus 1984). Nevertheless, this method requires the assumption of an instantaneous steady-state temperature (referred to as temperature jump) during the entire exposure. This is, however, not correct in the microsecond and millisecond regime and it introduces a bias. A simulation run with typical time–temperature histories for retinal damage calculated by the authors shows the extent of this error (Figure 15.10b). In view of this discrepancy and the fact that temperature measurements often suffer from significant errors (response delay in the microsecond regime, superficial measurement, and probe positioning), the discrepancies observed in Figure 15.10a are easily put into perspective.

References

Atchison, D.A. and G. Smith. 2000. *Optics of the Human Eye*. Edinburgh: Butterworth-Heinemann.

Atchison, D.A. and G. Smith. 2005. Chromatic dispersions of the ocular media of human eyes. *J Opt Soc Am A* 22(1):29–37.

Bargeron, C.B., O.J. Deters, R.A. Farrell and R.L. McCally. 1989. Epithelial damage in rabbit corneas exposed to CO_2 laser radiation. *Health Phys* 56(1):85–95.

Berendschot, T.T.J.M., P.J. DeLint and D. van Norren. 2003. Fundus reflectance: Historical and present ideas. *Prog Retin Eye Res* 22:171–200.

Birngruber, R., F. Hillenkamp and V.-P. Gabel. 1978. Experimentelle und theoretische Untersuchungen zur thermischen Schädigung des Augenhintergrundes durch Laserstrahlung. Report AO 251. Munich: Gesellschaft für Strahlen- und Umweltforschung (German).

Birngruber, R., E. Drechsel, F. Hillenkamp and V.-P. Gabel. 1979. Minimal spot size on the retina formed by the optical system of the eye. *Int Ophthal* 1(3):175–178.

Birngruber, R., V.-P. Gabel and F. Hillenkamp. 1983. Experimental studies of laser thermal retinal injury. *Health Phys* 44(5):519–531.

Birngruber, R., F. Hillenkamp and V.-P. Gabel. 1985. Theoretical investigations of laser thermal retinal injury. *Health Phys* 48(6):781–796.

Birngruber, R. 1991. Choroidal circulation and heat convection at the fundus of the eye. In *Laser Applications in Medicine and Biology*, ed. M.L. Wolbarsht, Vol. 5, pp. 277–361. New York: Plenum.

Boettner, E.A. and D. Dankovic. 1974. Ocular absorption of laser radiation for calculating personnel hazards. Final report. Brooks City-Base, TX: USAF School of Aerospace Medicine.

Borland, R.G., P.A. Smith and G.P. Owen. 1992. A model for the prediction of eye damage from pulsed lasers. *Laser Light Ophthalmol* 5(2):61–67.

Bradley, D.V., A. Fernandes, M. Lynn, M. Tigges and R.G. Boothe. 1999. Emmetropization in the rhesus monkey (*Macaca mulatta*): Birth to young adulthood. *Invest Ophthalmol Vis Sci* 40(1):214–229.

Bresnick, G.H., G.D. Frisch, J.O. Powell, B.M. Landers, G.C. Holst and A.G. Dallas. 1970. Ocular effects of argon laser radiation; I: Retinal damage threshold studies. *Invest Ophthal* 9(11):901–910.

Buitelveld, H., J.M. Hakvoort and M. Donze. 1994. The optical properties of pure water. In *Proceedings of SPIE, Ocean Optics XII*, ed. J.S. Jaffe, pp. 174–183.

Byer, H.H., E. Carpino and B.E. Stuck. 1972. Determination of the thresholds of CO_2 laser corneal damage to Owl monkeys, Rhesus monkeys and Dutch-belted rabbits. Final report. Frankford Arsenal, PA: US Army.

Cain, C.P., C.A. Toth, R.J. Thomas, et al. 2000. Comparison of macular versus paramacular retinal sensitivity to femtosecond laser pulses. *J Biomed Opt* 5(3):315–320.

Chen, B., S.L. Thomsen, R.J. Thomas and A.J. Welch. 2006. Modeling thermal damage in skin from 2000-nm laser irradiation. *J Biomed Opt* 11(6):064028.

Connolly, J.S., H.W. Hemstreet and D.E. Egbert. 1978. Ocular hazards of picosecond and repetitive-pulsed lasers. Vol. II: Argon-ion laser. Report SAM-TR-78-21. Brooks City-Base, TX: USAF School of Aerospace Medicine.

Coogan, P.S., W.F. Hughes and J.A. Molsen. 1974. Histologic and spectrophotometric comparisons of the human and rhesus monkey retina and pigmented ocular fundus. Final report. Brooks City-Base, TX: USAF School of Aerospace Medicine.

Criado, J.M., L.A. Pérez-Maqueda and P.E. Sánchez-Jiménez. 2005. Dependence of the preexponential factor on temperature. *J Therm Anal Calorim* 82:671–675.

Davis, T.P. and W.J. Mautner. 1969. Helium-Neon laser effects on the eye. Report C106–59223. Fort Detrick, MD: US Army Medical Research & Development Com.

Day, R., B.J. Bennion, S. Ham and V. Daggett. 2002. Increasing temperature accelerates protein unfolding without changing the pathway of unfolding. *J Mol Biol* 322:189–203.

Deaton, M.A., D.G. Odom, A.M. Dahlberg, P. Lester, B.L. Cowan and D.J. Lund. 1990. Increased synthesis of heat shock proteins and partial protection of the retina against the damaging effects of argon laser irradiation. *Laser Life Sci* 3(3):177–185.

Delori, F.C. and K.P. Pflibsen. 1989. Spectral reflectance of the human ocular fundus. *Appl Opt* 28(6):1061–1077.

Desmettre, T., C.-A. Maurage and S. Mordon. 2001. Heat shock protein hyperexpression on chorioretinal layers after transpupillary thermotherapy. *Invest Ophthalmol Vis Sci* 42(12):2976–2980.

Dewhirst, M.W., B.L. Viglianti M. Lora-Michiels, M. Hanson and P.J. Hoopes. 2003. Basic principles of thermal dosimetry and thermal thresholds for tissue damage from hyperthermia. *Int J Hyperthermia* 19(3):267–294.

Farrell, R.A., R.L. McCally, C.B. Bargeron and W.R. Green. 1985. Structural alterations in the cornea from exposure to infrared radiation. Technical report. Fort Detrick, MD: US Army Med Res & Dev Com.

Feeney-Burns, L., E.S. Hilderbrand and S. Eldridge. 1984. Aging human RPE: Morphometric analysis of macular, equatorial and peripheral cells. *Invest Ophthalmol Vis Sci* 25(2):195–200.

Fine, B.S., S. Fine, L. Feigen and D. MacKeen. 1968. Corneal injury threshold to carbon dioxide laser irradiation. *Am J Ophthalmol* 66(1):1–15.

Fine, I., E. Loewinger, A. Weinreb and D. Weinberger. 1985. Optical properties of the sclera. *Phys Med Biol* 30(6):565–571.

Gabel, V.-P., R. Birngruber and F. Hillenkamp. 1976. Die Lichtabsorption am Augenhintergrund. Report A 55. Munich: Gesellschaft für Strahlen- und Umweltforschung (German).

Gabel, V.-P., R. Birngruber and F. Hillenkamp. 1978. Visible and near infrared in pigment epithelium and choroid. In: *XXIII Concilium Ophthalmologicum*, ed. K. Shimuzu and J.A. Oosterhuis, Excerpta Medica, 658:62.

Geeraets, W.J., R.C. Williams, G. Chan, W.T. Ham, D. Guerry and F.H. Schmidt. 1962. The relative absorption of thermal energy in retina and choroid. *Invest Ophthalmol* 1(3):340–347.

Gerrard, A. and J.M. Burch. 1994. *Introduction to Matrix Methods in Optics*. New York: Dover.

Glenn, T.N., S. Rastegar and S.L. Jacques. 1996. Finite element analysis of temperature controlled coagulation in laser irradiated tissue. *IEEE Trans Biomed Eng* 43(1):79–87.

Glickman, R.D. 2002. Phototoxicity to the retina: Mechanisms of damage. *Int J Toxicol* 21:473–490.

Hammer, M., A. Roggan, D. Schweitzer and G. Müller. 1995. Optical properties of ocular fundus tissues: An *in vitro* study using the double-integrating-sphere technique and inverse Monte Carlo simulation. *Phys Med Biol* 40:963–978.

Hammer, M. and D. Schweitzer. 2002. Quantitative reflection spectroscopy at the human fundus. *Phys Med Biol* 47:179–191.

Hammond, B.R., B.R. Wooten and D.M. Snodderly. 1997. Individual variations in the spatial profile of human macular pigment. *J Opt Soc Am A* 14(6):1187–1196.

Henderson, R. and K. Schulmeister. 2004. *Laser Safety*. New York: Taylor & Francis.

Henriques, F.C. and A.R. Moritz. 1947. Studies of thermal injury. I: The conduction of heat to and through skin and the temperatures attained therein. A theoretical and an experimental investigation. *Am J Pathol* 23(4):531–549.

Herrmann, K., C. Flöhr, J. Stalljohann, et al. 2007. Influence of choroidal perfusion on retinal temperature increase during retinal laser treatments. In *Proceedings of SPIE, Therapeutic Laser Applications and Laser–Tissue Interactions III*, ed. A. Vogel, SPIE Publishing, 6632.

Hodgkinson, I.J., P.B. Greer and A.C.B. Molteno. 1994. Point-spread function for light scattered in the human ocular fundus. *J Opt Soc Am A* 11(2):479–486.

Iwata, S., M.A. Lemp, F.J. Holly and C.H. Dohlman. 1969. Evaporation rate of water from the precorneal tear film and cornea in the rabbit. *Invest Ophthalmol* 8(6):613–619.

Jacques, S.L. 2006. Ratio of entropy to enthalpy in thermal transitions in biological tissues. *J Biomed Opt* 11(4):041108.

Jacques, S.L., R.D. Glickman and J.A. Schwartz. 1996. Internal absorption coefficient and threshold for pulsed laser disruption of melanosomes isolated from retinal pigment epithelium. In *Proceedings of SPIE, Laser–Tissue Interaction VII*, ed. S.L. Jacques, SPIE Publishing 2681:468–477.

Jean, M. and K. Schulmeister. 2013. Validation of a computer model to predict laser induced thermal injury thresholds to the retina. In *ILSC 2013 Conf Proceedings, Laser Insitute of America* 1002:229–238.

Kandulla, J., H. Elsner, R. Birngruber and R. Brinkmann. 2006. Noninvasive optoacoustic online retinal temperature determination during continuous-wave laser irradiation. *J Biomed Opt* 11(4):041111.

Keilhauer, C.N. and F.C. Delori. 2006. Near-infrared autofluorescence imaging of the fundus: Visualization of ocular pigment. *Invest Ophthalmol Vis Sci* 47(8):3556–3564.

King-Smith, P.E., B.A. Fink, N. Fogt, K.K. Nichols, R.M. Hill and G.S. Wilson. 2000. The thickness of the human precorneal tear film: Evidence from reflection spectra. *Invest Ophthalmol Vis Sci* 41(11):3348–3359.

Lappin, P.W. 1971. Assessment of ocular damage thresholds for laser radiation. *Am J Optom Arch Am Acad Optom* 48(7):600–606.

Lee, H., C. Alt, C.M. Pitsillides and C.P. Lin. 2007. Optical detection of intracellular cavitation during selective laser targeting of the retinal pigment epithelium: Dependence of cell death mechanism on pulse duration. *J Biomed Opt* 12(6):064034.

Lepock, J.R. 2003. Cellular effects of hyperthermia: Relevance to the minimum dose for thermal damage. *Int J Hyperthermia* 19(3):252–266.

Lund, D.J., P.R. Edsall, B.E. Stuck and K. Schulmeister. 2007. Variation of laser-induced retinal injury thresholds with retinal irradiated area: 0.1-s duration, 514-nm exposures. *J Biomed Opt* 12(2):024023.

Lund, D.J., P. Edsall and B.E. Stuck. 2008a. Spectral dependence of retinal thermal injury. *J Laser Appl* 20(2):76–82.

Lund, B.J., D.J. Lund and P.R. Edsall. 2008b. Laser-induced retinal damage threshold measurements with wavefront correction. *J Biomed Opt* 13(6):064011.

Maher, E.F. 1978. Transmission and absorption coefficients for ocular media of the rhesus monkey. Final report. Brooks City-Base, TX: USAF School of Aerospace Medicine.

Mapstone, R. 1968. Determinants of corneal temperature. *Br J Ophthal* 52:729–741.

Marshall, J., A.M. Hamilton and A.C. Bird. 1975. Histopathology of ruby and argon lesions in human and monkey retina. *Br J Ophthal* 59:610–629.

Matylevitch, N.P., S.T. Schuschereba, J.R. Mata, et al. 1998. Apoptosis and accidental cell death in cultured human keratinocytes after thermal injury. *Am J Pathol* 153(2):567–577.

McCally, R.L., R.A. Farrell and C.B. Bargeron. 1992. Cornea epithelial damage thresholds in rabbits exposed to Tm:YAG laser radiation at 2.02 μm. *Laser Surg Med* 12:598–603.

Milsom, P.K., S.J. Till and G. Rowlands. 2006. The effect of ocular aberrations on retinal laser damage thresholds in the human eye. *Health Phys* 91(1):20–28.

Moritz, A.R. and F.C. Henriques. 1947. Studies of thermal injury. II: The relative importance of time and surface temperature in the causation of cutaneous burns. *Am J Pathol* 23(5):695–720.

Neumann, J. and R. Brinkmann. 2005. Boiling nucleation on melanosomes and microbeads transiently heated by nanosecond and microsecond laser pulses. *J Biomed Opt* 10(2):024001.

Ng, E.Y.K. and E.H. Ooi. 2007. Ocular surface temperature: A 3D FEM prediction using bioheat equation. *Comput Biol Med* 37:829–835.

Ooi, E.H. and E.Y.K. Ng. 2008. Simulation of aqueous humor hydrodynamics in human eye heat transfer. *Comput Biol Med* 38:252–262.

Ooi, E.H., W.T. Ang and E.Y.K. Ng. 2008. A boundary element model of the human eye undergoing laser thermokeratoplasty. *Comput Biol Med* 38:727–737.

Pflibsen, K.P., F.C. Delori, O. Pomerantzeff and M.M. Pankratov. 1989. Fundus reflectometry for photocoagulation dosimetry. *Appl Opt* 28(6):1084–1096.

Prydal, J.I. and F.W. Campbell. 1992. Study of precorneal tear film thickness and structure by interferometry and confocal microscopy. *Invest Ophthalmol Vis Sci* 33(6):1996–2005.

Reddy, J.N. and D.K. Gartling. 2001. *The Finite Element Method in Heat Transfer and Fluid Dynamics*, 2nd edn. Boca Raton, FL: CRC.

Rockwell, B.A., D. Hammer, P. Kennedy, et al. 1997. Retinal spot size with wavelength. In *Proceedings of SPIE, Laser–Tissue Interaction VIII*, ed. S.L. Jacques, SPIE Publishing, 2975:148–154.

Roider, J. and R. Birngruber. 1995. Solution or the heat conduction equation. In *Optical–Thermal Response of Laser-Irradiated Tissue*, eds. A.J. Welch and M.J.C. van Gemert, pp. 385–409. New York: Plenum.

Sanders, V.E. 1974. Wavelength dependence on threshold ocular damage from visible laser light. Report. Brooks City-Base, TX: USAF School of Aerospace Medicine.

Sarna, T. 1992. Properties and functions of the ocular melanin: A photobiophysical view. *J Photochem Photobiol B* 12:215–258.

Schüle, G., M. Rumohr, G. Huettmann and R. Brinkmann. 2005. RPE damage thresholds and mechanisms for laser exposure in the microsecond-to-millisecond time regimen. *Invest Ophthalmol Vis Sci* 46(2):714–719.

Schulmeister, K., B.E. Stuck, D.J. Lund and D.H. Sliney. 2011. Review of thresholds and recommendations for revised exposure limits for laser and optical radiation for thermally induced retinal injury. *Health Phys* 100(2):210–220.

Schulmeister, K., J. Husinsky, B. Seiser, F. Edthofer, H. Tuschl and D.J. Lund. 2006. Ex-plant retinal laser induced threshold studies in the millisecond time regime. In *Proceedings of SPIE, Optical Interactions with Tissue and Cells XVII*, eds. S.L. Jacques and W.P. Roach, SPIE Publishing, 6084.

Scott, J. 1988. A finite element model of heat transport in the human eye. *Phys Med Biol* 33(2):227–241.

Scott, J. 1988. The computation of temperature rises in the human eye induced by infrared radiation. *Phys Med Biol* 33(2):243–257.

Segelstein, D.J. 1981. The complex refractive index of water. PhD. thesis, University of Missouri-Kansas City. Data compiled by S.A. Prahl. http://omlc.ogi.edu/spectra/water/data/segelstein81.dat (accessed March 28, 2011).

Sliney, D.H. 2005. What is the minimal retinal image size?: Implications for setting MPEs. In *ILSC Proceedings*, Orlando, Florida, pp. 43–47.

Sliney, D.H. and B.C. Freasier. 1973. Evaluation of optical radiation hazards. *Appl Opt* 12(1):1–24.

Sliney, D.H., J. Mellerio, V.-P. Gabel and K. Schulmeister. 2002. What is the meaning of threshold in laser injury experiments? Implications for human exposure limits. *Health Phys* 82(3):335–347.

Snodderly, D.M., G.J. Handelman and A.J. Adler. 1991. Distribution of individual macular pigment carotenoids in central retina of macaque and squirrel monkeys. *Invest Ophthalmol Vis Sci* 32(2):268–279.

Snodderly, D.M., M.M. Sandstrom, I.Y.-F. Leung, C.I. Zucker and M. Neuringer. 2002. Retinal pigment epithelial cell distribution in central retina of Rhesus monkeys. *Invest Ophthalmol Vis Sci* 43(9):2815–2818.

Spraul, C.W., G.E. Lang and H.E. Grossniklaus. 1996. Morphometric analysis of the choroid, Bruch's membrane and retinal pigment epithelium in eyes with age-related macular degeneration. *Invest Ophthalmol Vis Sci* 37(13):2724–2735.

Stolarski, D.J., J. Stolarksi, R.J. Thomas, G.D. Noojin, K.J. Schuster and B.A. Rockwell. 2002. Nonlinear absorption studies of melanin. In *Proceedings of SPIE, Laser–Tissue Interaction XIII*, eds. S.L. Jacques et al., SPIE Publishing, 4617.

Stuck, B.E. 1981. Ocular effects of holmium (2.06 µm) and erbium (1.54 µm) laser radiation. *Health Phys* 40:835–846.

Takata, A.N., L.P. Kuan, L. Goldfinch, N. Thomopoulis, J.K. Hinds and A. Weigandt. 1974. Thermal model of laser-induced eye damage. Final report. Brooks City-Base, TX: USAF School of Aerospace Medicine.

Thompson, C.R., B.S. Gerstman, S.L. Jacques and M.E. Rogers. 1996. Melanin granule model for laser-induced thermal damage in the retina. *Bull Math Biol* 58(3):513–553.

van der Berg, T.J.T.P. and H. Spekreijse. 1997. Near infrared light absorption in the human eye. *Vision Res* 37(2):249–253.

van Norren, D. and L.F. Tiemeijer. 1986. Spectral reflectance of the human eye. *Vision Res* 26(2):313–320.

Verheyen, A. 1996. Necrosis and apoptosis: Irreversibility of cell damage and cell death. In *Toxicology: Principles and Applications*, eds. R.J.M. Niesink, J. De Vries and M.A. Hollinger, pp. 473–501. Boca Raton, FL: CRC.

Vincelette, R.L., B.A. Rockwell, J.W. Oliver, et al. 2009. Trends in retinal damage thresholds from 100-millisecond near-infrared laser radiation exposures: A study at 1110, 1130, 1150 and 1319 nm. *Laser Surg Med* 41(5):382–390.

Vogel, A. and R. Birngruber. 1992. Temperature profiles in human retina and choroid during laser coagulation with different wavelengths ranging from 514 to 810 nm. *Laser Light Ophthalmol* 5(1):9–16.

Wang, Z., J. Dillon and E.R. Gaillard. 2006. Antioxidant properties of melanin in retinal pigment epithelial cells. *Photochem Photobiol* 82:474–479.

Weiter, J.J., F.C. Delori, G.L. Wing and K.A. Fitch. 1986. Pigment epithelial lipofuscin and melanin and choroidal melanin in human eyes. *Invest Ophthalmol Vis Sci* 27(2):145–152.

Welch, A.J. and G.D. Polhamus. 1984. Measurement and prediction of thermal injury in the retina of the Rhesus monkey. *IEEE Trans Biomed Eng* 31(10):633–644.

Welch, A.J. and L.A. Priebe. 1980. Significance of blood flow in calculations of temperature in laser irradiated tissue. *IEEE Trans Biomed Eng* 27(3):164–166.

Welch, A.J. and J.C. van Gemert. 1995. *Optical–Thermal Response of Laser-Irradiated Tissue*. New York: Plenum.

Welch, A.J., L.A. Priebe, L.D. Forster, R. Gilbert, C. Lee and P. Drake. 1979. Experimental validation of thermal retinal models of damage from laser radiation. Final report. Brooks City-Base, TX: USAF School of Aerospace Medicine.

Wikler, K.C. and P. Rakic. 1990. Distribution of photoreceptor subtypes in the retina of diurnal and nocturnal primates. *J Neurosci* 10(10):3390–3401.

Wright, N.T. 2003. On a relationship between the Arrhenius parameters from thermal damage studies. *J Biomech Eng* 125:300–304.

Zagers, N.P.A. and D. van Norren. 2004. Absorption of the eye lens and macular pigment derived from the reflectance of cone photoreceptors. *J Opt Soc Am A* 21(12):2257–2268.

Zhang, R., W. Verkruysse, B. Choi, et al. 2005. Determination of human skin optical properties from spectrophotometric measurements based on optimization by genetic algorithms. *J Biomed Opt* 10(2):024030.

Zuclich, J.A., H. Zwick, S.T. Schuscheraba, B.E. Stuck and F.E. Cheney. 1998. Ophthalmoscopic and pathologic description of ocular damage induced by infrared laser radiation. *J Laser Appl* 10(3):114–120.

Zuclich, J.A., P. Edsall, D.J. Lund, et al. 2008. New data on the variation of laser induced retinal-damage threshold with retinal spot size. *J Laser Appl* 20(2):83–88.

16

Automatization of Dry Eye Syndrome Tests

Manuel G. Penedo, Beatriz Remeseiro, Lucía Ramos, Noelia Barreira,
Carlos García-Resúa, Eva Yebra-Pimentel, and Antonio Mosquera

CONTENTS

Dry eye is a symptomatic disease that affects activities of daily living, adversely impacting important tasks such as computer use, driving, and others. Based on data from the largest studies of dry eye to date, the Physicians' Health Study (PHS) and other studies, it has been estimated that about 3.23 million women and 1.68 million men (a total of 4.91 million Americans) 50 years and older have dry eye. In practice, there are several clinical tests to diagnose this syndrome by means of analyzing tear film quality. This chapter describes automatic image-processing methodologies to perform two clinical tests: analysis of the interference lipid pattern and the tear film breakup time test.

16.1 Tear Film

The tear film is a complex layer of liquid covering the anterior surface of the eye. Classically, it is described as a trilaminar structure consisting of a thin anterior lipid layer (0.1–0.05 µL), an intermediate aqueous layer (7 µL) and an innermost mucous layer (0.02–0.04 µL) [1] (Figure 16.1). All of these layers must work properly to keep the eye moist and free from dry eye [2]. The tear film is not evenly distributed over the ocular surface. The total volume of the tear film is 7.0 ± 2.0 µL, with a thickness ranging from 6 to 10 µm. Along the upper and lower lids it forms a tear meniscus or marginal tear strips. This represents 70% of the total volume of tear fluid within the palpebral aperture [1]. A small proportion lies beneath the eyelids between the palpebral and bulbar conjunctivae, and the remainder covers the cornea and the exposed bulbar conjunctiva [2].

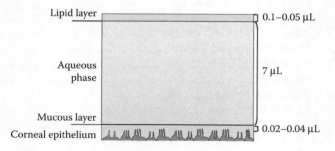

FIGURE 16.1
Trilaminar structure of the tear film.

16.1.1 Structure and Function

The structure of the tear film is classically described as a trilaminar structure comprising a superficial lipid layer, an intermediate aqueous phase, and an underlying mucous layer.

16.1.1.1 Lipid Layer

This is the outermost and thinnest layer of the tear film and is mainly secreted by the meibomian glands, embedded in the upper and lower tarsal plates [3]. The normal lipid layer is divided into two layers: the anterior and posterior lipid layers. The anterior lipid layer is formed by nonpolar lipids, mainly mixed wax esters and sterol esters (more than 60% of the total lipids). The posterior lipid layer is formed by highly polar lipids: free sterols, free fatty acids, and phospholipids [2]. The main function of the lipid layer is the reduction of evaporation from the aqueous phase. Furthermore, the nonpolar structure of the lipid layer is important in preventing surface contamination of the film with highly polar skin lipids, which could disrupt the tear film.

16.1.1.2 Aqueous Phase

The aqueous phase is the major component of the film, comprising around 98% of its total thickness. It is a complex dilute solution of both inorganic electrolytes and low- and high-molecular-weight organic substances. This is the major, intermediate phase of the tear film and is approximately 6.5–7.5 μm thick [1]. This phase is mainly secreted by lacrimal glands situated in the superior temporal angle of the orbit. This phase contains many ions and molecules such as electrolytes, hydrogen ions, proteins, enzymes, and metabolites, which provide the proper functions of the tear film.

16.1.1.3 Mucous Layer

The preocular tear film of the human eye is dependent on a constant supply of mucus, which must be of adequate chemical and physical quality to maintain the corneal and conjunctival surfaces in the proper state of hydration [2]. Secreted by goblet cells (sited in the conjunctiva), it represents 0.2% of the whole tear film, is formed by glycoproteins, and performs several functions. The main function of these mucous glycoproteins is to lower the surface tension of tears from about 70 dynes/cm to about half of that value. Lubrication of the cornea is also an important function, allowing the lids to slide smoothly with minimal friction during blinking and wetting the ocular surface to maintain a stable tear film [1].

The tear film is an essential component of the eye that fulfils some important functions [1,2]. The first function is the lubrication of the eyelids, which allows the eyelid margins and palpebral conjunctiva to slide smoothly over one another with minimal friction during blinking. The visual function is another role of the tear film. The corneal epithelium is a rough surface and the tear film fills the small irregularities in the corneal epithelium, providing a smooth, regular optical surface to guarantee high optical quality. The tear film also has a cleaning function. It takes desquamated epithelial cells, debris, and so forth from the epithelium and, due to the action of the lids, these are "washed" from the surface of the eye. In addition, since the corneal surface is avascular, the nutrition is driven by the tear film. Oxygen dissolves in the tear fluid and nutrients, such as glucose, are passed from the palpebral conjunctival vessels into the tear film. Finally, the tear film contains proteins (such as lysozyme or lactoferrin) that inhibit microbiological contamination.

16.1.2 Composition

The tear film is a matrix-like structure composed of water, electrolytes, immunoglobulins, antimicrobial molecules, mucins, and so on. The composition of the tear film is distributed into the three layers. The lipid layer comprises polar and nonpolar lipids secreted by meibomian glands. The major, intermediate watery phase of the tear film contains dissolved ions, organic solutes, and other metabolites. Finally, the mucous layer is made up of glycoproteins secreted by goblet cells of the conjunctiva. The concentration of each layer is as follows:

- *Lipid layer*: The major lipid classes are wax esters, sterol esters (mainly cholesterol), diesters, triglycerides, free sterols, and polar lipids. Hydrocarbons and free fatty acids, both straight and branched chain, are also present [1].

- *Aqueous phase*: This layer contains many ions and molecules including electrolytes (sodium, potassium, calcium, chloride, bicarbonate, and phosphate ions), proteins (lysozyme, lactoferrin, albumin, lipocalin, secretory immunoglobulin A), enzymes (lactate dehydrogenase, malate dehydrogenase, pyruvate kinase), and metabolites (glucose, urea) [2].

- *Mucous layer*: This layer mainly comprises O-linked glycoproteins. The principal sugars in crude ocular mucus are sialic acid, galactose, glucose, and N-acetylglucosamine [2].

16.2 Dry Eye Syndrome

Commonly, the term "dry eye" has been used to describe a variety of conditions of diverse origin that affect the tear film, the ocular surface, or both. However, there has always been a lack of consensus on the main characteristics of dry eye syndrome (DES), leading to confusion between clinicians.

To solve this, the international committee of the Dry Eye WorkShop (DEWS) clarified the main aspects of DES and established a complete definition as follows [4]:

> Dry Eye is a multifactorial disease of the tears and ocular surface that results in symptoms of discomfort, visual disturbance, and tear film instability with potential damage to the ocular surface. It is accompanied by increased osmolarity of the tear film and inflammation of the ocular surface.

From this definition, some factors can be elucidated. First, DES is a multifactorial disease, which means that several factors are responsible for the condition. Therefore, in order to establish an accurate DES diagnosis, a battery of clinical tests may be necessary. Second, a stable tear film covering the ocular surface is essential to maintain eye physiology, otherwise the ocular surface will be damaged. Third, a poor tear film shows increased osmolarity. This hyperosmolarity is considered to be the primary cause of ocular surface damage and inflammation. Thus, DES represents an inflammatory status.

16.2.1 Semiology

Nichols et al. have reported that the most common symptom of DES is dryness (98.7%), followed by ocular fatigue (85.1%), grittiness (78.5%), redness (71.6%), and soreness (64.8%) [3].

However, other studies have found ocular fatigue to be the most frequent symptom, followed by dryness [2]. Irritation, foreign-body sensation, burning, the presence of stringy mucous discharge, and transient blurring of vision also can affect dry eye patients [2]. DES cannot be diagnosed based on symptoms alone, since most of them can be caused by other conditions.

16.2.2 Epidemiology

One of the main problems in obtaining data on prevalence (the proportion with the disease within a population at a given point in time) is the different criteria of DES diagnosis between studies. There is consensus, however, that the prevalence of DES has increased, mainly due to current lifestyles [5]. Several factors can disrupt the tear film such as harmful environments (pollution, smoke, etc.), increased visual tasks that decrease the blink rate (especially when done with a computer), and increased use of antihistamines, antihypertensives, and so on [6]. These environmental and work factors, together with the ageing of the population (tear stability and secretion decrease with age) have increased the proportion of the population with DES [7]. Taking into account the lack of consensus discussed above, prevalence data found in the literature ranks from 10% to 35% [5]. If only contact lens wearers are considered, this prevalence is even greater [4]. Despite this discrepancy of data prevalence between studies, the weight of the evidence from large epidemiological studies indicates that female sex and older age (greater than 50 years) increase the risk for dry eye [2].

16.2.3 Classification

From an etiopathogenic point of view, DES can be mainly classified as aqueous tear-deficient dry eye (ADDE) and evaporative dry eye (EDE). Dry eye can be initiated in either of these classes, but they are not mutually exclusive [4,8].

16.2.3.1 ADDE

ADDE implies that dry eye is due to a failure of lacrimal tear secretion. In any form of dry eye due to lacrimal acinar destruction or dysfunction, dryness results from reduced lacrimal tear secretion and volume. This causes tear hyperosmolarity and stimulates a cascade of inflammatory events. ADDE has two major subclasses: Sjogren's syndrome dry eye and non-Sjogren's syndrome dry eye. Sjogren's syndrome is an exocrinopathy in which the exocrine glands (such as lacrimal and salivary glands) are targeted by an autoimmune process. Non-Sjogren's syndrome dry eye does not present those systemic autoimmune features. The most common form of non-Sjogren's syndrome dry eye is age-related dry eye, although other factors can contribute to ADDE, such as lacrimal gland infiltration, sarcoidosis, lymphoma, obstruction of the lacrimal gland ducts, and reflex hyposecretion [4,8].

16.2.3.2 EDE

EDE is caused by excessive water loss from the exposed ocular surface in the presence of normal lacrimal secretory function. The volume and composition of the lacrimal fluid are adequate, with tear abnormality created by other periocular diseases, usually leading to increased tear evaporation. This is the type of dry eye most commonly found in young to middle-aged people, and related to ambient conditions (air conditioning), contact lens wear, or both [4,8]. Current work conditions, such as computer use, have increased the proportion of people with EDE [4]. The main cause of EDE is meibomian gland dysfunction [9]. Meibomian glands, embedded in the upper and lower tarsal plates, are responsible for lipid secretion, which is essential to retard tear film evaporation [9].

Blink rate is an important factor in tear film stability. If the blink rate is reduced, the period between blinks is lengthened (the ocular surface is exposed to water loss), increasing tear film evaporation [10]. This mainly occurs during the performance of concentration tasks, such as reading, but most remarkably when using a computer. Contact lens wear may cause tear instability and dry eye because the contact lens disrupts the tear film. In fact, the primary reasons for contact lens intolerance are discomfort and dryness [4].

16.3 Morbidity of Dry Eye

The high prevalence of dry eye among older people, together with the ageing of the population, makes DES a public health problem to be considered.

Dry eye is a prevalent condition with the potential for a high economic burden. From a public health point of view, dry eye supposes an economic impact derived from costs due to health-care system utilization, including health-care professional visits, nonpharmacological therapies, pharmacological treatments, and surgical procedures, with the latter two categories being the major cost drivers. Other costs include complementary and alternative therapeutics [11], purchase of specialized eyewear, and other therapeutics, such as humidifiers. Given the prevalence of the condition, indirect costs derived by DES may be large [11]. These can include pharmacological therapies other than tear replacements, complementary medicine use, and the cost of complications of surgical procedures. Additionally, costs derived from impacts on daily capacity can include lost work time and productivity, alterations in work type or environment, decreased work time, and days off work with dry eye symptoms. Intangible costs include decreased leisure time, impaired physical functioning and quality of life, and impact on social interactions and mental and general health.

In a survey designed to ascertain how much a patient's everyday activities were limited by symptoms of dry eye, it was found that patients with DES were significantly more likely to report problems with reading, carrying out professional work, using a computer, watching television, driving during the day, and driving at night [12]. Overall, patients with DES were about three times more likely to report problems with common activities than those without DES. With increased severity, patients also reported deficits in general health perception and vitality, and the most severely affected patients reported worse health-related domains [12].

Dry eye is associated with contact lens intolerance and discontinuation of contact lens wear, can adversely affect refractive surgery outcomes, and may be associated with increased risk of infection and complications with ocular surgery. Severe dry eye may lead to ocular damage [13], although the natural history of dry eye remains to be determined.

16.3.1 Impact of Dry Eye on Visual Function and Quality of Life

Dry eye limits and degrades visual performance and affects common vision-related daily activities. Visual complaints are highly prevalent among dry eye patients and are usually described as disturbed vision or blurry, foggy vision that clears temporarily with blinking. These transient changes can be profound, resulting in marked drops in contrast sensitivity and visual acuity, thus affecting workplace productivity and vision-related quality of life [14].

In this sense DES affects quality of life in different ways. Pain and irritative symptoms negatively disrupt the welfare of the patient. Also, DES affects ocular and general health. Perception and visual function may be reduced, which impacts visual performance. For example, the irritative symptoms of dry eye can be debilitating and result in both psychological and physical effects that impact quality of life. Dry eye also limits and degrades performance of common vision-related daily activities, such as driving. The need for frequent instillation of lubricant eye drops can affect social and workplace interactions.

From an ocular surface health point of view, corneal surface irregularity due to epithelial desiccation, tear film instability, and evaporation can occur. An uneven, disrupted tear film in the central cornea can result in transient vision changes in the dry eye patient. Optical aberrations created by tear film breakup between blinks contribute to a decline in retinal image quality that can be measured by both objective and subjective methods [14].

16.4 Tear Film Assessment

DES diagnosis is very difficult to achieve, mainly because this is a multifactorial syndrome, so several tests are necessary to obtain a clear diagnosis. Fortunately, there are a wide number of tests to evaluate different aspects of the tear film. Some clinical tests measure the quality and quantity of tears, but most have high variability and demonstrate poor to fair diagnosis repeatability [4].

16.4.1 Biomicroscopic Examination

This is an essential part of the protocol of eye examination, consisting of a biomicroscope (designed to view the anterior eye with high magnification) and a slit lamp to change the illumination technique (Figure 16.2a). It is not exclusive to tear film assessment and

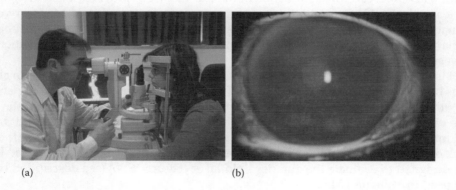

(a) (b)

FIGURE 16.2
(a) Eye examination by biomicroscopy. (b) Appearance of anterior eye dyed with fluorescein under biomicroscopic observation with cobalt blue and yellow filters. Light dots indicate damage of corneal epithelium surface.

provides information about the health of the ocular surface. Furthermore, biomicroscopy is essential during the performance of various tear film tests.

Biomicroscopic examination is essential for grading ocular surface staining, which is a sign of epithelial damage. Various stains are used, sodium fluorescein and lissamine green being the most common. Sodium fluorescein is a dye indicated to observe the corneal epithelium. Under biomicroscopic observation with cobalt blue and yellow filters, we can see potential corneal epithelium damage as green dots (Figure 16.2b) that, in severe cases, can form a confluent path. Lissamine green dye is used to observe the conjunctival epithelium, but in this case filters are not necessary.

Dry eye is a symptomatic disease, so the presence and status of symptoms need to be ascertained. Symptoms vary in severity according to the state of instability of the tear film and damage of the ocular surface [2]. One problem that can arise is the subjective interpretation of symptoms by the patient. In order to solve this, standardized symptom questionnaires have been developed for use in dry eye diagnosis. The aim of these questionnaires is to offer objective symptom evaluation and guarantee comparisons. Various questionnaires are available but the most used are McMonnies questionnaire, the Ocular Surface Disease Index (OSDI) questionnaire, and the Dry Eye Questionnaire (DEQ).

16.4.2 Clinical Tests

Clinical tests are those that can be performed in clinical settings as part of a routine eye-care examination. Classically, these tests have been divided into two groups: quantitative tests and qualitative tests. Quantitative tests assess quantity of tear film and are related to tear secretion, whereas qualitative tests assess the stability of tear film [8].

16.4.2.1 Quantitative Tear Film Tests

Quantitative tear film tests are related to the lacrimal gland secretion function. Defective lacrimal function is usually demonstrated by showing reduced aqueous tear volume and tear flow. The most used quantitative tear film tests are listed here.

16.4.2.1.1 Tear Meniscus Assessment

It has been estimated that the tear meniscus holds 75%–90% of the total volume of the tear film. Therefore, careful examination of the tear meniscus provides a useful indication of the tear volume [15]. Tear meniscus parameters most commonly used for tear volume examination are tear meniscus height, tear meniscus radius of curvature, and subjective examination of the meniscus. The main advantage of this tear meniscus examination is its noninvasive nature.

TMH is the parameter most used for assessing tear menisci. It can be assessed in clinical settings but biomicroscopy with high magnification is necessary to obtain enough resolution. With the aid of a graticule eyepiece, it is possible to measure TMH, from the lid to the top of the meniscus [15] (Figure 16.3a). The cutoff point between normal and dry eye is ≤0.1 mm. However, measuring the TMH with these settings could be difficult due to the lack of contrast to distinguish the highest limit of the meniscus [12]. Tearscope Plus, a device designed to evaluate the anterior lipid layer (Figure 16.3b) (see description below), can be used to evaluate TMH.

Subjective assessment of the TMH is frequently used by clinicians and has been advocated as part of routine ocular assessments, where the main features evaluated

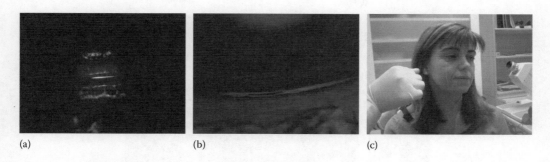

(a)   (b)   (c)

FIGURE 16.3
(a) Appearance of tear meniscus height by slit lamp biomicroscopy. (b) Appearance of tear meniscus height by Tearscope Plus. (c) Phenol red thread test in use.

qualitatively were the presence/absence of debris or foaming in the tear meniscus and its regularity. However, the reliability of this evaluation is affected by subjective criteria of the observer [15].

16.4.2.1.2 Schirmer Test

The Schirmer test estimates tear flow stimulated reflexly by insertion of a filter paper into the conjunctival sac. The strip is placed at the junction of the middle and lateral thirds of the lower eyelid and the patient is told to keep the eyes closed. After 5 min, the strip is replaced and the length of wetted strip is measured. The cutoff value to distinguish normal and dry eye subjects is established at 5 mm. Although this is a test widely employed, it is affected by a wide variability [2]. This test is very uncomfortable for the patient.

16.4.2.1.3 Phenol Red Thread Test

The phenol red thread test consists of a thread impregnated with phenol red, which is pH sensitive and changes from yellow to red over the pH range of normal tears (Figure 16.3c). This test only needs to be hooked over the lower lid for 15 sec and is more comfortable than the Schirmer test (it is barely noticeable for the patient). The cutoff value between controls and dry eye is 10 mm [4].

16.4.2.2 Qualitative Tear Film Tests

Qualitative tear film tests are related to the ability of the tear film to remain stable, which is essential to cover the anterior eye and perform its functions (optical, nutritive, antimicrobial, and cleaning). Secretion of the lacrimal gland may be normal and the volume and composition of the lacrimal fluid adequate, but there could be tear abnormality driven by other factors that can lead to increased tear evaporation. The most used qualitative tear film tests are listed here.

16.4.2.2.1 Lipid Layer Pattern Assessment

Tear film quality and lipid layer thickness can be assessed by noninvasively imaging the superficial lipid layer with interferometry. The Tearscope Plus, designed by Guillon, is the instrument of choice for rapid assessment of lipid layer thickness [16] (Figure 16.4a). With this instrument, a qualitative analysis of the lipid layer structure can be made.

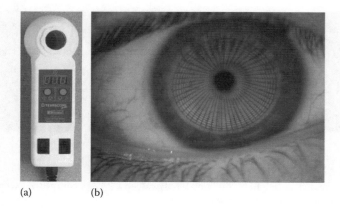

(a)   (b)

FIGURE 16.4
(a) Tearscope Plus. This device projects a cylindrical source of cool white fluorescent light onto the lipid layer. (b) NIBUT test with Tearscope Plus. Grid pattern projected onto the precorneal tear film for the observation of distortion and/or abnormality in the image.

16.4.2.2.2 *Tear Breakup Time (BUT)*

Tear BUT consists of measuring the time that the tear film remains stable without blinking. After fluorescein instillation, the patient is asked to keep the eye open until a sign of tear film rupture (dark spot) appears. This is the most commonly used test of tear film stability and the cutoff for dry eye diagnosis most used is <5 sec [10].

16.4.2.2.3 *Noninvasive Tear Breakup Time (NIBUT)*

NIBUT uses a grid or other pattern directed onto the precorneal tear film for the observation of distortion and abnormality in the image. The time interval in seconds following a blink to the first change of the image is defined as the NIBUT. This method avoids the need for fluorescein instillation and eliminates physical disturbance to the tear film. The Tearscope Plus is commonly used for NIBUT testing by utilizing accessory removable grids [4] (Figure 16.4b).

16.4.2.3 *Osmolarity of Tear Film*

Hyperosmolarity of tear fluid has been recognized as a common feature of all types of DES. It is considered that the osmolarity of the normal tear film is 302 ± 6.3 mOsm/L [17], while in DES it reaches values of 325–340 mOsm/L [17]. The measurement of tear film osmolarity provides a powerful tool that has even been labeled the "gold standard for DES diagnosis" [4].

Unfortunately, the measurement of tear film osmolarity requires very expensive instruments or laboratory equipment that is difficult to use. These difficulties have hindered the application of this procedure in daily practice. There are several types of osmometers based on different physicochemical procedures. The most used clinical technique is based on the electrical conductivity of fluids [18].

Conductivity osmometry is based on electrical conductivity of fluids to measure tear film osmolarity, for example, the TearLab™ osmometer (Figure 16.5a). TearLab™ is specifically designed to measure tear osmolarity. This instrument only needs 0.5 μL of tear sample, using capillary action to collect it directly from the lateral meniscus (Figure 16.5b).

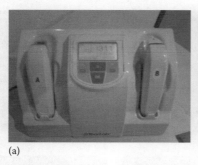
(a)

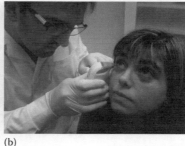
(b)

FIGURE 16.5
(a) TearLab osmometer, based on electrical conductivity technique. (b) TearLab in use.

16.4.3 Laboratory Tests

The composition of proteins in tears plays an important role in ocular surface diseases. Several studies have demonstrated changes in the tear protein patterns of dry eye patients compared with controls, so proteins are useful dry eye biomarkers. The most used biomarkers are lysozyme and lactoferrin [4]. Around 20%–30% of the total tear protein is made up of lysozyme, the most alkaline protein in the tears. Lysozyme levels decrease with dry eye, so their estimation could be useful in DES diagnosis. Although this test is reliable, it is expensive and cumbersome [8]. The lactoplate test determines the concentration of lactoferrin. The lactoplate uses circular discs of filter paper that are placed in the inferior conjunctival. They are placed on agar and incubated for 3 days. The size of the ring is proportional to the lactoferrin concentration of the sample collected. This method, although accurate, is also too expensive to be recommended for use in clinical trials [8].

16.5 Evaluation of Interference Lipid Pattern

The lipid layer of the tear film plays a major role in limiting evaporation during the inter-blink period and also affects tear film stability [3]. Tear film quality and lipid layer thickness can be assessed by noninvasively imaging the superficial lipid layer by interferometry and these two variables are correlated. The lipid layer may be evaluated by slit lamp examination, but the region observed is restricted to a small area (Figure 16.6a).

The Tearscope Plus, designed by Guillon, is the instrument of choice for rapid assessment of lipid layer thickness. It projects a cylindrical source of cool white fluorescent light onto the lipid layer, allowing observation of the superficial layer by thin-film interferometry. The instrument used in conjunction with a nonilluminated biomicroscope provides adequate magnification of the image. With this instrument, a qualitative analysis of the lipid layer structure (which reflects lipid layer thickness) can be made.

Guillon proposed five main grades of lipid layer thickness interference patterns for observations made using the Tearscope Plus [16]: open meshwork, closed meshwork, wave, amorphous, and color fringe (Figure 16.6b–f). This author also described abnormal lipid layer patterns (LLPs) and phenomena. The Tearscope Plus is based on interferential

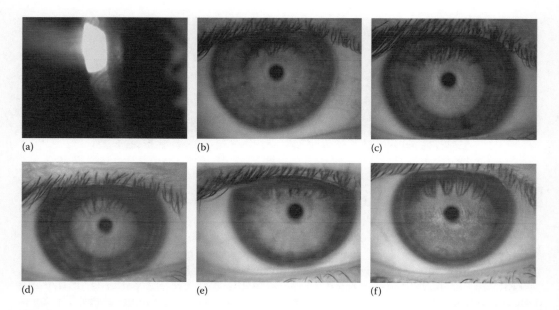

FIGURE 16.6

(a) Appearance of lipid layer by slit lamp examination. The region observed is restricted to a small area. (b) Open meshwork pattern. This represents a very thin, poor, and minimal lipid layer stretched over the ocular surface, which indicates a poor tear film prone to evaporative dry eye. (c) Closed meshwork pattern. More lipid than open meshwork (less stretching of the lipid film). (d) Wave pattern. Thicker than meshwork with wavy, gray streak effect. This represents average tear film stability. (e) Amorphous pattern. A thick, white, even, and well-mixed lipid layer that may show colors during the blink. Ideal candidate for contact lens fitting. (f) Color fringe pattern. Thicker lipid layer with mix of brown and blue color fringes well spread out over the surface. Good candidate for contact lens wear with possible tendency for greasing problems or lipid deposits if a contact lens is fitted.

phenomena. The thickness and regularity of the lipid layer are categorized by observing the appearance and color of the interference pattern between the lipid layer and the under-lying layers. The thicker lipid layers (>90 nm) are readily observed since they produce color and wave patterns. However, thin lipid layers (<60 nm) are difficult to visualize, since color fringes and other distinct morphological features are not present and observa-tions are affected by the subjective interpretation of the observer. Although the Tearscope has proven its validity, some amount of training is needed to interpret LLPs. This difficulty in interpreting LLPs (especially the thinner patterns) and the lack of a huge bank of LLP images for reference purposes have meant that many eye-care professionals have aban-doned this test. However, there is no doubt that the examination of the structure of the tear lipid layer is a useful technique that provides the clinician with valuable information about the stability of the tear film by noninvasive procedures.

Experts classify the tear film lipid layer into one of Guillon's categories through a man-ual process. This clinical task is not only difficult and time-consuming, but also affected by the subjective interpretation of the observers.

In García-Resúa et al. [18] and Ramos et al. [19], it was demonstrated that the manual evaluation of the interference lipid pattern can be automated, with the benefits of being faster and unaffected by subjective factors. The idea lies in characterizing the interference phenomena as a color texture pattern, using image-processing techniques. On the one hand, texture is used to characterize the interference patterns of Guillon's categories, since thick lipid layers show clear patterns while thinner layers are more homogeneous. On the other hand, color is another discriminant feature because some patterns show distinctive color characteristics.

In a similar way, a representative set of texture analysis methods and three color spaces were proposed in Remeseiro et al. [20] to characterize Guillon's patterns, presenting a wide comparative study between all of them. Regarding machine learning algorithms, the behavior of five popular classifiers was analyzed in [21] and a statistical comparison between them was presented.

16.5.1 Extraction of the Region of Interest

Before analyzing the texture corresponding to the interference pattern, it is necessary to extract the region where it appears. These images contain several parts of the eye that lack information for the automatic evaluation, such as the sclera, eyelids, and eyelashes (Figure 16.7a). Experts usually analyze just the bottom part of the iris, ignoring these irrelevant areas and focusing on the area where the tear has higher contrast. This leads to the first step, which consists in preprocessing the images to extract the region of interest (ROI) [22], where the automatic classification will take place.

The bottom part of the iris, where the ROI will be located, corresponds to the most illuminated area of the image due to the acquisition procedure. To detect this most illuminated area, the input image in RGB is transformed to the Lab color space and its luminance component L is selected (Figure 16.7b). Next, it is necessary to create a set of ring-shaped templates that cover the different shapes the ROI can have. Using the L component of the image and these templates, the ROI will be located using the *normalized cross-correlation technique* [23]. Thus, the ROI is selected as the area with maximum normalized cross-correlation value. As a result, a subtemplate is produced and the ROI is located as a rectangle inside it (Figure 16.7b). This final region is where texture and color analysis is performed to generate the final descriptor of the image, which will be classified into Guillon's categories.

16.5.2 Texture Analysis

Extracting texture features of the ROI image involves the application of a texture analysis method over the ROI image in grayscale. Thus, this image has to be transformed from RGB to grayscale, color information being considered later. To deal with this stage, five popular

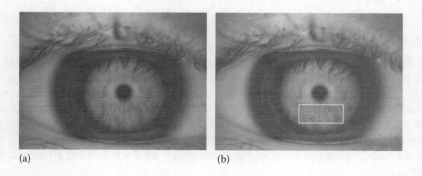

(a)   (b)

FIGURE 16.7
Extraction of the ROI. (a) Original image acquired with the Tearscope Plus. (b) Luminance component L of the original image converted to the Lab color space and delimited ROI.

texture analysis methods [24] were proposed in Remeseiro et al. [20]: *Butterworth filters, Gabor filters,* and *the discrete wavelet transform* as signal-processing methods; *Markov random fields* as a model-based method; and *co-occurrence features* as a statistical method.

16.5.2.1 Butterworth Filters

Butterworth band-pass filters [25] are frequency domain filters that have a flat response in the band-pass frequency, which gradually decays in the stopband. In general, to create a band-pass filter, the cutoff and the center frequencies must be defined. In this particular case, it is also necessary to determine the order n of the filter, which defines the slope of the decay. Note that the higher the order, the faster the decay.

Using Butterworth filters entails creating a bank of nine second-order filters, so that the whole frequency spectrum is covered by the band-pass frequencies used. Thereby, the filter bank maps each input image into nine filtered images, one per frequency band. Next, the feature vector associated to each image must be created. Thus, the results of each frequency band have to be normalized and the histograms of their output images have to be computed. Instead of the traditional histograms, uniform histograms with nonequidistant bins are used. The process consists of, given all the filtered images in a frequency band, sorting their pixels and defining the limits of the histogram so that each bin contains a maximum of N/N_{bins} pixels, N being the number of pixels in the corresponding frequency and N_{bins} the number of histogram bins.

Using 16-bin histograms, the descriptor of an input image has 16 components per frequency band. In this manner, the nine individual descriptors can be combined with just concatenating them.

16.5.2.2 Gabor Filters

Gabor filters are complex exponential signals modulated by Gaussians [26], which can have different shapes and different locations in the spatial and domain frequencies.

Using the same idea as in Butterworth filters, a bank of filters is created with 16 Gabor filters centered at four frequencies and four orientations. Thus, the filter bank maps each input image to 16 filtered images, one per frequency–orientation pair. The creation of the feature vector also follows the previous idea, generating the uniform histogram with nonequidistant bins. Once again, the individual descriptor associated to each filter can be combined with the other by means of their concatenation.

16.5.2.3 Discrete Wavelet Transform

The discrete wavelet transform [27] is a function defined in both the spatial and frequency domains that generates a set of wavelets by scaling and translating a *mother wavelet*. The scale and the translation of the mother wavelet control the band pass of the filter, generating high-pass (H) or low-pass (L) filters. The wavelet decomposition of an image consists of applying this set of wavelets horizontally and vertically, generating four subimages called LL, LH, HL, and HH. It is an iterative method that consists of repeating the process on the LL subimage, resulting in the standard pyramidal wavelet decomposition.

A generalized Haar algorithm [27] is the mother wavelet selected for the problem at hand. Using two scales, eight subimages are generated. On the other hand, some statistical measures are used to create the descriptor from the input image and the eight subimages.

Specifically, it contains 12 features: the mean and the absolute average deviation of the input and the LL images; and the energy of the LH, HL, and HH images.

16.5.2.4 Markov Random Fields

A Markov random field (MRF) [28] is a two-dimensional (2-D) lattice of points where each point has a value that depends on its neighboring values. Therefore, an MRF generates a texture model by expressing the gray value of each pixel in an image as a function of the gray values in its neighborhood. The values that define this function are called parameters of the model.

For the matter at hand, the neighborhood of a pixel is defined as the set of pixels within a distance d, using the *Chebyshev distance*. According to that, the parameters of the model have to be calculated for each input image. Using them, the directional variances proposed by Çesmeli and Wang [29] are obtained resulting in the feature vector. For a distance d, the descriptor comprises $4d$ features. The vector of each distance can be combined with the vectors of any other distances by means of their concatenation.

16.5.2.5 Co-Occurrence Features

Haralick et al. introduced co-occurrence features [30], a method based on the computation of the conditional joint probabilities of all pairwise combinations of gray levels, given an interpixel distance d and an orientation θ. In this sense, a set of gray-level co-occurrence matrices are generated and several statistics can be calculated from their elements. As in the above method, the *Chebyshev distance* is used. Consequently, for a distance $d = 1$, there are four orientations to consider and so four matrices are generated. In general, for a distance d the number of orientations and, therefore, the matrices is $4d$.

After obtaining the matrices, a set of 14 statistics proposed by Haralick et al. [30] have to be computed from each of them. These statistics represent features such as contrast and entropy. The feature vector of an input image is constructed calculating the mean and the range of these statistics across matrices, obtaining a total of 28 features per distance. Different distances can be considered and combined in different ways, by only concatenating them.

16.5.3 Color Analysis

Besides grayscale images, the use of Lab and RGB images is proposed in Ramos et al. [19] so as to consider not only texture features, but also color information. Next, these two color spaces are presented and how the previous texture extraction methods operate in color is explained.

16.5.3.1 Lab Color Space

The CIE 1976 $L^*a^*b^*$ color space [31] (Lab) is a chromatic color space that describes all the colors visible to the human eye. It is defined as a 3-D model with coordinates as follows: L, the lightness of the color; a, the position between magenta and green; and b, the position between yellow and blue. CIE recommends its use in images with natural illumination. Additionally, its colorometric components, which are differences of colors, make it appropriate in texture analysis. These reasons motivated its use in Ramos et al. and Remeseiro et al. [19,20].

Analyzing the texture in the Lab color space entails transforming the input image from RGB to Lab. Next, texture features are extracted from each component separately, generating three descriptors per image that correspond to the *L*, *a*, and *b* components. The final feature vector is created by their concatenation.

16.5.3.2 RGB Color Space: Opponent Colors

The RGB color space [32] (RGB) is an additive color space defined by three chromacities: red, blue, and green. It is one of the most commonly used color spaces for image processing. However, it is not perceptually uniform and, for this reason, the opponent process theory of human color vision, proposed by Hering [33] in the 1800s, is used in Ramos et al., Remeseiro et al., and Calvo et al. [19,20,22]. This theory states that there are three pairs of colors that are never seen together at the same place at the same time. These pairs, called opponent colors, are red versus green, green versus red, and blue versus yellow.

Using opponent colors to analyze the texture entails calculating the three opponent channels from the input image in RGB, which are defined as:

$$R_G = R - p \times G$$
$$G_R = G - p \times R \tag{16.1}$$
$$B_Y = B - p \times (R + G)$$

where *p* is a low-pass filter.

Finally, texture features are extracted from each opponent channel individually and the final descriptor is their concatenation.

16.5.4 Results

After performing previous stages, an input image leads to a feature vector containing texture and color information. These features should be distinctive in order to classify the vector into one of Guillon's categories. For this purpose, machine learning provides algorithms that improve automatically through experience based on data, in a process called training. Data can be seen as examples that represent relations between features and classes. In this context, the images of the training data set are the examples with their descriptors as features; while the classes correspond to Guillon's categories.

In Ramos et al. [19] and Remeseiro et al. [21], several machine learning algorithms applied to the problem at hand were statistically analyzed. Next, these six popular algorithms [34] are briefly explained:

- *Naïve Bayes*: A simple probabilistic classifier based on the Bayesian theorem and the maximum *a posteriori* hypothesis that can predict class membership probabilities.
- *Logistic model tree*: An algorithm for supervised learning tasks that consists of a decision tree with logistic regression functions in the leaves.
- *Random tree*: A decision tree formed by a stochastic process, which means that it is randomly selected from a set of trees with the same probability of being sampled.

- *Random forest*: An ensemble of individual decision trees where each one depends on the values of a random vector sampled independently and with the same distribution for all trees in the forest.
- *Multilayer perceptron*: A feedforward artificial neural network composed of simple neurons called perceptrons and trained by a supervised learning technique called back propagation.
- *Support vector machine (SVM)*: A supervised learning method that, based on the statistical learning theory, constructs an n-dimensional hyperplane that optimally separates the data in classes.

Both works [19,21] performed several experiments using these classifiers and the different texture extraction methods in three color spaces. After exhaustive statistical analysis, the same general conclusion was reached in both, selecting the SVM as the most competitive method.

In Remeseiro et al. [20], several experiments were performed using the five texture extraction methods in the three color spaces presented above, with the SVM as classifier due to its statistical outperformance. All these experimental results were obtained using a data set composed of 105 images from healthy subjects between 19 and 33 years old. This data set, labeled for experts, includes 29 open meshwork, 29 closed meshwork, 25 wave, and 22 color fringe images. A tenfold cross-validation [35], widely used to validate a model, was performed to generalize the results to larger data sets.

Regarding texture extraction methods, the different experiments performed can be summarized as follows:

- *Butterworth filters*: Using the nine frequency band filters and 16-bin histograms, each frequency band was analyzed separately. Additionally, the adjacent frequency bands were combined by means of the concatenation of their individual descriptors.
- *Gabor filters*: 3-bin, 5-bin, 7-bin, and 9-bin histograms were analyzed using the bank of 16 Gabor filters.
- *Discrete wavelet transform*: Each feature was analyzed individually to determine its relevance. Then, two alternative descriptors were created: one composed of the 12 features presented above and the other composed of the six best-performing features according to the previous analysis.
- *Markov random fields*: Each distance from 1 to 10 was analyzed individually in order to compare different neighborhoods.
- *Co-occurrence features*: Each distance from 1 to 7 was analyzed individually, as well as the combination of adjacent distances through the concatenation of their descriptors.

Each of these experiments was performed in grayscale, Lab, and opponent colors. Table 16.1 shows the best result for each pair texture–color, where the best result per color space is highlighted. These results are shown in terms or percentage accuracy, a measure that represents the rate percentage of the images that are correctly classified according to their category. Also, the parameter configuration of each pair is specified.

From Table 16.1, it can be concluded that, in general, the use of color information improves the accuracy obtained in grayscale. This can be explained because color is one

TABLE 16.1

Comparison of Different Feature Extraction Methods

	Grayscale	Lab	Opp. Colors
Butterworth filters	83.81 (freqs. 1–9)	93.33 (freqs. 5–7)	90.48 (freqs. 2–4)
Gabor filters	88.57 (3 bins)	95.24 (7 bins)	88.57 (5 bins)
Discrete wavelet transform	85.71 (12 feats.)	89.52 (6 feats.)	85.71 (6 feats.)
Markov random fields	83.81 (dist. 4)	83.81 (dist. 3)	84.76 (dist. 1)
Co-occurrence features	*92.38* (dist. 7)	*96.19* (dist. 6)	*92.38* (dists. 3–4)

Note: Best SVM categorization accuracy (%) and parameter configuration in the three color spaces.

of the distinctive features of Guillon's patterns. Regarding texture information, co-occurrence features produce best results, closely followed by Gabor filters, providing both classification results with maximum accuracy over 95%. These results demonstrate that it is possible to precisely evaluate the interference lipid pattern through a completely automatic process that eliminates the subjectivity of the manual test.

16.6 Evaluation of the Tear Film Breakup Time

The preocular tear film does not remain stable for long periods of time. Normal blinking guarantees that a stable tear film covers the anterior eye to maintain its adequate physiology. When blinking is prevented, the tear film ruptures and dry spots appear over the cornea. A lipid film is seldom stable for long periods of time; some of the superficial lipids will migrate to the epithelium interface, contaminating the adsorbed mucin layer and converting it into a hydrophobic surface.

The breakup time (BUT) test consists of measuring the time that the tear film remains stable without blinking. To perform this test, instillation of fluorescein dye into the anterior surface of the eye is needed. Then, with the help of a cobalt blue filter attached to a slit lamp biomicroscope and a yellow filter (Wratten #8 filter; Eastman Kodak Company, Rochester, NY) to improve the visibility of the fluorescein emission, the tear film appears green (Figure 16.8a). The procedure consists of asking the patient to blink three times to spread the fluorescein evenly and then keep the eye open for as long as possible until a dark spot appears in the fluorescent tear film (which indicates tear film disruption) (Figure 16.8b). The BUT is the time in seconds from a full blink to the appearance of the first dark spot in the tear film. This is the most commonly used test of tear film stability. Reduced BUT or limited ocular surface wetting is one of the main signs of an abnormal tear film. Classically the cutoff value between normal and dry eyes is considered as <10 sec, but this cutoff value has been questioned by many authors. In this sense, Abelson et al. [10] have found that the mean BUT for normal subjects is 7.1 sec (range 4.7–11.4 sec) and for dry eye patients 2.2 sec (range 0.9–5.2 sec). On the basis of this, a cutoff for dry eye diagnosis of <5 sec is recommended. However, this test is affected by low repeatability mainly driven by subjective appreciation of the dark spot and the technique of fluorescein instillation.

The automation of the breakup time measure is a little explored field. In the literature there are two approaches to achieve this goal, proposed by Yedidya et al. [36,37] and Cebreiro et al. [38]. The two alternatives consist of a multistep algorithm that shares the

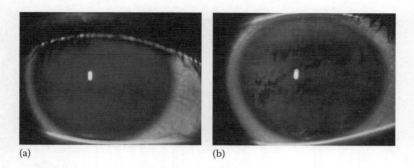

FIGURE 16.8
(a) Tear film with fluorescein. (b) The formation of dark spots points out tear film disruptions.

main stages but is conducted differently by the authors. First, the different measurement areas contained in a tear film video are delimited. Then, the ROI is extracted and the consecutive frames are aligned through the video. Finally, the BUT test is performed in each measurement area.

16.6.1 Location of Measurement Areas

A tear film video is composed of different measurement areas separated by blinks (Figure 16.9). Both approaches need to delimit the beginning and the end of each measurement area to perform the BUT separately in each.

This process can be automated by detecting the blinks when consecutive frames present a big difference in intensity. The proposal of Cebreiro et al. [38] performs this automation by calculating symmetric finite differences to consecutive frames. On these differences, a negative peak represents the beginning of a blink, since there is a transition from a lighter frame (open eye) to a darker frame (closed eye). Similarly, a positive peak represents the end of a blink, since there is a transition from a darker frame to a lighter frame. A range is used to identify these peaks so that values outside this range correspond to blinks and values inside are related to frames where the eye is open. Therefore, a measurement area is identified as an interval between a positive difference and a negative difference. Furthermore, the measurement area should exceed a minimum of frames. Sometimes the lamp is off during an interval of the sequence or there are semiblinks in the measurement area. In these cases, there could be two consecutive differences with the same sign. In order to discard these occurrences, the lowest absolute values are removed until all pairs of consecutive blinks have opposite signs. The delimited zones constitute the measurement areas (Figure 16.10).

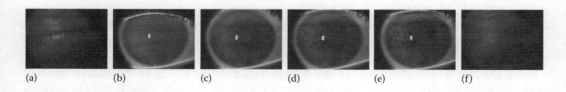

(a) (b) (c) (d) (e) (f)

FIGURE 16.9
Several frames within a measurement area: (a) blink at the beginning of the area, (b) stable tear film before breakup, (c) breakup, (d,e) evolution after the breakup, and (f) blink at the end of the area.

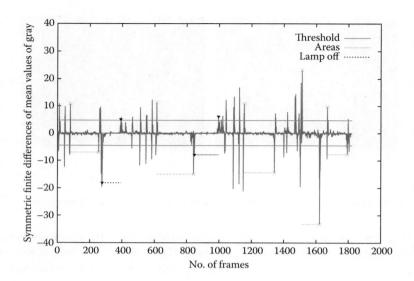

FIGURE 16.10
Measurement areas automatically detected. The intervals between peaks with opposite signs correspond to the correct measurement areas and the other two areas are discarded because the lamp is off.

16.6.2 Extraction of the ROI

Once the measurement areas are identified, the next step is to extract the ROI within each frame since it includes regions that do not contain relevant information and could mislead the results of the methodology.

Yedidya et al. [36,37] carry out this stage assuming the shape of the ROI is a perfect circle. First, an edge map of the image immediately after a blink is created using the Canny edge detector [39]. In these videos, the pupil is not visible at all and the edges of the eyelids are usually stronger than the iris borders, due to the fluorescein spreading. The ratio between the iris pixels and everything else is too high so it is impractical to perform a fitting to the iris directly. For this reason, three threshold images are created over the edge image: one of the iris (I_{iris}) and the others (I_{low}, I_{up}) of the lower and upper eyelids. Then RANSAC [40] is used to fit a polynomial of degree 2 to I_{low} and I_{up}. Therefore, the upper and lower eyelids are segmented and then all pixels above and below them, respectively, are discarded in I_{iris}. After this, RANSAC is applied in order to fit a circle model to the remaining pixels.

After the detection of the iris, a fine tuning is performed using Levenberg–Marquardt (LM) [40] minimization. The initial guess (x_0, y_0, r_0) is the circle found by the RANSAC. A maximum error e of a few pixels is defined to compute the gradient magnitude for all pixels in the annulus formed by the circles with center (x_0, y_0) and radii $r_0 - e$ and $r_0 + e$. The main idea is to minimize the sum of distances of pixels with strong magnitudes to the circle. The ROI will be the intersection between the eyelids and the iris (Figure 16.11).

Once the iris is well delimited in the first image, the extraction of the ROI in the rest of the sequence is done in a similar way. For each frame, the LM algorithm is computed using the previous result as an initial guess. Thus, for every image, only the fast LM algorithm is conducted, so the time-consuming RANSAC is computed only once, for the first image.

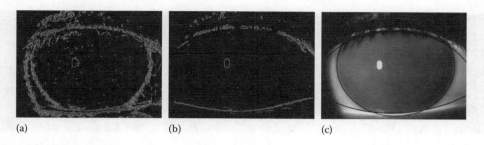

(a)   (b)   (c)

FIGURE 16.11
Steps for locating the ROI. (a) Cropped edge map. (b) Cropped edge map for locating the eyelids. (c) Curves fitted for the eyelids and the iris.

The eye can move through the sequence, so it is necessary to register it in each frame. Thus, the methodology is independent of slight motions of the ROI since the iris appears in the same location in the aligned video. To this end, the circles representing the iris are aligned from the center of the ROI detected in the consecutive frames. Moreover, a second alignment is performed based on minimizing differences of intensities in an area surrounding the iris. In order to avoid cumulative error, the sequence is treated as a set of blocks composed of a few consecutive images. The first image of each block is aligned with an image of the previous block and the remaining frames within the block are aligned with the first one.

The approach proposed by Cebreiro et al. [38] begins this step with the estimation of the size of the iris. Assuming its circular shape, a bank of circular masks with different radii covering the typical eye sizes is selected. To this end, the Canny edge detector [39] is applied to the green component of the frames placed at 25%, 50%, and 75% of each measurement area. Then, the maximum correlation in the frequency domain among the three edge images and the different masks is analyzed to determine the best fit. The largest value of these correlations corresponds to the optimal radius and, therefore, the size of the eye. This size is fixed throughout the sequence and the center of the circle is used to align the successive frames.

Sometimes the eye is not fully open and the ROI includes outer parts like eyelids or eyelashes. These elements can disrupt the results so the authors proposed to crop the region where the measure will take place. Therefore, the top and the bottom of the circular ROI are cropped in order to discard the eyelids. Moreover, the radius of the ROI is reduced to get rid of noise due to eyelashes (Figure 16.12).

16.6.3 BUT Measurement

The last step of the methodology consists of scanning the aligned video to compute the BUT measure. The breakup of the tear film is characterized by the appearance of dark spots on the surface of the eye. In order to detect the emergence of these points the evolution in intensity of each pixel is examined through the video sequence.

The proposal of Yedidya et al. [36,37] in addition to measuring the breakup time creates an image that shows the degree of dryness for each pixel in the iris area. The dryness image is initialized with no breakup for all pixels. In order to estimate the degree of thinning of each pixel, three terms are calculated. First, the $D(x, y)$ term corresponds to the average difference in intensities between the four last images and the four first images. This term is made relative to the iris average intensity to be more sensitive to small

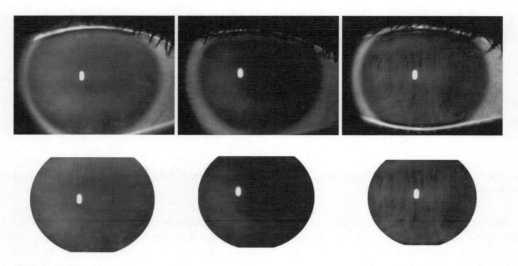

FIGURE 16.12
Adjustment of the ROI. (*top*) Original frames of eyes in different positions. (*bottom*) Adjusted regions of interest.

changes in intensity through the video. Then, the $B(x, y)$ term relates the initial intensity of the pixel to the initial average intensity of the iris. It is used to compensate those pixels with initial value outside the average value. Finally, the $R(x, y)$ term provides information about the evolution of the intensity of each pixel throughout the sequence. It is mainly used for refinement and also to include or discard pixels near the boundaries whose intensities fluctuate for small misalignments. Therefore, the intensity value for each pixel of the dryness images is calculated as the sum of the terms weighted by a factor selected according to the importance of each of them. This value corresponds to the degree of thinning, so that higher values relate drier areas.

The computation of the breakup time is directly related to the creation of the dryness image, since the intensity values are calculated in the same way but using only values from the first frame to the current frame. A breakup threshold B_T is chosen arbitrarily to be close to the maximum possible pixel intensity in the iris. This threshold represents the minimum intensity for a pixel to be considered as a break. If the intensity of a pixel (x, y) is above B_T, this means a break is suspected. A break is considered when a small number of pixels are over the breakup threshold. The minimum number of pixels is chosen to compensate for cases where there are some misaligned pixels.

Yedidya et al. also proposed dividing the ROI into five areas according to the Contact Lens Research Unit (CCLRU) standards [41] (Figure 16.13). For this course, the area of thinning and the breakup time are calculated in each subarea to get more elaborate results related to the degree of dryness and the location.

The dryness image produces good segmentation results but it has a few disadvantages. For example, small errors in alignment can bias the degree of dryness for a pixel. Otherwise, the spatial relationships between neighboring pixels and the knowledge regarded from the temporal changes are not considered. For these reasons, Yedidya et al. propose a new approach based on a three-dimensional (3-D) volume to segment the dry regions [42]. In this new version, each aligned frame in the sequence is considered as a 3-D slice so the video is transformed into a spatiotemporal volume. The volume is modeled as a 3-D multilabel Markov Random Field (MRF) in which each voxel has a label related to

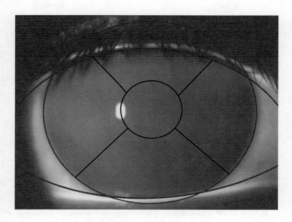

FIGURE 16.13
ROI divided into five local areas in a similar way to the CCLRU standards.

its degree of dryness. The 3-D volume is created as a graph based on temporal and spatial changes. Therefore, the first slice corresponds to the first image after the blink and the last slice is the last image in the measurement area. The remaining slices are related to the time elapsed since the blink. The structure of the graph is based on a 6-connectedness neighborhood. Therefore, each voxel in the MRF is connected to its four direct neighbors in the same image and to the equivalent pixel in the previous and next frames. In this way, the spatial smoothness and the temporal knowledge are considered. The segmentation goal consists of assigning a label to each voxel of the MRF. The label set represents the estimated thickness from no thinning of the tear film to a complete absence of fluid of the tear film. Labels must change gradually so a monotonic dryness constraint is enforced to the cost function. The details of the 3-D MFR segmentation are explained in Yedidya et al. [42].

The breakup time is measured in the 3-D approach in the same way as in the previous version but considering a break of pixels when it has the highest label of the MRF.

The approach of Cebreiro et al. [38] is based on building evolution curves to analyze the intensity through the sequence. Each tear film video presents variations in the illumination and the amount of fluorescein instilled, so not all measurement areas have the same intensity levels. Moreover, the dark pixels at the breakup vary in a range of values close to zero according to lighting conditions, but not exactly zero. For these reasons, this proposal establishes a threshold to determine the range of black level in each measurement area. To this end, a histogram of the first frame of each measurement area is created and the gray levels of a percentage of the darkest pixels are analyzed. The black level threshold corresponds to the largest value of these gray levels, that is, pixels with values below this threshold area are considered as black (Figure 16.14).

A black level evolution curve for each measurement area is built from the percentage of points considered as black in the consecutive frames. In some cases, this curve is virtually zero because the tear does not break up in the interval. On the contrary, if there is a measure, the percentage of black increases with time since the fluorescein is not regenerated (Figure 16.15).

Another threshold obtained as a percentage of the total height of the black level curve evolution is used to determine the breakup time. The BUT is measured as the time elapsed since the blink at the beginning of the measurement area to the moment when the curve exceeds this threshold (Figure 16.15).

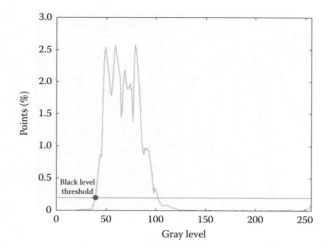

FIGURE 16.14

Calculation of the black threshold from the histogram of a frame at the beginning of the measurement area. The value is obtained as the highest gray level of a percentage of the darkest pixels.

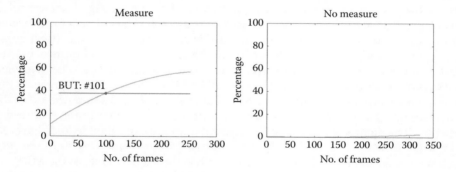

FIGURE 16.15

Black evolution curves. (*left*) The black area increases with time. (*right*) There is no measure.

16.6.4 Results

The automatic approaches related were tested over several tear film videos from healthy patients of different age groups varying from very dry eye to an eye with no visible dryness. In all cases, the patients were instructed to keep their eyes open as long as possible.

Table 16.2 shows the results of the automatic detection of the different measurement areas conducted in the work of Cebreiro et al. [38]. As can be seen, this methodology works well in detecting areas where there is BUT measurement as well as those where there is no measure.

In order to assess the accuracy of BUT detection, the results obtained by the proposed methodologies were compared with values provided by different clinical experts. Differences between the values annotated by each expert and the average of them all have been analyzed. This error is located mainly in an interval of ±2.5 sec due to the subjectivity of this measure.

Table 16.3 summarizes the error in seconds of each approach as well as the error produced between the experts themselves. These results show that the estimation of the BUT by these automatic approaches is in agreement with the manual detection. As can be seen,

TABLE 16.2

Confusion Matrix between Measurement Areas
Identified by Experts and Detected Automatically

		System	
		Measure (%)	No Measure (%)
Expert	Measure	91	9
	No measure	25	75

TABLE 16.3

Differences between Both Approaches and Each Individual
Expert with Respect to the Average Expert BUT Measurement

BUT Estimation Error	Yedidya et al. (%)	Cebreiro et al. (%)	Experts (%)
<1 s	66.67	45	84
1–2 s	19.04	40	11.25
2–3 s	9.52	10	2.5
>3 s	4.77	5	1.25
Total	21	40	160
Average error	1.06 s	1.55 s	0.78 s

Source: Data from Cebreiro, E., Ramos, L., Mosquera, A., Barreira, N., and Penedo, M.G., Automation of the tear film break-up time test, In *Proceedings of the 4th International Symposium on Applied Sciences in Biomedical and Communication Technologies (ISABEL)*, Barcelona, ACM, New York, 2011: Yedidya, T., Hartley, R., and Guillon, J.P., Automatic detection of pre-ocular tear film break-up sequence in dry eyes, In *Proceedings of Digital Image Computing: Techniques and Applications (DICTA)*, Canberra, IEEE Computer Society, Los Alamitos, CA, pp. 442–448, 2008.

most of the measures have an error in an interval of ±2.5 sec. This value is acceptable since it is in the same range as among the experts so it is not significant.

The results obtained by both approaches demonstrate that automation of BUT measurement is possible, since the average difference between these proposals and the experts' measures was within the acceptable range considering the high interobserver variance.

References

1. J.R. Larke. *The Eye in Contact Lens Wear*. Butterworth-Heinemann, Oxford, 1997.
2. D.R. Korb. *The Tear Film: Structure, Function and Clinical Examination*. Butterworth-Heinemann, London, 2002.
3. K.K. Nichols, J.J. Nichols, and G.L. Mitchell. The lack of association between signs and symptoms in patients with dry eye disease. *Cornea*, 23(8):762–770, 2004.
4. M.A. Lemp, C. Baudouin, J. Baum, M. Dogru, G.N. Foulks, S. Kinoshita, P. Laibson, et al. The definition and classification of dry eye disease: Report of the definition and classification subcommittee of the international dry eye workshop (2007). *Ocul Surf*, 5(2):75–92, 2007.
5. S.C. Pflugfelder. Prevalence, burden, and pharmacoeconomics of dry eye disease. *Am J Manag Care*, 14(3 Suppl.):S102–S106, 2008.

6. C. Fenga, P. Aragona, A. Cacciola, R. Spinella, C. Di Nola, F. Ferreri, and L. Rania. Meibomian gland dysfunction and ocular discomfort in video display terminal workers. *Eye*, 22(1):91–95, 2008.

7. S. Patel and I. Wallace. Tear meniscus height, lower punctum lacrimale, and the tear lipid layer in normal aging. *Optom Vis Sci*, 83(10):731–739, 2006.

8. M.A. Lemp. Report of the national eye institute/industry workshop on clinical trials in dry eyes. *CLAO J*, 21(4):221–232, 1995.

9. A.J. Bron, F.M. Sci, and J.M. Tiffany. The contribution of meibomian disease to dry eye. *Ocul Surf*, 2(2):149–165, 2004.

10. M.B. Abelson, G.W. Ousler III, L.A. Nally, D. Welch, and K. Krenzer. Alternative reference values for tear film break up time in normal and dry eye populations. *Adv Exp Med Biol*, 506(Pt B):1121–1125, 2002.

11. P. Reddy, O. Grad, and K. Rajagopalan. The economic burden of dry eye: A conceptual framework and preliminary assessment. *Cornea*, 23(8):751–761, 2004.

12. B. Miljanovic, R. Dana, D.A. Sullivan, and D.A. Schaumberg. Impact of dry eye syndrome on vision-related quality of life. *Am J Ophthalmol*, 143(3):409–415, 2007.

13. W. Stevenson, S.K. Chauhan, and R. Dana. Dry eye disease: An immune mediated ocular surface disorder. *Arch Ophthalmol*, 130(1):90–100, 2012.

14. R. Tutt, A. Bradley, C. Begley, and L.N. Thibos. Optical and visual impact of tear break-up in human eyes. *Invest Ophthalmol Vis Sci*, 41(13):4117–4123, 2000.

15. C. García-Resúa, J. Santodomingo-Rubido, M. Lira, M.J. Giraldez, and E. Yebra-Pimentel. Clinical assessment of the lower tear meniscus height. *Ophthalmic Physiol Opt*, 29:487–496, 2009.

16. J.P. Guillon. Non-invasive tearscope plus routine for contact lens fitting. *Cont Lens Anterior Eye*, 21(Suppl. 1):S31–S40, 1998.

17. A. Tomlinson, S. Khanal, K. Ramaesh, C. Diaper, and A. McFadyen. Tear film osmolarity: Determination of a referent for dry eye diagnosis. *Invest Ophthalmol Vis Sci*, 47(10):4309–4315, 2006.

18. C. García-Resúa, M.J. Giráldez-Fernández, M.G. Penedo, D. Calvo, M. Penas, and E. Yebra-Pimentel. New software application for clarifying tear film lipid layer patterns. *Cornea*, 32(4):538–546, 2013.

19. L. Ramos, M. Penas, B. Remeseiro, A. Mosquera, N. Barreira, and E. Yebra-Pimentel. Texture and color analysis for the automatic classification of the eye lipid layer. In *LNCS: Advances in Computational Intelligence (International Work Conference on Artificial Neural Networks IWANN 2011)*, vol. 6692, pp. 66–73, 2011.

20. B. Remeseiro, L. Ramos, M. Penas, E. Martínez, M.G. Penedo, and A. Mosquera. Colour texture analysis for classifying the tear film lipid layer: A comparative study. In *International Conference on Digital Image Computing: Techniques and Applications (DICTA)*, pp. 268–273, Noosa, Australia, 2011.

21. B. Remeseiro, M. Penas, A. Mosquera, J. Novo, MG. Penedo, and E. Yebra-Pimentel. Statistical comparison of classifiers applied to the interferential tear film lipid layer automatic classification. *Comput Math Methods Med*, 207315, 2012.

22. D. Calvo, A. Mosquera, M. Penas, C. García-Resúa, and B. Remeseiro. Color texture analysis for tear film classification: A preliminary study. In *Lecture Notes in Computer Science: International Conference on Image Analysis and Recognition (ICIAR)*, vol. 6112, pp. 388–397, 2010.

23. J.C. Russ. *The Image Processing Handbook* (3rd edn). CRC, Boca Raton, FL, 1999.

24. C.H. Chen, L.F. Pau, and P.S.P. Wangs. *The Handbook of Pattern Recognition and Computer Vision* (2nd edn). World Scientific, Singapore, 1998.

25. R. Gonzalez and R. Woods. *Digital Image Processing*. Pearson/Prentice Hall, Upper Saddle River, NJ, 2008.

26. D. Gabor. Theory of communication. *J Inst Electric Eng*, 93:429–457, 1946.

27. S.G. Mallat. A theory for multiresolution signal decomposition: The wavelet representation. *IEEE Trans Pattern Analysis Machine Intelligence*, 11:674–693, 1989.

28. J. Besag. Spatial interaction and the statistical analysis of lattice systems. *J R Statistic Soc B*, 36:192–236, 1974.

29. E. Çesmeli and D. Wang. Texture segmentation using Gaussian–Markov random fields and neural oscillator networks. *IEEE Trans Neural Netw*, 12:394–404, 2001.
30. R.M. Haralick, K. Shanmugam, and Its'Hak Dinstein. Texture features for image classification. *IEEE Trans Syst Man Cybernet*, 3:610–621, 1973.
31. K. McLaren. The development of the CIE 1976 (L*a*b) uniform colour-space and colour-difference formula. *J Soc Dyers Colourists*, 92(9):338–341, 1976.
32. S.J. Sangwine and R.E.N. Horne. *The Colour Image Processing Handbook*. Chapman & Hall, London, 1998.
33. E. Hering. *Outlines of a Theory of the Light Sense*. Harvard University Press, Cambridge, MA, 1964.
34. T. Mitchell. *Machine Learning*. McGraw Hill, New York, NY, 1997.
35. J. Rodriguez, A. Perez, and J. Lozano. Sensitivity analysis of k-fold cross-validation in prediction error estimation. *IEEE Trans Pattern Analysis Machine Intelligence*, 32:569–575, 2010.
36. T. Yedidya, R. Hartley, and J.P. Guillon. Automatic detection of pre-ocular tear film break-up sequence in dry eyes. *Proceedings of Digital Image Computing: Techniques and Applications (DICTA)*, Canberra, IEEE Computer Society, Los Alamitos, CA, pp. 442–448, 2008.
37. T. Yedidya, R. Hartley, J.P. Guillon, and Y. Kanagasingam. Automatic dry eye detection. *Med Image Comput Comput Assist Interv*, 10:792–799, 2007.
38. E. Cebreiro, L. Ramos, A. Mosquera, N. Barreira, and M.G. Penedo. Automation of the tear film break-up time test. In *Proceedings of the 4th International Symposium on Applied Sciences in Biomedical and Communication Technologies (ISABEL)*, Barcelona, October, ACM, New York, 2011.
39. C. Canny. A computational approach to edge detection. *IEEE PAMI*, 8:679–698, 1986.
40. R.I. Hartley and A. Zisserman. *Multiple View Geometry in Computer Vision* (2nd edn). Cambridge University Press, Cambridge, 2004.
41. T. Terry, C. Schnider, and B.A. Holden. The CCLRU standards. *Optician*, pp. 18–23, 1993.
42. T. Yedidya, P. Carr, R. Hartley, and J.P. Guillon. Enforcing monotonic temporal evolution in dry eye images. *Med Image Comput Comput Assist Interv*, pp. 976–979, 2009.

17

Thermal Modeling of the Ageing Eye

Anastasios Papaioannou and Theodoros Samaras

CONTENTS

17.1 The Healthy Ageing Eye

Like the rest of the human body, the human eye undergoes several changes due to ageing. These anatomical and physiological processes follow either a gradual decrease or a gradual increase. There is a difference between disease and the changes that occur due to eye ageing, although the visual impairments caused by the latter may be similar to but less important than the ones caused by the former. It is widely acknowledged that the scientific community has placed more emphasis on understanding and treating diseases that cause blindness, such as glaucoma, than on studying the effects of ageing on the eye.

17.1.1 Anatomical Changes

The anatomical changes in the eye have a significant impact on visual performance. Several alterations take place in the anterior segments of the eye as it grows, with a significant process being the shallowing of the anterior chamber depth, which in turn affects the development and anterior displacement of the lens. In their study, Lim et al. (1992) measured the dimensional changes in anterior chamber depth (ACD), lens thickness (LT), and relative lens position (RLP) in the healthy ageing eye. Dubbelman et al. (2002) determined the posterior and anterior radii of the corneal surface in healthy eyes of subjects in the age range 16–62 years, using corrected-for-distortion Scheimpflug photography.

In this chapter we consider three different age groups (20–29, 40–49, and 60–69 years) in order to construct models which describe the dimensional changes in the healthy eye due to ageing. Table 17.1 shows the values for different parts of the eye per age group.

The ACD, the RLP, the corneal radius (R_{cornea}, radius of corneal curvature), and the radius of the anterior chamber (R_{AC}) decrease with age, in contrast with the LT, which increases during eye growth. Another fact is that the axial length (AXL) and the vertical length (VL) initially decrease, until about the age of 50 years, but in older eyes they increase again, even surpassing the value of the 20-year-old eye. Figure 17.1 illustrates the different parts of the human eye with the geometrical dimensions denoted on them.

Liu (2006) studied the mechanism of the formation of the anterior chamber angle in normal adult eyes. In both sexes and in various populations, the ACD decreases with increasing age. On the contrary, the LT increases as the eye grows and this may contribute to the decrease of the ACD. Figure 17.2 shows the shallower ACD as well as the augmentation of the LT in the older age groups in the numerical models used later in this chapter.

TABLE 17.1

Geometrical Dimensions of Parts in the Human Eye Model (Figure 17.1) per Age Group

Models	Cornea Thickness (mm)	Anterior Chamber Depth (mm)	Lens Thickness (mm)	Relative Lens Position (mm)	Axial Length (mm)	Vertical Length (mm)	R_{cornea} (mm)	R_{AC} (mm)
20–29	0.57[a]	3.43[b]	3.93[b]	5.392[b]	24.22	23.07	7.902[c]	6.478[c]
40–49	0.57[a]	3.26[b]	4.124[b]	5.342[b]	23.87	22.73	7.822[c]	6.378[c]
60–69	0.57[a]	3.01[b]	4.53[b]	5.285[b]	24.27	23.11	7.742[c]	6.278[c]

[a] Karampatzakis, A., Samaras, T. *Phys. Med. Biol.* 55, 5653–5665, 2010.
[b] Lim, K. J., Hyung, S. M., Youn, D. H. *Korean J. Ophthalmol.* 6, 19–31, 1992.
[c] Dubbelman, M., Weeber, H. A., van der Heijde, R. G. L., Volker-Dieben, H. J. *Acta Ophthalmol. Scand.* 80, 379–383, 2002.

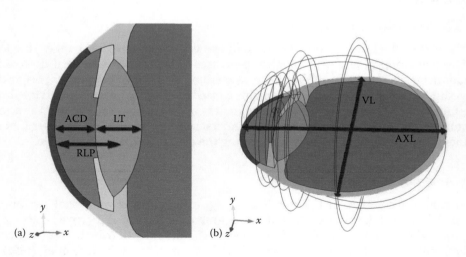

FIGURE 17.1

Dimensions of (a) the anterior segments and (b) the eyeball. (a) ACD, anterior chamber depth; LT, lens thickness; RLP, relative lens position; (b) AXL, axial length; VL, vertical length.

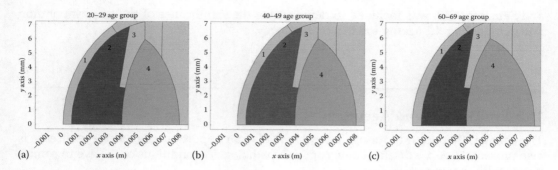

FIGURE 17.2
(a–c) The anatomical changes in the anterior chamber and lens: decrease of the ACD and increase of LT, respectively. 1, cornea; 2, anterior chamber; 3, iris; 4, lens.

17.1.2 Functional Changes

The tear film is a complex, rather unstable structure which covers the corneal surface. It consists of proteins, lipids, and mucins and is divided into three layers: the lipid, the aqueous, and the mucous. The lipid layer sits on the top and creates an oily membrane, the role of which is to protect and cover the tear film. The middle aqueous layer retains moisture in the eye and supplies oxygen and other nutrients to the cornea. It comprises 98% water with small amounts of salt, proteins, and other compounds. The mucus layer provides a cover directly on top of and in contact with the cornea, acting like an adhesive between the latter and the tear film, in order to keep it fixed on the eye.

Moss et al. (2000) have shown that age, along with a history of arthritis, thyroid disease or gout, smoking, caffeine use, and diabetes, is a risk factor for dry eye syndrome. The rate of oil production by the human body decreases with age, a fact that affects the tear film by increasing the evaporation rate of the aqueous layer. In their study Mathers and Lane (1998) calculated the mean tear film values of normal eyes by age decade. Tan et al. (2010) developed a novel technique to measure tear evaporation and monitor its variation with respect to time. The evaporation rate was determined to be 58.9 and 55.82 W/m^2 for older (above 35) and younger (below 35) subjects, respectively.

In this chapter, in order to study the effect of the changing evaporation rate of the tear film with age, three models were created with different values for the evaporation rate, as summarized in Table 17.2. The model with the constant evaporation rate (Karampatzakis

TABLE 17.2

Summary of Different Evaporation Rates Used in the Eye Models (W/m^2)

Model	20–29 Years	40–49 Years	60–69 Years
Reference model[a]	30.68	33.85	47.32
New model[b]	55.82	58.90	58.90
Constant rate[c]	40.00	40.00	40.00

[a] Mathers, W. D., Lane, J. A. Meibomian gland lipids, evaporation, and tear film stability. In: Sullivan, D. A., Dartt, D. A., Meneray, M. A. (eds), *Lacrimal Gland, Tear Film, and Dry Eye Syndromes* 2, pp. 349–360. Plenum, New York, 1998.
[b] Tan, J. H., Ng, E. Y. K., Acharya, R. U. *Med. Phys.* 37, 6022–6034, 2010.
[c] Karampatzakis, A., Samaras, T. *Phys. Med. Biol.* 55, 5653–5665, 2010.

and Samaras 2010) was included to demonstrate the significance of the tear evaporation rate in modeling the ageing eye in a realistic way.

17.2 Eye Disease and Ageing

The changes that occur in the ageing eye may play an important role when eye disease is also present. Here we discuss some common pathological conditions of the eye in combination with the impact of ageing.

17.2.1 Contact Lens

The most common eye problems are refractive errors, such as myopia, presbyopia, astigmatism, and hyperopia. Of the above conditions, presbyopia is inextricably associated with age and signifies a difficulty in vision of close up objects, due to the loss of the lens capability to accommodate increasing age. Eyeglasses, contact lenses, and surgery are ways of correcting refractive errors.

A contact lens is placed on the external surface of the cornea to correct vision. Its advantages, in comparison with eyeglasses, are the provision of better peripheral vision and the prevention of moisture collection. Older people often complain that they find it difficult to wear contact lenses, the reason being that the lens greatly increases the tear evaporation rate. Mathers (2004) studied evaporation in subjects wearing various types of contact lenses. An increase in evaporation was found with old contact lenses. In particular, an evaporation rate of 55.82 W/m^2 was estimated for contact lenses worn daily for 6 weeks.

Ooi et al. (2007) simulated a two-dimensional model of heat transfer in the human eye wearing a contact lens using finite element analysis. Three types of contact lenses were studied. However, in this chapter we consider only one type: Lotrafilcon A (conventional hydrogel). Because of the different curvature of the cornea and the contact lens, a gap is created between them. This gap was modeled by Ooi et al. (2007) as a new domain, called POLTF (post-lens tear film) (Figure 17.3). The above evaporation rate proposed by Mathers (2004) was assumed for the calculations in our model. The properties and specifications of the specific type of contact lens and POLTF used in the model are listed in Table 17.3.

17.2.2 Intraocular Lens

In the case of natural crystalline lens destruction (cataract), it is necessary to replace the damaged lens with an artificial intraocular lens (IOL). Cataract is another condition associated with age (Glynn et al. 2009). Exactly the same as the healthy mature lens, the IOL focuses light onto the retina. There is wide variety in the design and material of an IOL (plastic, silicone, or acrylic). Its small diameter and softness make it easy to place an IOL in the eye through a very small incision.

In this chapter we assumed an IOL made of polymethyl methacrylate (PMMA). The evaporation rate for every age group was the same as that for the reference models (Mathers and Lane 1998). Table 17.4 shows the physical and thermal properties of PMMA used for modeling. Due to the smaller value in thermal conductivity from the natural lens, an IOL provides a kind of insulation between the vitreous humor and the anterior chamber (Karampatzakis and Samaras 2010).

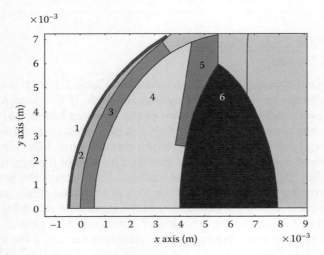

FIGURE 17.3
The insertion of a contact lens in the model of the human eye results in new parts in the model. 1, Contact lens (Lotrafilcon A); 2, POLTF; 3, cornea; 4, anterior chamber; 5, iris; 6, lens.

TABLE 17.3

Properties and Specifications of the Specific Type of Contact Lens and POLTF Used in the Models

Parameter	Contact Lens (Type: Lotrafilcon A)	Post-Lens Tear Film (POLTF)
Base curve (mm)	8.4[a]	—
Diameter (mm)	13.8[a]	—
Center thickness (mm)	0.08[a]	—
Thermal conductivity (W/m K)	0.281[b]	0.6232[b]
Specific heat (J/kg K)	2259.9[b]	4178[b]
Density (kg/m³)	1080[b]	1000[b]
Emissivity	0.955[b]	—

[a] Ooi, E. H., Ng, E. Y. K., Purslow, C., Acharya, R. *Proc. Inst. Mech. Eng. H.* 221, 337–349, 2007. (Data obtained from Purslow, C., Wolffsohn, J. S., Santodomingo-Rubido, J. *Cont. Lens Anterior Eye.* 28, 29–36, 2005.)

[b] Ooi, E. H., Ng, E. Y. K., Purslow, C., Acharya, R. *Proc. Inst. Mech. Eng. H.* 221, 337–349, 2007.

TABLE 17.4

Physical Properties of a Natural Lens and an Artificial IOL

Parameter	Natural Lens	IOL
Thermal conductivity (W/m K)	0.4[a]	0.2[b]
Specific heat (J/kg K)	3000[a]	1500[b,c]
Density (kg/m³)	1000[a]	1185[b]

[a] Lagendijk, J. J. W. *Phys. Med. Biol.* 27, 1301–1311, 1982.

[b] Matbase. Mechanical, physical and environmental properties of materials: PMMA. http://www.matbase.com/material/polymers/commodity/pmma/properties. 2012.

[c] National Physical Laboratory. Kaye and Laby tables of physical and chemical constants: Specific heat capacities. http://www.kayelaby.npl.co.uk/general_physics/2_3/2_3_6.html. 2012.

17.3 Methodology

17.3.1 Numerical Models

In this chapter, we use three detailed, anatomically realistic 3D models of the human eye, which correspond to the geometrical dimensions of Table 17.1, representing three different age groups. In all models the circulation of the aqueous humor (AH) in the anterior chamber is taken into account, together with blood perfusion and metabolic heat generation in the rest of the eye tissues, as in the finite element model (FEM) model presented in Karampatzakis and Samaras (2010). The modeled regions of the eye include the cornea, the anterior chamber, the iris, the lens, the vitreous humor, and the sclera. The choroid and the retina are omitted in the models since they are relatively thin compared with the sclera and are considered as being embedded in the latter. The posterior chamber behind the iris and in front of the lens is also neglected since in the 3D case it would result in a huge number of finite elements because of its narrow aperture to the anterior chamber. All biological materials assigned to the various regions are assumed to be homogeneous and isotropic; their physical properties can be found in Table 17.5. In all three models the inflow and outflow of the AH in the anterior chamber are not taken into account; neither is blinking, which leads to almost instantaneous temperature changes on the corneal surface.

In the case that a model involves a contact lens or an artificial IOL, the physical properties of the regions concerned (shown in Figure 17.3 for the contact lens) are given in Tables 17.3 and 17.4 respectively.

17.3.2 Mathematical Formulation

In order to calculate the temperature distribution in the eye tissues we solved the steady-state general heat transfer equation, including the effects of blood perfusion in the iris and the sclera and mass transfer in the anterior chamber:

$$\nabla(-k\nabla T) = A - B(T - T_b) - \rho c(\bar{v} \cdot \nabla T) \tag{17.1}$$

TABLE 17.5

Thermal Properties of the Biological Materials Present in the Eye

Material	Thermal Conductivity k (W/m K)	Density ρ (kg/m)	Specific Heat Capacity c (J/kg K)	Blood Perfusion Power Equivalent (W/m K)	Basal Metabolism (W/m)
Cornea	0.58	1,050	4,178	–	–
Aqueous humor	0.58	996	3,997	–	–
Iris	0.52	1,050	3,600	35,000	10,000
Lens	0.4	1,000	3,000	–	–
Vitreous humor	0.603	1,100	4,178	–	–
Sclera	0.58	1,050	3,800	8,000	22,000

Note: The original references of values are reported in Karampatzakis, A., Samaras, T. *Phys. Med. Biol.*, 55, 5653–5665, 2010.

where:
  T is the temperature
  ρ is the mass density
  c is the specific heat capacity
  k is the thermal conductivity
  T_b is the blood temperature
  A is the metabolic heat generation rate
  B is the term associated with the blood perfusion rate (Table 17.5 contains the values and units of these quantities)

The vector $\vec{v}$ represents AH velocity in the anterior chamber and is associated with heat exchange, due to fluid convection, described by the solution of the three-dimensional, incompressible Navier-Stokes equation

$$\rho(\vec{v}\cdot\nabla)\vec{v} = \nabla\left[-p\vec{I} + \eta\left(\nabla\vec{v} + (\nabla\vec{v})^T\right)\right] + \vec{F} \tag{17.2}$$

where:
  p is the pressure
  η is the dynamic viscosity (assigned a value of 0.00074 N s/m^2 according to Ooi and Ng (2008))
  $\vec{F}$ is a volume force field exerted on the fluid, such as gravity

Fluid convection was included in Equation 17.2 through the effect of buoyancy, originating from the temperature difference between the back surface of the cornea and the front surface of the lens (pupil) at the bottom of the anterior chamber. Therefore, the Boussinesq approximation was introduced in the volume force term of Equation 17.2:

$$\vec{F} = \rho\,\vec{g}\,\beta(T - T_{\text{mean}}) \tag{17.3}$$

where:
  ρ is a reference density for the AH (Table 17.5)
  g is the gravity acceleration
  β is the volume expansion coefficient of AH (set at 3×10^{-4}/K according to Kumar et al. (2006))
  T_{mean} is a reference temperature, calculated during the simulation as the mean temperature on the back surface of the cornea

The solution of Equations 17.2 and 17.3 requires the introduction of boundary conditions in the computational domain. The ones used here were similar to those applied by Karampatzakis and Samaras (2010), that is, there was heat exchange between the cornea and the ambient environment, as well as between the sclera and the surrounding tissue. The former was modeled by the boundary equation:

$$-k\frac{\partial T}{\partial \hat{n}} = h_c(T - T_a) + \varepsilon\sigma(T^4 - T_a^4) + E \tag{17.4}$$

where:

h_c is the heat transfer coefficient between the cornea and the environment

T_a is the ambient temperature

ε is the corneal surface emissivity

σ is the Stefan–Boltzmann constant

E is the heat loss due to tear evaporation

$\hat{n}$ is the unit normal vector pointing away from the cornea

The latter was imposed on the sclera boundary, and the heat transfer due to convection was described by

$$-k\frac{\partial T}{\partial \hat{n}} = h_s\left(T - T_b\right) \tag{17.5}$$

where h_s is the heat transfer coefficient between the sclera and the surrounding tissues and T_b is the blood temperature.

The values of the quantities included in the boundary conditions for the general heat transfer equation, namely Equations 17.4 and 17.5, are given in Table 17.6. The evaporation rate is missing from this table because it was assumed to be dependent on age (Table 17.2). The boundary for the calculations of the AH fluid dynamics was set to no-slip ($\bar{v} = 0$) at the walls of the anterior chamber.

17.3.3 Numerical Solution

The coupled problem at the steady state of general heat transfer with fluid convection was solved by FEM implemented in the software Comsol Multiphysics 3.5a (COMSOL AB, Stockholm, Sweden). The mesh consisted of about 60,000–350,000 tetrahedral elements. The elements were quadratic in the case of the heat transfer problem and linear for solving the fluid dynamics equation. A direct algorithm (SParse Object Oriented Equations Solver or SPOOLES) was used for solving the equation system. The stopping (convergence) criterion was a relative tolerance of 10^{-5}. The time required for the solution reached up to 15 h on a server with two quad-core Intel Xeon E5520 at 2.27 GHz and 24 GB of RAM, of which the various models used up to 20 GB of RAM. The largest number of elements and longer simulation times were necessary for the contact lens models, where the lens itself and the POLTF region (Figure 17.3) required a considerable number of elements to be modeled adequately.

TABLE 17.6

Values of the Quantities Used in Boundary Conditions

Quantity	Description	Value
T_b	Blood temperature (°C)	37
T_a	Ambient temperature (°C)	23
h_s	Body heat transfer coefficient (W/m² K)	65
h_c	Ambient heat transfer coefficient (W/m² K¹)	10
σ	Stefan–Boltzmann constant (W/m² K⁴)	5.67×10^{-8}
ε	Emissivity of cornea surface	0.975

17.4 Results and Discussion

17.4.1 The Healthy Ageing Eye

In the following we present the numerical results on the temperature distribution in the tissues, but mainly on the cornea, for the numerical models of the human eye for three different age groups, that is, 20–29, 40–49, and 60–69 years. The evaporation rate used in each age group was that proposed by Mathers and Lane (1998) (Table 17.2).

Figures 17.4 and 17.5 show the distribution of the ocular surface temperature (OST) for the three age groups in supine and standing positions, respectively. The latter presents greater interest than the former due to its asymmetrical pattern.

It is clear from Figure 17.5 that the coolest point on the cornea surface does not correspond to its geometric center. This fact has partly been attributed to the flow of the AH, which pushes colder masses to the lower part of the anterior chamber (Karampatzakis and Samaras 2010).

However, as is shown more clearly in Figure 17.6, the coolest point appears to be lower in younger than in older subjects. In particular, the minimum temperature of the OST is

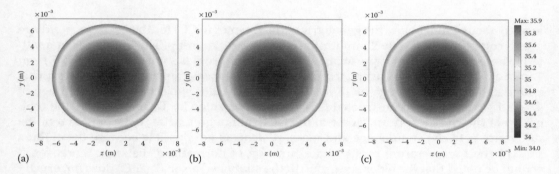

FIGURE 17.4
Distribution of the OST for supine position of the subject and for different age groups: (a) 20–29 years, (b) 40–49 years, and (c) 60–69 years.

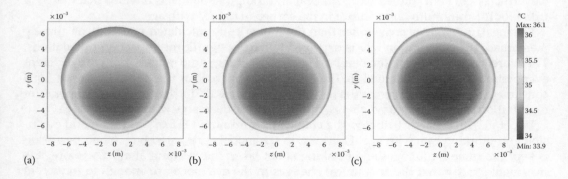

FIGURE 17.5
Distribution of the OST for standing position of the subject and for different age groups: (a) 20–29 years, (b) 40–49 years, and (c) 60–69 years.

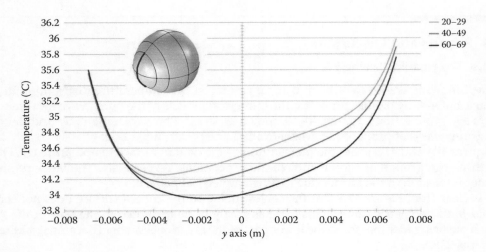

FIGURE 17.6
Profile of the OST along the sagittal midline of the eye (see inset) for the three numerical models corresponding to the three age groups.

located about 4 mm below the geometric corneal center (GCC) for the 20–29 year-old age group compared with only 2 mm for the 60–69-year-old group. This finding is in qualitative agreement with the approximate temperature profiles shown in Figure 17.7 from Tan et al. (2011), which were created based on actual measurements of two age groups: young subjects with an age of 18.9 ± 0.8 years and older subjects with a mean age of 47 ± 8.4 years. In the reconstructed OST profiles presented by Tan et al. (2011), the coolest tip of the cornea appears closer to the GCC, although a better determination of the difference between simulations and measurements is not possible because the authors present their temperature profiles as a function of normalized distance. Moreover, it should be noted that the older age group in the study by Tan et al. (2011) does not exactly correspond to the second age group presented here (40–49 years of age) since it had a large variation.

There is a discrepancy between the calculated and the measured values of the minimum OST. The values reported by Tan et al. (2011) are lower than those estimated in this study. Nevertheless, in both studies (experimental and computational) it is obvious that there is a trend for the minimum temperature in the cornea to reduce with age.

The measured values are smaller than the numerically calculated ones, but, as already mentioned, the evaporation rate is expected to have a significant impact on calculations. Therefore, we present here the results (Figure 17.7) of the same models, but with different evaporation rates, as explained in Table 17.2. It is apparent in the figure that even for a constant evaporation rate across the various ages (Figure 17.7b), the pattern of temperature distribution remains the same, that is, minimum OST decreases with age.

Tan et al. (2011) have attributed the change in minimum OST to reduced blood perfusion and blinking rate with age. However, in the models presented here blood perfusion is kept the same for all ages and blinking is not taken into account at all. Therefore, it is reasonable to say that the anatomical changes in the eye alone are enough to induce, at least partly, the drop of minimum OST in the ageing eye. It is possible, then, that an underlying mechanism which contributes to the observed effect is the change in AH flow in the anterior chamber.

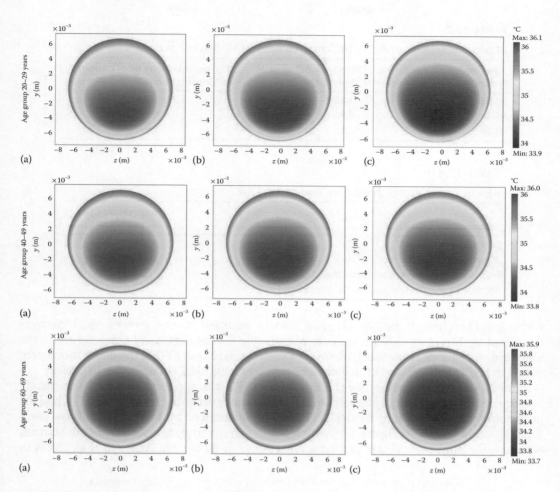

FIGURE 17.7
Distribution of the OST for standing position of the subject for different age groups and different evaporation rates of the tear film (see Table 17.2): (a) reference model; (b) constant rate; and (c) new model.

It has already been mentioned (Table 17.1) that the depth of the anterior chamber reduces with age. This results in an increased velocity (Table 17.7) of the AH calculated with the numerical model. An increased maximum velocity of the AH in the standing position is also expected, if we use the formula introduced by Canning et al. (2002):

$$u_{max} = \Delta T \times 1.98 \times 10^{-4} \, m/(sK) \tag{17.6}$$

The value of the coefficient 1.98×10^{-4} m/(s K) was derived by Canning et al. (2002) for an ACD of 2.75 mm. If we scale this value to the ACDs of Table 17.8 and use as ΔT, the difference in temperature between the front and back surfaces of the anterior chamber (Figure 17.8), we can derive the theoretical values for the maximum velocity (Table 17.7). These are lower than the numerically calculated values, but they still show an increment

TABLE 17.7

Maximum Velocity of AH in the Three Numerical Models of the Eye

Age Group (years)	Maximum Velocity of AH from Numerical Model ($\times 10^{-4}$ m/s)	Maximum Velocity of AH According to Canning et al. (2002) ($\times 10^{-4}$ m/s)
20–29	3.89	2.57
40–49	3.94	2.60
60–69	4.10	2.64

TABLE 17.8

Rate of Temperature Change per Year for the OST

Source	Temperature Change per Year (°C)
Morgan et al. (1999)	−0.010
Acharya et al. (2009)	−0.038
Numerical calculations, reference model (this study)	−0.006
Numerical calculations, new model (this study)	−0.004

with age. Therefore, it can be claimed that in addition to the physiological changes described by Tan et al. (2011) which are responsible for the decreased temperature in the older eye, another possible mechanism for the observed lower OST is the faster movement of AH in the anterior chamber, which is caused by anatomical changes due to ageing.

In terms of absolute values for the minimum OST, it is apparent that the numerically predicted values are in better agreement with those measured by Tan et al. (2011) when the new evaporation rates ("new model" in Table 17.2) introduced by Tan et al. (2010) are used. This is clearly shown in Figure 17.9, which depicts the average temperature of the cornea with age; the values are closer to the measurements of figure 9 in Acharya et al. (2009) or

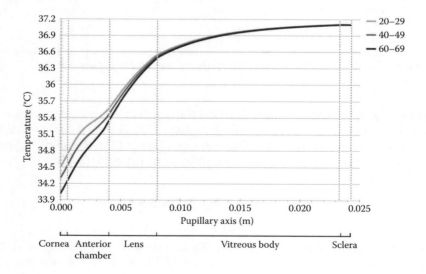

FIGURE 17.8

Temperature distribution along the pupillary axis for the three numerical models corresponding to the different age groups (evaporation rate of reference model).

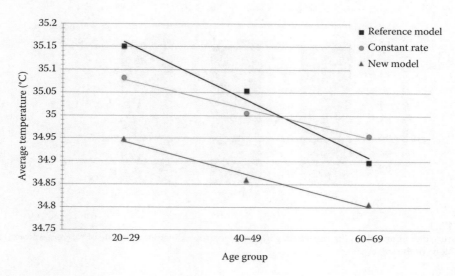

FIGURE 17.9
Change in average OST for different age groups.

figure 2 in Morgan et al. (1999) than for the other two models of evaporation. However, there is great uncertainty in the rate of temperature change per year: as shown in Table 17.8, the numerically estimated values are closer to the measured value of Morgan et al. (1999) although the OST from calculations is higher in absolute values compared with the measured OST from that study.

Another interesting point is the variation of temperature on the corneal surface. In the present study, the calculated minimum and maximum values of OST differed by less than 2°C (Figure 17.10). The deviation between the two temperature extremes on the cornea was

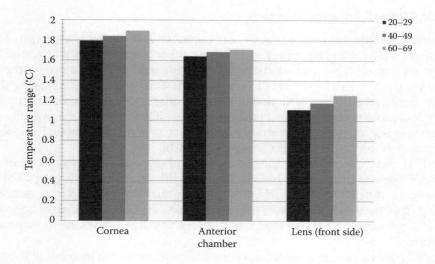

FIGURE 17.10
Temperature deviation across the cornea, the anterior chamber, and the front surface of the lens for different age groups (evaporation rate of reference model).

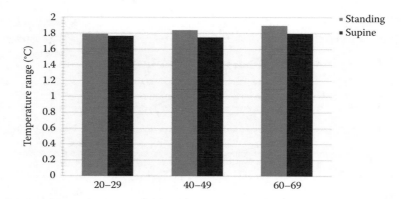

FIGURE 17.11

Temperature deviation across the cornea for different age groups (evaporation rate of reference model) and for two positions of the subject.

larger in the older group, and this fact was also observed for the anterior chamber and the front surface of the lens. Of course, the deeper we get into the model (that is, comparing the corneal surface with the lens surface) the smaller this deviation becomes, since the heating from the surrounding tissue (expressed in the form of the boundary condition on the sclera in the models) helps to smooth the temperature distribution. Nevertheless, the pattern of higher temperature deviation in older subjects holds for the lens as well. The contribution of AH flow to this pattern is evident from Figure 17.11, which shows that when the subject is in the supine position, the increase in temperature deviation with age disappears. Therefore, the anatomical changes in the eye due to ageing and their consequences on the AH flow must contribute to the asymmetry of OST distributions.

17.4.2 Contact and Intraocular Lenses

In this section, we present results that were obtained with the reference models of the first two age groups (20–29 and 40–49 years), in which either a contact lens was placed in front of the cornea (Figure 17.3) or an artificial IOL was inserted at the position of the natural lens. The purpose of this study was to compare the OST and eye temperature distribution in the healthy ageing eye with that of the eye under treatment for visual impairment. Although it is more probable to find patients with an IOL in the older age group (60–69), this group was not included in the study because discomfort from contact lens wearing is more common among older people (Young et al. 2002).

Figure 17.11 clearly shows that wearing any kind of corrective lens (contact lenses or an artificial IOL) results in a change in OST that resembles the effect of ageing. This is better understood from Figure 17.12, where it is shown that the corneal temperature profile of a young (20–29 years) IOL wearer is similar to that of a healthy subject who is 20 years older. It still remains to be discovered whether this physical condition has any biological implications.

Contrary to the above effect, wearing a contact lens inverses the increase of temperature range between maximum and minimum OST with age. Figure 17.13 indicates that the contact lens plays an important role in making the OST distribution more uniform with age, which does not hold for patients with an IOL.

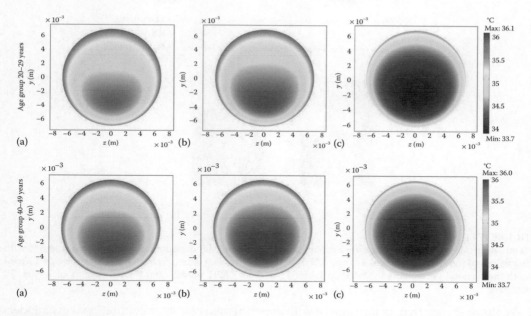

FIGURE 17.12
Distribution of the OST for standing position of a subject: (a) reference model, no corrective lenses; (b) IOL; and (c) contact lens.

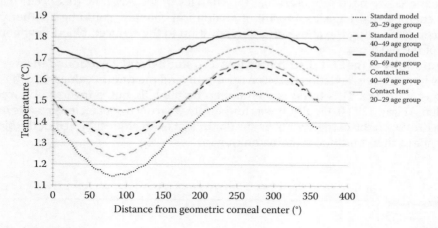

FIGURE 17.13
Temperature deviation profile on the cornea for standing position of a subject with and without a contact lens; "standard model" has been implemented with the values of the reference model in Table 17.2, whereas the "contact lens" model calculations were performed with the physical parameters included in Table 17.3.

17.5 Conclusions

In this chapter, we calculated the OST distributions for different age groups and conditions and compared them with experimentally obtained measurements wherever possible.

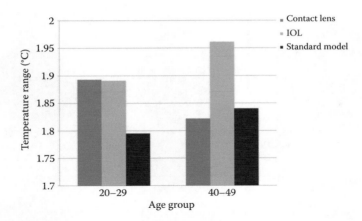

FIGURE 17.14
Temperature deviation across the cornea for different age groups; "standard model" has been implemented with the values of the reference model in Table 17.2, whereas the "contact lens" model calculations were performed with the physical parameters included in Table 17.3 and the "IOL" model used the parameters of Tables 17.2 and 17.4.

We have shown that, in agreement with experimental results, computational eye models that consider the physiological and anatomical changes due to ageing and are constructed accordingly could predict the decrease in the minimum temperature of the cornea with age, as well as the approach of its location to the GCC. Moreover, based on the numerical simulations, we have proposed that the changes in the AH flow that occur inside the anterior chamber with age, as a result of anatomical changes, could be another possible mechanism explaining the above effect, in addition to the reduced blood flow and blinking rate of the older eye.

The uniformity of the OST distribution was also studied and it was found that the frontal eye parts have a large deviation between minimum and maximum values, which becomes even larger with age. This trend is maintained by the IOL, but is inversed by wearing a contact lens (Figure 17.14). Finally, it was found that wearing a contact lens results in a temperature profile on the cornea which is similar to that of an older subject, but the biological significance of this condition remains unknown.

References

Acharya, U. R., Ng, E. Y. K., Yee, G. C., Tan, J. H., Kagathi, M. (2009) Analysis of normal human eye with different age groups using infrared images. *J. Med. Syst.* 33: 207–213.

Canning, C. R., Greaney, M. J., Dewynne, J., Fitt, A. D. (2002) Fluid flow in the anterior chamber of a human eye. *IMA J. Math. Appl. Med. Biol.* 19: 31–60.

Dubbelman, M., Weeber, H. A., van der Heijde, R. G. L., Volker-Dieben, H. J. (2002) Radius and asphericity of the posterior corneal surface determined by corrected Scheimpflug photography. *Acta Ophthalmol. Scand.* 80: 379–383.

Glynn, R. J., Rosner, B., Christen, W. G. (2009) Evaluation of risk factors for cataract types in a competing risks framework. *Ophthalmic Epidemiol.* 16: 98–106.

Karampatzakis, A., Samaras, T. (2010) Numerical model of heat transfer in the human eye with consideration of fluid dynamics of the aqueous humour. *Phys. Med. Biol.* 55: 5653–5665.

Kumar, S., Acharya, S., Beuerman, R., Palkama, A. (2006) Numerical solution of ocular fluid dynamics in the rabbit eye: Parametric effects. *Ann. Biomed. Eng.* 34: 530–544.

Lagendijk, J. J. W. (1982) A mathematical model to calculate temperature distributions in human and rabbit eyes during hyperthermic treatment. *Phys. Med. Biol.* 27: 1301–1311.

Lim, K. J., Hyung, S. M., Youn, D. H. (1992) Ocular dimensions with ageing in normal eyes. *Korean J. Ophthalmol.* 6: 19–31.

Liu, L. (2006) Development of the anterior chamber. In: Weinreb, R. N., Friedman, D. S. (eds), *Angle Closure and Angle Closure Glaucoma*, Appendix A, pp. 65–69. Kugler, The Hague.

Matbase (2012) Mechanical, physical and environmental properties of materials: PMMA. http://www.matbase.com/material/polymers/commodity/pmma/properties; accessed on 1 July 2012.

Mathers, W. D. (2004) Evaporation from the ocular surface. *Exp. Eye Res.* 78: 389–394.

Mathers, W. D., Lane, J. A. (1998) Meibomian gland lipids, evaporation, and tear film stability. In: Sullivan, D. A., Dartt, D. A., Meneray, M. A. (eds), *Lacrimal Gland, Tear Film, and Dry Eye Syndromes 2*, pp. 349–360. Plenum, New York.

Morgan, P. B., Soh, M. P., Efron, N. (1999) Corneal surface temperature decrease with age. *Cont. Lens Anterior Eye*. 22: 11–13.

Moss, S. E., Klein, R., Klein, B. K. (2000) Prevalence of and risk factors for dry eye syndrome. *Arch. Ophthalmol.* 118: 1264–1268.

National Physical Laboratory (2012) Kaye and Laby tables of physical and chemical constants: Specific heat capacities. http://www.kayelaby.npl.co.uk/general_physics/2_3/2_3_6.html; accessed on 1 July 2012.

Ooi, E. H., Ng, E. Y. K. (2008) Simulation of aqueous humor hydrodynamics in human eye heat transfer. *Comput. Biol. Med.* 38: 252–262.

Ooi, E. H., Ng, E. Y. K., Purslow, C., Acharya, R. (2007) Variations in the corneal surface temperature with contact lens wear. *Proc. Inst. Mech. Eng. H.* 221: 337–349.

Purslow, C., Wolffsohn, J. S., Santodomingo-Rubido, J. (2005) The effect of contact lens wear on dynamic ocular surface temperature. *Cont. Lens Anterior Eye*. 28: 29–36.

Tan, J. H., Ng, E. Y. K., Acharya, R. U. (2010) Evaluation of tear evaporation from ocular surface by functional infrared thermography. *Med. Phys.* 37: 6022–6034.

Tan, J. H., Ng, E. Y. K., Acharya, U. R. (2011). Evaluation of topographical variation in ocular surface temperature by functional infrared thermography. *Infrared Phys. Technol.* 54: 469–477.

Young, G., Veys, J., Pritchard, N., Coleman, S. (2012) A multi-centre study of lapsed contact lens wearers. *Ophthalmic Physiol. Opt.* 22: 516–527.

18

A Perspective Review on the Use of In Vivo Confocal Microscopy in the Ocular Surface

Sze-Yee Lee, Andrea Petznick, Shakil Rehman, and Louis Tong

CONTENTS

18.1 Introduction

Optical microscopy is a vital tool in life science investigations with the aim of imaging at subcellular resolution. Confocal microscopy is used for obtaining three-dimensional (3-D) images of thick objects (Wilson 1990; Pawley 1995; Masters 1996). This is possible by what is known as the optical sectioning property of the confocal microscope, in which images of very thin sections of an object can be obtained and a 3D image can be produced by properly arranging these slices.

The principle of confocal microscope is fundamentally different from that of a conventional wide-field microscope, in which the image is collected by illuminating the whole object. In confocal microscopy, a tightly focused spot of light is scanned in a raster manner on the sample and scattered light is collected by a point detector. This set of points is then interlaced to obtain a 2-D image. Finally, lateral scanning in the depth and collection of these 2-D scans is used to make a 3-D image of the sample.

The development of the confocal microscope is attributed to a patent by Minsky in 1961 that was basically a stage scanning system that led to a spinning disc confocal microscope in 1968 (Minsky 1961; Petran et al. 1968). This was achieved by scanning multiple points on a stationary sample using a rotating Nipkow disc. A sound theoretical understanding was developed for the image formation in a confocal microscope in 1978 (Sheppard and Choudhury 1977; Sheppard and Wilson 1979). Confocal imaging was applied for fluorescent biological specimens around the same time (Amos and White 2003). The first application of the confocal microscope in imaging human and rabbit corneas was reported in 1985 (Lemp et al. 1985). A slit scanning confocal microscope was developed in 1969 by employing an oscillating two-sided mirror for simultaneous scanning and de-scanning of the sample. This microscope helped to image living neural tissue (Svishchev 1969; Masters and Thaer 1994). The first commercial confocal microscope was developed in 1987. Later advances in stable laser sources, high-efficiency scanning mirrors, high-quality filters, low-noise detectors, and faster computers have added to the improvement of the confocal microscope. Presently, slit scanning *in vivo* confocal microscopes (IVCMs) and laser scanning IVCMs are commercially available from a number of providers.

There are two distinct modes of imaging in a confocal microscope. A confocal microscope can be used in reflection or transmission mode depending on the application. The transmission type of confocal imaging is used for thin samples that otherwise cannot be imaged *in vivo*. The reflection mode of confocal imaging is used for live tissue and *in vivo* imaging and can provide 3-D images of samples at a higher resolution than is possible with wide-field microscopes. Changes in the index of refraction or fluorophores are used as contrast agents for obtaining information at cellular levels.

The ability of a confocal image to provide histological information without prior staining and excising of the tissue gives clinicians extra control over diagnosis. A confocal microscope in ophthalmology is used for obtaining useful information about the structure and function of the cornea and retina. The specificity of confocal imaging has been established for providing quantitative diagnosis of cell morphology, cell count, and infections.

Recent advances in optical and electronics technology have significantly improved the confocal imaging methods. The availability of stable lasers that provide full coverage of the ultraviolet, visible, and near-infrared spectral regions; improved interference filters such as dichroic beam splitters, excitation and emission filters, and acousto-optic tunable filters for excitation laser intensity and wavelength control; and sensitive low-noise detectors and faster computers all have contributed toward the development of a modern confocal microscope.

There are various types of confocal microscopes for applications in the field of biomedicine. An early confocal microscope based on a Nipkow disc was a tandem scanning microscope providing video-rate imaging (Xiao et al. 1988; 1990). This confocal microscope has the ability to image live samples at faster rates, thereby allowing direct observation of the sample along with true color imaging. But the poor image quality due to low intensity of the reflected light constrained the use of this microscope in clinical settings. Faster imaging can also be achieved by using a slit for scanning in which the slit width can be adjusted to allow variation of the thickness of the optical sections. However, the use of a slit also renders the microscope to be confocal only in one dimension, that is, perpendicular to the slit width. A slit scanning confocal microscope has low contrast and limited improvement in imaging properties (Masters 1996).

A laser is used as a coherent high-intensity light source in a point scanning confocal microscope in which the laser beam is focused to a small spot with the help of a microscope objective. This focal spot is scanned by two mirrors providing fast scanning in a plane. The reflected light refocused by the microscope objective is de-scanned by the scanning mirrors again and imaged on a pinhole aperture before a photomultiplier detector (Young and Roberts 1951; Davidovits and Egger 1973; Webb et al. 1980). Such a confocal microscope has been introduced into imaging human eyes in clinical applications and is termed a scanning laser ophthalmoscope (Webb et al. 1980; 1987; Webb 1990).

IVCM has been historically used in clinical practice for evaluation of the back of the eye, specifically the optic disc and the retina. Recently, IVCM has greatly enhanced our understanding of the structure and function of the ocular surface. It is anticipated that the there is a promising future for IVCM imaging.

18.2 Imaging of Various Structures in the Ocular Surface

Detailed and in-depth observation of specific ocular surface components in health and disease can be carried out using IVCM (Figure 18.1). This section will elaborate on the capabilities of IVCM in observing various aspects of the cornea and conjunctiva.

18.2.1 Examination of the Cornea

IVCM has been a very useful tool in providing information of the anatomical structure of the cornea. The cornea is an avascular, transparent tissue and its unique structure, together with the tear film, provides the majority of optical power that refracts the light entering into the eye. Roughly, the cornea consists of several layers: the epithelium, stroma, and endothelium. The stroma is separated from the epithelium and endothelium by Bowman's membrane and Descemet's membrane, respectively. IVCM enables the investigator to measure the thickness of each layer and observe changes that may occur with corneal diseases or ageing (Zhivov et al. 2006).

The outermost layer is the epithelium and consists of five to six cell layers: a single layer of cylindrical basal cells, two to three rows of wing-shaped cells, and two rows of superficial cells. The basal cells secrete collagen that form Bowman's membrane and can also undergo mitosis to produce fresh epithelial cells. The size and shape of cells as well as cell densities can be determined using IVCM. The stroma, which accounts for approximately 90% of the cornea, consists of many layers of regularly arranged collagen fibers. Stellate-shaped cells called keratocytes that help to maintain the structure of the stroma are scattered within this layer. During inflammation, keratocytes may become activated and their activity can be evaluated using IVCM. Activated keratocytes show a greater cellular metabolic activity, as noted by an increased nuclear reflectivity within the stroma (Chiou et al. 2006). Furthermore, the number and distribution of keratocytes can vary according to the health status of the cornea (Table 18.1). For example, during inflammation a greater density of keratocytes may be found close to a wound site (Snyder et al. 1998; West-Mays and Dwivedi 2006).

The innermost layer of the cornea is the single-layered endothelium. Unlike the epithelial layer, these cells do not regenerate even in the event of injury, and the number of cells

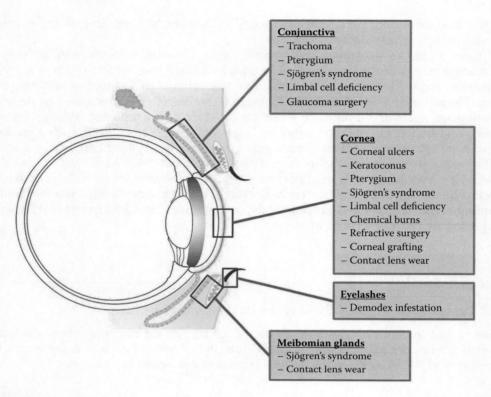

FIGURE 18.1
Overview of the utility of IVCM within the ocular surface system. Various structures of the ocular surface can be examined in healthy and diseased eyes. IVCM may assess long-term changes associated with the condition.

TABLE 18.1

Corneal Stromal Keratocyte Changes in Various Conditions as Reported by IVCM Imaging

Condition	Activated	Density	Distribution
	Changes		
Keratoconus	Yes	–	–
Pterygium	Yes	Decreased	–
LASIK	–	Decreased	–
PRK	–	–	Irregular
Corneal grafts			
Short term	Yes	Decreased	–
Long term	–	Increased[a]	–
CL wear (mucin balls)	Yes	–	–

Note: CL, contact lens.
            –, not previously evaluated.
[a] Increased numbers from period of time after operation, but not to the original levels.

decreases with age at an average rate of 0.6% per year (Bourne et al.1997). The endothelial cells are vital in maintaining corneal transparency. These cells have a pump function and actively transport water from the cornea. IVCM can easily detect areas of endothelial cell loss, called guttata, that occur in degenerative diseases such as Fuchs dystrophy (Chiou et al. 1999). The ability of IVCM to analyze endothelial cell density makes it a useful tool in monitoring corneal diseases (Guthoff et al. 2009).

The cornea is the most densely innervated structure and therefore the most sensitive part of the human body. A stimulus of small magnitude to the corneal surface will cause an immediate involuntary protective reaction to blink or close the eye. Corneal sensitivity diminishes with age, along with the nerve density, by approximately 0.9% per year (Millodot 1977; Roszkowska et al. 2004; Niederer et al. 2007a). In addition, corneal nerves may be affected by certain types of eye surgery, for example laser *in situ* keratomileusis (LASIK), or diseases, such as keratoconus (Calvillo et al. 2004; Patel et al. 2006; Darwish et al. 2007; Niederer et al. 2008). Systemic diseases such as diabetes and peripheral autoimmune neuropathy also have manifestations in the corneal nerves (De Cilla et al. 2009; Lalive et al. 2009). Table 18.2 shows a summary of corneal nerve fiber changes in the various ocular and systemic conditions that were reported using IVCM imaging. Since all these changes are long-term processes, IVCM allows monitoring of patients over prolonged periods of time for possible deterioration of the condition.

Normally, the cornea is avascular to maintain its transparency, but in a state of chronic inflammation, blood vessels may invade the corneal tissue and these may be viewed by IVCM. Some of the chronic ocular surface diseases with new blood vessel formation, also known as vascularization, will be described in the next section. Blood vessels exhibit hyperreflective walls and hyporeflective lumen in IVCM-acquired images (Chiou et al. 2006). The abnormal vessel growth is a response to a lack of oxygen, which the ocular system aims to compensate for with blood vessels that transport oxygen and nutrients to the deprived part of the cornea. Although this produces no symptoms in the early stages, in the later stages it can be devastating for the vision. An additional imaging modality for identification of corneal vascularization may be useful.

TABLE 18.2

Corneal Nerve Fiber Changes in Various Conditions as Reported by IVCM Imaging

Condition	Corneal Nerve Fiber Changes				
	Numbers	**Density**	**Thickness**	**Tortuosity**	**Others**
HSV keratitis	Decreased	–	–	–	Increased prominence
Keratoconus	–	Decreased	Increased	Increased	–
Pterygium	–	–	–	Increased	Localized bulges and breakages
Dry eye	–	Decreased	–	Increased	Increased and irregular patterns of branching
SS	Increased	–	–	Increased	–
LSCD	–	Decreased[a]	–	–	–
LASIK	–	Decreased	–	–	Decreased length and width
Corneal grafts	Decreased	–	–	–	Gradual, random, and disorderly regeneration

Note: SS, Sjögren's syndrome.

–, not previously evaluated.

[a] Questionable as to whether it is a true decrease or merely undetectable.

In addition to the stromal keratocytes, dendritic cells, called Langerhans cells, can become activated and serve as potent markers for severity of inflammation. These cells can be located among the suprabasal and basal cells and nerve plexus of the cornea. They present as large cells with longer processes or smaller cells without cellular extensions in IVCM images (Jalbert et al. 2003). These are resident antigen-presenting cells involved in the activation of other immune cells or lymphocytes, which can propagate inflammation (Wakamatsu et al. 2008).

Apart from visualizing alterations in the cornea, including deposits and changes of morphology, IVCM has the ability to detect novel structures that have not been identified previously. For example, the limbal lacuna, a well-concealed and protected structure consisting of normal limbal epithelial cells deep inside the limbal stroma, was very recently detected with IVCM (Zarei-Ghanavati et al. 2011). Its role within the ocular surface system is still unclear and needs to be further investigated. Furthermore, IVCM can be used to diagnose easily missed pathologies such as limbal stem cell deficiency, which will be discussed in detail later in the chapter (Parrozzani et al. 2011; Miri et al. 2012).

18.2.2 Examination of the Conjunctiva

The conjunctiva is a thin, transparent tissue that lines the inner surface of the eyelids (tarsal conjunctiva) and the scleral surface (bulbar conjunctiva). The conjunctiva functions as an additional immunological defense system from microbes and lubrication of the eye. It contains mucus-producing goblet cells that facilitate stability and spreading of tears over the ocular surface.

Analysis of the conjunctival cells was commonly done with impression cytology. The most superficial cell layer of the conjunctiva is collected with a filter membrane and prepared for histological staining to visualize the epithelial cells, goblet cells, and inflammatory cells of the conjunctiva. Unfortunately, this method only allows for the assessment of the most superficial cell layer while IVCM can evaluate deeper cell layers without the need to take a tissue sample. Thus, many clinicians have chosen the use of IVCM over impression cytology to examine the conjunctiva. Although the assessment of goblet cells within the conjunctiva using IVCM is still controversial, some authors defining them as dark round structures or oval white bodies, IVCM has some advantages over impression cytology (Murube and Rivas 2003; Wakamatsu et al. 2010). As well as being able to visualize deeper layers of the conjunctiva, IVCM images can be immediately and directly viewed, whereas impression cytological samples have to be sent to a laboratory to be processed and analyzed.

IVCM has been a key instrument in discovering conjunctiva-associated lymphoid tissues (CALT), which are lymphatic aggregates embedded in the palpebral conjunctiva (Knop and Knop 2000). CALT are composed of T and B lymphocytes, macrophages, plasma cells, and dendritic cells and serve as an induction site for immune defense responses of the ocular surface (Astley et al. 2003; Knop and Knop 2005; Liang et al. 2010).

Recently, IVCM has been used to further investigate the eyelid margins. Their functional anatomy is of utmost importance for optimal distribution of the tear film. The IVCM method determined two distinctive sections of the palpebral conjunctiva: the lip wiper and the mucocutaneous junction (MCJ) or line of Marx (Knop et al. 2011b). Abnormalities of the MCJ can be viewed with fluorescein dye staining. For example, patients with dry eye show greater epithelial cell keratinization in this area than normal volunteers (Korb et al. 2010).

In summary, IVCM can be used to examine the conjunctiva and analyze the amount of inflammation. This would be complementary to traditional slit lamp biomicroscope examination, which observes the ocular surface at a lower magnification.

18.2.3 Examination of the Meibomian Glands and Eyelashes

Meibomian glands are the oil-secreting glands in the upper and lower eyelids. Their secretions, commonly known as meibum, form the outermost lipid layer of the tear film, which helps to reduce excessive tear evaporation. Meibum is produced in secretory acini. From there, it travels through connecting ductules and ducts until it reaches the meibomian gland openings or orifices to finally be released into the tear film (Bron et al. 1991).

Due to their anatomical locations within the tarsal plates, the glands are generally difficult to visualize using commonly available clinical instruments. The slit lamp biomicroscope, for example, can only evaluate gland openings. A transillumination technique, meibography, can visualize the meibomian glands from the inner eyelid surface at relatively lower magnification (Nichols et al. 2005; Arita et al. 2008; Pult 2012). This way, qualitative and quantitative analysis of the glandular changes including loss and twistedness can be observed (Arita et al. 2008; Pult et al. 2012; Srinivasan et al. 2012). However, this technique cannot provide information on the microanatomy of the individual acini.

The visualization of meibomian glands using IVCM was pioneered fairly recently, in 2005 (Kobayashiet al. 2005). A high image resolution made the evaluation of the microstructure of individual meibomian glands possible. In 2008, two novel parameters for the investigation of meibomian glands, diameter and density of the glandular acinar units, were described (Matsumoto et al. 2008). This study also analyzed morphological gland changes in meibomian gland dysfunction (MGD). In MGD, the glands are obstructed and the integrity of the lipid layer is compromised due to either a decrease in the ability to deliver meibum efficiently or a change in the biochemistry of the meibum, or both (Knop et al. 2011a). MGD is a leading cause for evaporative dry eye and is extremely common, with prevalence rates in the general population ranging from 8.6% to 69.3% (McCarty et al. 1998; Foulks and Bron 2003; Lin et al. 2003; Bron and Tiffany 2004; Bron et al. 2004; Lekhanont et al. 2006; Uchino et al. 2006; Jie et al. 2009; Viso et al. 2012).

This method of meibomian gland evaluation has since been used in various other studies. Acinar density and diameter have been reported to average from 100 to 119 units/mm^2 and 41–53 µm, respectively, in normal patients (Matsumoto et al. 2008; Villani et al. 2011a; Villani et al. 2011b). In MGD patients, acinar densities were reduced to 47–57 units/mm^2 and the average diameter increased to 98–106 µm (Table 18.3) (Matsumoto et al. 2008; Villani et al. 2011a). Normal cut-off values of additional parameters, such as acinar longest diameter, acinar shortest diameter, inflammatory cell density, and acinar unit density, were later developed (Table 18.4) (Ibrahim et al. 2010). This technique may be promising for the evaluation of the efficacy of MGD treatments. For example, in a study involving 37 patients, there was a significant decrease in inflammatory cell density in patients receiving

TABLE 18.3

Proposed Diagnostic Criteria for MGD

Parameter	Normal Cutoff Values	Sensitivity (%)	Specificity (%)
Acinus			
• Longest diameter	<65 (µm)	90	81
• Shortest diameter	<25 (µm)	86	96
• Unit density	>70 (glands/mm^2)	81	81
Inflammatory cell density	<300 (cells/mm^2)	100	100

Source: Ibrahim, O.M., Matsumoto, Y. et al., *Ophthalmology*, 117, 665–672, 2010.

TABLE 18.4

Meibomian Gland Characteristics in Controls and MGD Patients

Study	Age Range		Acinar Unit Density (units/mm^2)		Acinar Unit Diameter (µm)	
	Controls	MGD Patients	Controls	MGD Patients	Controls	MGD Patients
Matsumoto et al., 2008	66 ± 15	68 ± 14	101 ± 34	48 ± 27	42 ± 12	98 ± 53
Villani et al., 2011a	50 ± 15	52 ± 10	110 ± 31	57 ± 21	53 ± 14	106 ± 41
Villani et al., 2011b	25 ± 4	–	119 ± 22	–	45 ± 9	–

anti-inflammatory treatment for MGD over a 12-week period, but not in the group receiving conventional treatment (Matsumoto et al. 2008).

Using IVCM, the understanding of the pathology in some ocular surface diseases has changed. Traditionally, in Sjögren's syndrome, a systemic autoimmune condition, inflammation primarily involves the exocrine salivary and lacrimal glands. IVCM showed microscopic changes in the meibomian glands, which suggests meibomian gland inflammation as part of the pathology of Sjögren's syndrome (Villani et al. 2011a). Another area is the relationship of MGD with contact lens wear. Recent meta-analysis revealed that MGD is not associated with contact lens wear in epidemiological studies (Schaumberg et al. 2011). The growing interest in imaging modalities, such as IVCM and meibography, has challenged this point of view and indicated the need for further studies. In IVCM, the meibomian acinar units in 20 contact lens wearers were found to be smaller in size and higher in density than 20 age-matched non-contact-lens-wearing controls. This study focused only on patients who wore soft contact lens for at least 1 year (Villani et al. 2011b). A longitudinal study may be warranted to observe the chronological changes in meibomian gland morphology in contact lens wear.

Demodex mites are common commensals found in the sebaceous glands of the eyelashes and ducts of the meibomian glands. Excessive numbers of these mites can cause inflammation of the eyelids and may contribute to blockage of the meibomian glands, leading to dry eye symptoms (Czepita et al. 2007). To assess the presence of demodex mites, eyelashes of a patient are usually epilated from the upper and lower lids in order to count the number of mites present (Lee et al. 2010). However, this method can only be used as a representation of the real situation, as storage and transportation of the eyelashes may alter the number of mites. A more suitable alternative of counting demodex mites is the use of IVCM. The number of mites on the eyelashes can be counted without epilation and these mites can even be seen among the dandruff of the lashes (Kojima et al. 2011). This method has also been used for other parts of the face, scalp, and chest (Longo et al. 2012).

IVCM will now play a bigger role in the management of patients with inflammatory eye diseases, such as Sjögren's syndrome and demodex infestations.

18.3 Clinical Applications

The high magnification and resolution of IVCM images have allowed the technique to emerge as a powerful tool for the study of ocular surface structures at the cellular level. Reports on the use of IVCM in disease diagnosis and monitoring of disease progression have been extremely valuable as it can provide information that conventional clinical examination tools are unable to offer. For instance, analysis of cell densities in each layer of the cornea and conjunctiva has been used to determine normal values for the general population in order to identify abnormalities associated with disease or changes with age.

A further strength of IVCM is its ability to make differential diagnoses of diseases that may be manifest in ambiguous clinical signs, such as corneal edema. Building on the example of corneal edema, IVCM allows the clinician to decide whether the edema is due to inflammation (identified by the presence of excessive inflammatory cells) or endothelial cell dropout (identified by a diminished number of endothelial cells). Pre- and postoperative assessments can also be performed. For example, the regeneration process of damaged corneal nerves following refractive surgery can be observed and compared with preoperative states.

18.3.1 Assessment of Corneal and Conjunctival Disease

Corneal disease is a major cause of blindness worldwide (Smith and Taylor 1991; Whitcher et al. 2001). The main causes of corneal blindness are usually infectious in nature, with a higher prevalence in developing countries (Taylor and Taylor 1999). Corneal infections, when left untreated, lead to corneal melting, scarring, and vascularization (Whitcher et al. 2001). This may result in loss of corneal transparency and subsequent loss of vision.

18.3.1.1 Trachoma

Trachoma is the most common cause of corneal blindness and originates from a conjunctival infection by the bacteria *Chlamydia trachomatis* (Smith and Taylor 1991; Taylor and Taylor 1999). Without timely treatment, chronic inflammation may occur, resulting in conjunctival scars, as well as vascularization, scarring, and opacification of the cornea (Thylefors et al. 1987; Whitcher et al. 2001).

Recently, Hu et al. reported on cellular changes that were only noted in the conjunctiva of patients with trachoma as compared with patients without the disease. IVCM imaging showed abnormal follicular structures, black cystic spaces indicating tissue swelling, and structures typical of scarring in patients with active disease. Additionally, inflammatory cells in the form of dendritiform cells were seen more frequently and numerously in patients with trachoma (Hu et al. 2011a). In a second report, the authors observed that inflammatory cells in trachomatous scars mainly resided within the most superficial portion (within 30 μm of the conjunctival surface) (Hu et al. 2011b). This discovery suggested a close interaction between these inflammatory dendritiform cells and the epithelium and implies a bacteria-induced cellular response rather than an acquired cell-mediated response.

Based on IVCM images, a grading system for conjunctival inflammation was developed. The system evaluates features in the palpebral conjunctiva that are characteristic for trachoma, such as the presence of inflammatory infiltrates, inflammatory dendritiform cells, tissue edema, and papillae. The extent of conjunctival scarring was also gradable using a four-point grading system. This ranges from normal homogenous and amorphous appearance (grade 0) to well-defined bands or sheets of tissue and visible striations in more than half of the area of the scan (grade 3) (Hu et al. 2011a).

Unfortunately, trachoma is more prevalent in developing countries, where access to health care is limited and the availability of IVCM is scarce. Therefore, the use of IVCM for diagnosis and disease monitoring may not be suitable in those countries. Nevertheless, a clinical setting that utilizes IVCM may allow clinicians to better document the level of inflammation of the disease. For research purposes, IVCM will enable us to investigate the pathophysiology of trachoma and broaden our knowledge of the disease.

18.3.1.2 Corneal Ulcers

Ulcerative corneal infections, also known as ulcerative keratitis, are caused by four main types of microorganisms—viruses, bacteria, fungi, and amoeba. Common risk factors of ulcerative keratitis include ocular trauma, contact lens wear, and certain systemic diseases (Stehr-Green et al. 1987; Dart 1988; Stehr-Green et al. 1989; Liesegang 1997; Radford et al. 1998; Schaefer et al. 2001).

Viral keratitis is usually caused by the herpes simplex virus (HSV). This infection cannot be completely eradicated and can recur after the initial infection has apparently resolved. This is attributed to the virus's ability to survive in a latent state in the trigeminal nerve or corneal tissue (Stevens et al. 1972; Rock et al. 1987; Kaye et al. 1991; Shimomura 2008).

The characteristic wire netting of the dendritic cells and presence of Langerhans cells in active HSV keratitis can be imaged with IVCM, which facilitates the diagnosis of the infection (Guthoff et al. 2009). Monitoring of treatment can be achieved by analyzing the Langerhans cells, where a decrease in number is a sign of recovery, and the corneal endothelium (Guthoff et al. 2009; Hillenaar et al. 2009). In patients with previous HSV keratitis, corneal epithelial cell and nerve fiber changes were also observed (Table 18.5) (Rosenberg et al. 2002). These changes would not be detectable by slit lamp examination and could be useful in predicting recurrence of the infection.

Bacterial keratitis is more commonly seen in contact lens wearers. When bacterial keratitis is suspected, initial treatment is commenced with broad-spectrum antibiotics. Upon isolation of the class of bacteria involved, that is, gram negative or gram positive, a more specific treatment can be implemented to target the pathogenic species.

On examination with a slit lamp biomicroscope, the ulcer caused by bacterial infection is usually recognizable as a central or paracentral white lesion on the cornea. IVCM studies on bacterial keratitis demonstrated this lesion as a hyperreflective structure surrounded by edematous epithelium with an indistinct posterior border. At the basal cell layer and subbasal nerve plexus, inflammatory activity can be visualized by the presence of Langerhans cells and leukocytes (Guthoff et al. 2009). Unfortunately, differentiation of the bacterial species involved in this type of keratitis is not possible with IVCM and corneal scraping and culture remain the only way to identify the responsible bacteria (Vaddavalli et al. 2006).

Fungal keratitis can be caused by contact of the eye with a sharp end of a plant, excessive steroid use, and inappropriate hygiene conditions (Thomas 2003). The trauma introduces fungal microspores and the wound enables the microspores to penetrate into deeper layers (Rosa et al. 1994; Houang et al. 2001).

Even in the early stages of the infection, the fungi can be depicted by IVCM as hyperreflective elements in the anterior corneal stroma, along with the infiltration of inflammatory cells (Table 18.5). IVCM images have shown differential physical characteristics of various fungal agents (Table 18.5), providing a way to instantly identify the species of fungus involved in the disease (Brasnu et al. 2007).

Amoebic keratitis, although rare, is the most devastating of corneal infections. The amoebic genus that causes the greatest concern is *Acanthamoeba*. It causes intense eye pain and can have devastating consequences for vision (Duguid et al. 1997). Patients with *Acanthamoeba* keratitis present with subtle signs (usually only a mild to moderate red eye) in spite of intense pain, which often befuddle clinicians (Clarke and Niederkorn 2006).

TABLE 18.5

IVCM Findings in Corneas with the Four Types of Infectious Keratitis

Organism	Appearance/Findings

Viruses (HSV)	Active state:
	• Characteristic wire netting of the dendritic cells
	• Presence of Langerhans cells within the cornea
	• Corneal endothelium:
	  • Increased spaces between cells
	  • Undefined cell borders
	  • Guttata
	  • Infiltration of inflammatory cells
	Previous infection
	• Larger cornea surface epithelial cells
	• Presence of highly reflective structures found at the level of the basal epithelial cells, particularly around areas of stromal fibrosis
	• Areas with increased abnormal extracellular matrix
	• Subbasal nerve fiber bundles undetectable
	• Reduced long nerve fiber bundles

Bacteria	• Ulcer structure:
	  • Hyperreflective
	  • Undistinguishable border at the bottom
	  • Surrounded by edematous epithelium
	• Presence of Langerhans cells and leukocytes

Fungi	• Hyperreflective elements in the anterior corneal stroma • Corneal epithelial and stromal disorganization (corneal fibroblast activation) • Dendritiform and round inflammatory cells present at the epithelial level and area of stromal infiltrates
• *Fusarium solani*	• High contrast lines 200–300 × 3–5 μm • Branches at right angles in the anterior stroma
• *Candida albicans*	• High contrast elongated particles 10–40 × 5–10 μm
• *Aspergillus fumigatus*	• High contrast lines 200–300 × 3–5 μm • Branches at 45° in the anterior stroma
Protozoa (*Acanthamoeba*)	Cysts: • 10–28 μm in size • Characteristic hyperreflective round particles in the corneal epithelium and stroma Trophozoites: • 24–40 μm in size • Highly reflective and surrounded by edematous surrounding tissue in the corneal epithelium and stroma

Identification of *Acanthamoeba* keratitis using IVCM was first described in 1992 and was suggested to be used as a tool for rapid and successful diagnosis (Chew et al. 1992). The characteristic round structure of the *Acanthamoeba* cysts (its inactive form) and hyperreflective trophozoites (its active form) are easily recognized in IVCM images (Guthoff et al. 2009; Kumar et al. 2010).

Identification of the causative microorganism for an infection is usually determined by corneal scraping and culture. However, this process requires special culture media and may take weeks. Time is crucial as ulcerative keratitis can lead to significant loss of vision in a matter of weeks. Most importantly, only 30%–67% of the collected samples produce positive cultures (O'Day et al. 1979; Keay et al. 2006; Yeh et al. 2006; Kanavi et al. 2007). In addition, the different types of ulcerative keratitis share similar clinical features (e.g., a central corneal lesion). The ambiguous signs complicate diagnosis and management.

Without recognizing the microorganism responsible for the infection, misdiagnosis and delayed implementation of appropriate treatment are fairly common (Berger et al. 1990).

IVCM's accuracy in the microbiological diagnosis of ulcerative keratitis is generally high in terms of identifying the class of organism (Table 18.6) (Kanavi et al. 2007; Vaddavalli et al. 2011). Tu et al. demonstrated IVCM's superiority to corneal cultures and smears. In that study, IVCM identified that 90.6% of patients had keratitis caused by *Acanthamoeba*, while a positive result could only be achieved in 73.2% and 54.8% of corneal smears and corneal cultures, respectively (Tu et al. 2008). In another remarkable example, a case of combined fungal and *Acanthamoeba* keratitis was detected by IVCM (Babu and Murthy 2007). IVCM is potentially a powerful tool in helping clinicians to identify the microorganism instantly and, thus, implement the correct treatment in time.

18.3.1.3 Keratoconus

Keratoconus is a degenerative disease characterized by thinning of the cornea, a typical conical shape that can be noted at the later stage of disease, and associated worsening of vision. The etiology of keratoconus remains unclear; nonetheless, excessive eye rubbing, contact lens wear, a positive family history, and various systemic diseases have been linked to the disease (Krachmer et al. 1984; Rabinowitz 1998; Edwards et al. 2001). Despite having well-established clinical features, early to moderate forms of the condition may go undetected due to the subtle signs that are commonly missed (Rabinowitz 1998).

IVCM observations of keratoconic eyes have revealed alterations in the arrangement of corneal nerves as well as in all layers of the cornea. Images of abnormal nerve fibers in affected corneas are consistent with findings of decreased corneal sensitivity in patients with keratoconus (Patel et al. 2009). Nerve fibers were noted to be increased in thickness, prominence, and tortuosity (Patel et al. 2006; Ucakhan et al. 2006). The density of nerve fibers was also decreased in keratoconic eyes. This decrease was greater in severe cases and in therapeutic contact lens wear. Patterns of nerve fiber arrangements seem to respect and parallel the contour of the cornea, forming closed loops at the apex (Patel et al. 2006; Niederer et al. 2008). Whether the nerve changes precede the condition or are induced by the corneal morphology change, the pathophysiology of corneal nerve changes in keratoconus remains unclear.

IVCM findings in the epithelial layer included elongated superficial cells, increased nuclei size of the winged-shaped cells, decreased basal cell density, and increased cell size (Hollingsworth et al. 2005; Ucakhan et al. 2006; Weed et al. 2007; Mocan et al. 2008; Niederer et al. 2008). Disruptions in Bowman's membrane may explain the abnormal advancement of epithelial cell processes into Bowman's membrane (Sherwin et al. 2002; Niederer et al. 2008). The main change in the stromal layer is a reduction in keratocyte cell

TABLE 18.6

Detection of Fungi and Amoeba in Keratitis Using IVCM*

Study	Microorganism	Sensitivity (%)	Specificity (%)
Tu et al., 2008	Acanthamoeba	90.6	100
Kanavi et al., 2007	Acanthamoeba	100	84
	Fungi	94	78
Vaddavalli et al., 2011	Fungi	89.2	92.7

*As judged against clinical diagnosis in suspected cases, confirmed cases, or both.

density, which is inversely correlated with disease severity (Hollingsworth et al. 2005; Ku et al. 2008; Mocan et al. 2008; Niederer et al. 2008). The keratocytes in keratoconus become irregularly arranged, explaining the corneal haze, and also show increased reflectivity in IVCM images (Hollingsworth et al. 2005; Mocan et al. 2008; Niederer et al. 2008). Descemet's membrane folds were also observed in one study (Ucakhan et al. 2006). In the endothelial layer, changes in cell density, enlargement of cells, changes in shape, and areas of cell loss have been reported that were correlated with severity of disease (Hollingsworth et al. 2005; Ucakhan et al. 2006; Mocan et al. 2008; Niederer et al. 2008).

Today, diagnosis and monitoring of keratoconus are routinely performed with the less invasive method of corneal topography. However, IVCM observations of microscopic cornea structure changes have given us additional important insights into the pathophysiology and etiology of the disease.

18.3.1.4 Pterygium

Pterygium is a noncancerous growth of the conjunctiva, forming a wing-shaped, commonly vascularized, and raised lesion over the cornea. Its etiology and pathophysiology are currently unclear. A greater incidence in the equatorial regions and in people with a highly active outdoor lifestyle strongly suggests high exposure to ultraviolet radiation as the main risk factor (McCarty et al. 2000).

Histopathological knowledge of pterygium is mostly obtained from laboratory studies on surgically excised pterygium tissue, which offers little information on its growth process in the living human tissue. The high magnification and excellent resolution of IVCM allow for real-time observation of pterygium at a cellular level and its effect on the surrounding corneal and conjunctival tissue.

Decreased central corneal epithelial cell density, increased dendritiform cells in the epithelium, and decreased stromal keratocytes have been observed in corneas with pterygia (Papadia et al. 2008). The density of the mucin-producing goblet cells in the conjunctiva was also found to rise with increasing pterygium activity (Labbe et al. 2010). In a conference proceeding, Martone et al. reported differences in progressive and nonprogressive pterygia based on IVCM images of the corneal area adjacent to the pterygium. The pterygia were classified as progressive and nonprogressive at 12 months postoperatively in a double-masked study. Generally, corneas in nonprogressive pterygia are relatively quiet, with little or no inflammatory activity and edema. In progressive cases, stromal edema was significantly increased together with keratocyte activation. Infiltration of inflammatory cells and the presence of numerous capillaries and hyperreflective structures at the pterygium head are indications of progressive pterygium (Martone et al. 2009). More studies are needed to validate these findings. This information could be extremely useful in predicting the progression rate of pterygium growth and, thus, the need for excision surgery.

In addition, even though pterygium growth occurs only over the superficial surface of the cornea, morphological abnormalities have been found in deeper layers, such as the subbasal nerve fibers. Wang et al. (2010) reported increased tortuosity, localized bulges, and breakages in corneal nerve fibers. The effects of pterygium growth on corneal sensation and corneal nerve fibers have not been reported elsewhere.

18.3.1.5 Dry Eye

Dry eye is a dysfunction of the tear film. The tear film becomes unstable and initiates a vicious cycle whereby the ocular surface is insufficiently lubricated. This causes increased inflammatory activity with subsequent cell damage to the surface and symptoms of dry eye. The prevalence of dry eye ranges widely from 5% to 35%, with higher incidence rates in the ageing population and women (McCarty et al. 1998; Lin et al. 2003). Other risk factors include contact lens wear, history of ocular surgery, presence of systemic disease, and use of medication (Smith et al. 2007).

The conventional method of dry eye diagnosis utilizes slit lamp biomicroscopy, which cannot directly assess the subtle inflammation in the corneal and conjunctival surface and IVCM may be a valuable additional tool, as elaborated on below.

Previous IVCM findings of corneal and conjunctival changes in dry eye were remarkable. Findings revealed that dry eye patients have a decreased epithelial cell density, a thinner cornea, and decreased nerve fiber density with irregular patterns of nerve fiber branching and increased tortuosity (Zhang et al. 2005; Erdelyi et al. 2007). Furthermore, the number of nerve fibers correlated positively with corneal fluorescein and rose bengal dye staining, which are conventional parameters of epithelial damage (Zhang et al. 2005).

18.3.1.6 Sjögren's Syndrome

Sjögren's syndrome is an autoimmune disease in which the body's own immune cells attack the salivary and tear glands. These patients often suffer from severe dry eye and IVCM has the potential to play a major role in the understanding of the cause–effect relationship of the disease. Sjögren's syndrome is a systemic condition but manifests itself in the ocular surface. IVCM investigations noted an accumulation of inflammatory cells in the cornea and conjunctiva in patients with the disease. Similar, but less marked, observations were also made in dry eye patients without the syndrome. IVCM found that a higher number of inflammatory cells worsen tear stability and surface damage. In addition, lower conjunctival epithelial cell densities and higher epithelial microcyst densities were found in patients with Sjögren's syndrome as compared with non-Sjögren's syndrome dry eye patients and normal controls (Wakamatsu et al. 2010). Corneal nerve fiber changes, such as increased number and tortuosity, were more pronounced in patients with Sjögren's syndrome (Zhang et al. 2005).

Although diagnosis and monitoring of dry eye using the routine clinical techniques such as slit lamp examination and Schirmer's test are generally sufficient, information on the microscopic changes in the ocular tissues that only IVCM can provide may be key in testing the efficacy of novel anti-inflammatory treatments.

18.3.1.7 Limbal Stem Cell Deficiency

The limbus forms the barrier between the cornea and conjunctiva. It harbors stem cells that are vital proliferative cells that help to maintain epithelial cells covering the cornea (Cotsarelis et al. 1989). These cells are situated in the limbal lacuna. In limbal stem cell deficiency (LSCD), the damage to the cells causes conjunctivalization of the cornea, which is an invasion of the conjunctival epithelium onto the cornea. This abnormal growth of the conjunctiva often triggers an inflammatory cell infiltration and vascularization of the cornea. The cornea becomes edematous and optically and morphologically irregular and its epithelium destabilizes. Blurring of vision, intermittent pain, sensitivity to light, twitching of the eyelids, and tearing are some of the symptoms patients might experience with LSCD.

On slit lamp presentation, the corneal surface may appear dull and irregular, varying in transparency. The demarcation of the conjunctival tissue on the cornea is usually clear.

In severe cases, vascularization of the cornea can be seen and because of the tendency of the epithelium to break down, erosions of the cornea may be observed with fluorescein dye staining (Holland and Schwartz 1997; Dua et al. 2000). For a firm diagnosis to be made when the slit lamp findings are questionable, impression cytology is the current method of choice. The filter is impressed upon the area of affected cornea and the detection of goblet cells and conjunctival epithelial cells confirms the diagnosis of LSCD (Dua and Azuara-Blanco 1999; Dua et al. 2000).

However, despite the fact that the presence of goblet cells in the cornea is indicative of LSCD, Miri et al. (2012) noted that goblet cells are not always present in the corneas of LSCD. In fact, out of 17 eyes in which corneas had been conjunctivalized, IVCM imaging only revealed six corneas with goblet cells present, although the authors admit that the corneas may not have been scanned thoroughly enough. In any case, the failure to detect goblet cells on the cornea using IVCM may suggest a lower density of goblet cells, possibly relating to the original etiology of the disease or extensive destruction of these cells (Miri et al. 2012). These clinical features of LSCD mentioned so far do not point to a single etiology.

It has been observed in LSCD, but not in normal corneas, that dendritic cells were located in the central cornea. The hypothesis is that in LSCD, cells have moved from the limbus to the central cornea (Mastropasqua et al. 2006; Miri et al. 2012). The conjunctival epithelial basal cells in LSCD had prominent nuclei and indistinct borders, as compared with hyporeflective cell bodies and well-defined bright borders in the normal conjunctiva. Intraepithelial cysts, ranging from 12 to 52 μm in diameter, were found in all conjunctivalized cornea epithelia surrounded by goblet cells. These cysts appear as dark spaces among the goblet cells. Where these cysts are larger in size, there were fewer goblet cells (Miri et al. 2012). It is not clear what these cysts represent and further investigations are warranted.

Corneal nerve density, like in most other ocular surface diseases, were reduced and even undetectable using IVCM, especially in severe LSCD where Bowman's membrane was not visible. Failure to visualize the corneal nerves may be attributed to a true destruction of the nerves or simple an inability to locate the nerves due to the thick conjunctiva tissue in between the objective lens and cornea.

18.3.1.8 Chemical Burns

Chemical burns to the ocular surface are classified as either acid or alkali burns. They are always considered as emergencies as they may threaten the vision of the patient (Tuft and Shortt 2009). Alkali burns cause more of a concern due to their ability to penetrate through the cornea more quickly than acids. Saponification of the cell membrane leads to further and deeper penetration into the eye and beyond the ocular surface in a matter of minutes; therefore urgent treatment is critical (Paterson et al. 1975; Wright 1982). Acid burns, on the other hand, coagulate corneal proteins in the corneal epithelium, which prevents further penetration into deeper layers and causes only superficial injury (Wright 1982).

Most cases of ocular chemical burns are not sight-threatening, but severe dry eye and limbal stem cell disease may occur due to the chemical that was introduced into the ocular surface system by the injury. The root cause for this lays in the potential damage to the conjunctival goblet cells by the chemical. The goblet cells are major producers of mucin, which enables the tear film to adhere to the epithelial surface.

Patients with a chemical injury to the eye have a significantly reduced number of conjunctival goblet cells (Le et al. 2010). This may then affect the tear film, leading to dry eye (Nelson and Wright 1984; Tiffany 2003).

Long-term effects of chemical burns can be monitored by either IVCM or impression cytology. Generally, the most commonly used technique to monitor the integrity of goblet cells in the conjunctiva is impression cytology. In recent years, however, some clinicians have shifted to IVCM methodology, as no cell sample collection is necessary. Using IVCM, goblet cells can be easily recognized. They appear as large hyperreflective ovals scattered among the epithelial cells (Kobayashi et al. 2005; Messmer et al. 2006). This makes IVCM an ideal tool for monitoring long-term effects of chemical burn, supporting a potentially wider use of this technique.

18.3.2 Corneal Surgery

The two main types of corneal surgery are refractive surgery and corneal grafting. As previously mentioned, the cornea is the most innervated structure of the human body, with the highest density of nerve fibers. Any surgical procedure that involves a cut into the stroma would inevitably affect the viability of nerves. Nerve regeneration is a lengthy process and IVCM has been essential in examining the extent of injury following surgery and recovery of nerves.

18.3.2.1 Refractive Surgery

Refractive surgery is one approach to permanently correct refractive errors by reshaping the cornea. Wearing glasses and contact lenses are usually effective ways to improve sight, but refractive surgery has become extremely popular as it allows patients to reduce or even cease their dependence on glasses or lenses (Sawet al. 1996; Solomon et al. 2009). LASIK surgery is one type of refractive surgery and remains the procedure of choice for most patients and surgeons when correcting short-sightedness.

IVCM examination of eyes that underwent the procedure show significantly decreased nerve fiber density, length, and width (Perez-Gomez and Efron 2003; Darwish et al. 2007). Corneal nerves are severed during flap creation and removal of tissue in the stromal bed by laser, leading to LASIK-induced dry eye (Calvillo et al. 2004, 2007). These changes can be monitored by IVCM pre- and postoperatively.

Clinicians are able to examine flap-related corneal complications after LASIK surgery in relatively gross detail by using the slit lamp biomicroscope, but changes at the cellular level can only be elucidated by IVCM. For example, IVCM can easily identify epithelial ingrowth at the flap site or a decrease in keratocyte cell count within the flap zone (Pisella et al. 2001; Perez-Gomez and Efron 2003; Kaufman and Kaufman 2006). Corneal flap thickness is also measureable and was noticed to be usually thinner than proposed (Pisella et al. 2001). Hyperreflective particles were detected in the zone between the flap and the underlying stroma (interface zone) (Pisella et al. 2001; Perez-Gomez and Efron 2003). It is believed that these particles are fine metallic debris from the flap-cutting blade (McCarty et al. 2000). If so, these particles may oxidize or degrade, triggering a possible immunological response, in a clinical entity called diffuse lamellar keratitis (Ku et al. 2008).

Microfolds within the flap at Bowman's membrane were also detected after surgery. These folds appear as long dark straight or slightly curved lines, varying in thickness, length, and orientation and a significant degree of microfolds may affect the visual outcome (Perez-Gomez and Efron 2003). They are believed to be a byproduct of the stretching of the flap during surgery or a result of an incompatibility of the flap to the surgically altered stroma (Vesaluoma et al. 2000).

Another technique to correct vision is photorefractive keratectomy (PRK). This method does not create a flap, but removes corneal epithelium to directly reshape the cornea from the top using the laser. However, LASIK is the preferred refractive surgical procedure today due to the relative discomfort and longer healing time associated with a PRK procedure. Long-term changes within the cornea have been observed by IVCM. Five years after the procedure, Moilanen et al. (2003) reported alterations in the corneal morphology that included irregular distribution of keratocytes in the anterior stroma with nuclei that appeared to be more reflective in PRK-operated eyes than normal unoperated eyes. In addition, Bowman's membrane that had been removed during surgery, and is normally located between the corneal epithelium and the stroma, had not been regenerated even 5 years after PRK. These variations did not interfere with visual performance. The nerve fiber density, posterior stroma, and endothelial layer had a similar appearance to those of unoperated eyes (Moilanen et al. 2003).

In summary, interface zone and flap thickness as well as haze development can be monitored using IVCM. Although it may not be advisable to perform IVCM in the first few days after surgery, especially for LASIK due to the possibility of flap displacement, IVCM is a helpful modality for monitoring long-term changes at the cellular level that would not be detectable with a slit lamp biomicroscope.

18.3.2.2 Corneal Grafting

Corneal grafting enables partial restoration of vision in patients who have suffered destructive corneal diseases, such as keratoconus, corneal dystrophies, and severe scarring due to keratitis or trauma. During this procedure, the diseased part of the cornea is replaced with a donor cornea. It is possible to either replace the diseased part of the cornea only (lamellar keratoplasty, deep anterior lamellar keratoplasty, endothelial keratoplasty) or perform a full thickness corneal graft (penetrating keratoplasty).

There is a chance of rejection of the transplanted tissue by the patient's body. Generally, the success rates of corneal grafting are high, being up to 90% in the first year. However, the host may develop an immunological response against the grafted tissue, causing the donor cornea to be rejected years after transplantation (Williams et al. 1997). On slit lamp examination, a rejection is characterized by blood vessel growth into the graft tissue, subepithelial infiltration of immune cells, haze, and corneal swelling (Cohen et al. 1995).

After corneal transplantation, the health of the donor cornea may depend on the viability and function of individual cell types within the graft. Unlike slit lamp biomicroscopy, IVCM has been shown to be useful for the follow-up of these cell types. The following changes can be observed. In the early phase (1 week) after full thickness corneal grafting, endothelial cells are lost rapidly, but numbers that are functional remain (Bourne 2001). The keratocytes become activated in the first week; their numbers drop, and then recover gradually, though not to the original numbers (Bourne 2001; Niederer et al. 2007b; Patel et al. 2007; Szaflik et al. 2007). Some corneal nerves do not survive, but sufficient nerves remaining became functional, which explains detectable corneal sensation in grafts (Bourne 2001; Imre et al. 2005; Patel et al. 2007). Other associated changes in the graft include stroma and descemet membrane folds (Szaflik et al. 2007). Donor epithelial tissue in the graft rapidly degenerates after surgery, and is replaced in time by host corneal epithelium (Szaflik et al. 2007).

The observations made with IVCM after corneal grafting have provided surgeons with a better understanding of causes of corneal graft failure. Short- and long-term postoperative follow-up using IVCM is possible and maybe even be advisable.

18.3.3 Contact Lens Wear

The use of contact lenses for the correction of vision is an attractive alternative to wearing spectacles. As mentioned in previous sections, contact lens wear can be a major risk factor for microbial keratitis and dry eye (Lemp 1995; Vajdic et al. 1999). It is known that contact lens wear introduces changes to the corneal curvature and thickness as well as regularity (Miller 1968; Liu and Pflugfelder 2000; Yeniad et al. 2003). Physiological alterations such as reduced oxygen intake, decreased corneal sensitivity, and infiltration of inflammatory cells may also occur (Millodot 1978; Donshik and Ballow 1983; Ang and Efron 1990; Thakur and Willcox 2000; Zhivov et al. 2007). These changes happen gradually when contact lenses are worn continuously for a month over 5 years, or worn for a few hours a day for 10 years (Holden et al. 1985; Patel et al. 2002).

The use of IVCM to investigate microscopic changes in the cornea and palpebral conjunctiva with contact lens wear has increased gradually over the past decade. Inflammatory cell changes can be observed with the IVCM but not the slit lamp biomicroscope. The density of Langerhans cells increases with number of years of contact lens wear, even before there are clinical discomfort and symptoms (Zhivov et al. 2007).

IVCM observations have revealed that the superficial corneal epithelial cells become smaller in size with prolonged contact lens wear and this subsequently increased the overall cell density of the epithelium (Efron 2007). It is not clear what implications this may have on the overall health of the cornea.

Contact lens wear can alter the size, shape, and distribution of endothelial cells due to lack of oxygen and IVCM can help in this assessment (Hollingsworth and Efron 2004; Zhivov et al. 2007). The endothelial cells act as hydration controls and pump fluid out of the corneal stroma, which tends to imbibe fluid. Any changes to the endothelial cell layer hence affect corneal clarity. Long-term contact lens (e.g., 5 years) wear may reduce the number of endothelial cells leading to cornea edema, loss of transparency, and eventually decrease in vision quality (Connor and Zagrod 1986; Hollingsworth and Efron 2004). This can be partially reversed when contact lens wear is discontinued.

Some corneal epithelial changes (reduced cell size, increased cell density) can be observed by IVCM but the clinical implications are not known. Excessive mechanical interaction between the lens and tear film creates translucent spheres of mucin called mucin balls. Originally it was thought that mucin balls are simply situated along the interface of the cornea and contact lens and do not migrate into the epithelium. IVCM investigations, however, revealed mucin balls within the entire thickness of the corneal epithelium with keratocytes being activated by their presence (Efron 2007). With slit lamp biomicroscopy, clinicians are usually able to identify superficial mucin balls, but when within the epithelium, their appearance is similar to that of microcysts, small vesicles containing fluid and debris. The distinction between cysts and mucin balls is important for their clinical management; mucin ball formation is attributed to an ill-fitting contact lens whereas microcysts are due to lack of oxygen. IVCM may be used to differentiate between these signs.

IVCM may play an essential role in detecting subtle ocular surface changes related to contact lens wear. The live viewing of highly magnified cells and tissue structures allow clinicians to immediately and accurately diagnose contact lens-associated complications and thus commence appropriate management.

18.3.4 Glaucoma Surgery

Frequently considered to be "the thief of sight," glaucoma is a major cause of blindness (Quigley 1996). Glaucoma is an eye disease that cannot be cured. The optical nerves in the eye responsible for the transmission of visual information to the brain are irreversibly damaged by high pressures in the eye (intraocular pressure), leading to loss of vision. However, disease progression can be controlled by medication, laser therapy, and surgery. There are several approaches to glaucoma surgery, but this section of the chapter will focus on trabeculectomy, one of the most commonly performed techniques (Cairns 1968). The procedure relieves some of the pressure inside the eye by creating a through-channel from the anterior chamber to the subconjunctival space. The draining of the aqueous fluid out of the eye reduces the intraocular pressure. The elevation of the conjunctiva postoperation is called the bleb.

The outcome of trabeculectomy surgery is judged by the intraocular pressure and bleb appearance. Thin diffuse blebs containing microcysts are generally considered more functional and more desirable. However, the bleb is loosely held in place by stitches and may collapse or become scarred over time, interrupting the outflow and raising the intraocular pressure. The short-term success rate of trabeculectomy is reasonable, but long-term outcomes are less optimistic (Inaba 1982; Singh et al. 1995; Giampani et al. 2008).

Clinicians today assess the bleb by slit lamp biomicroscopy (Park et al. 2009). For viewing cellular changes, IVCM is the most appropriate tool. IVCM is good to evaluate the density of the subepithelial connective tissue (thickness of the bleb) and number of microcysts. Functioning blebs should exhibit loosely arranged subepithelial connective tissue whereas densely packed tissue fibers indicate a failed bleb (Labbe et al. 2005; Ciancaglini et al. 2008). IVCM examinations of the conjunctival bleb have revealed different tissue patterns. The four different arrangements of the tissue fibers (trabecular, reticular, corrugated, and compacted) may each have a bearing on the function of the bleb. The trabecular pattern, straight and fine with large spaces in between, is seen only in functioning blebs. The reticular pattern is straight and crisscrossed with intermittent gaps. Corrugated patterns are curved, short, wide, and disorderly. Fibers with the compacted patterns are tightly packed, parallel, and hyperreflective. Future studies are indicated to establish the application of tissue fiber patterns in understanding bleb function (Guthoff et al. 2006).

IVCM is an excellent device for predicting bleb success in the long term as both the conjunctiva and cornea appear clinically normal regardless of the bleb function.

18.4 Operational Difficulties

The use of IVCM is mostly for research purposes and not routinely used in the clinic. The major reasons for this are the challenging nature of the procedure, the lack of universal reference values, the cost factor, and the relative invasiveness of IVCM.

Widespread use may also be hindered by the difficulty of handling the equipment. Imaging of the eye by IVCM may be challenging for the operator as well as for the patient. The patient has to remain motionless during the examination in order for the operator to locate the area of interest. The smallest of eye movements may result in a view that is not within the targeted area of interest. Furthermore, there may be some discomfort for the patient when the investigative cap is touching the eye. In order to change the depth of the scan within the tissue, the examiner needs to manually rotate the lens whilst in contact with the eye. Although topical anesthesia is applied to the eye, the patient will be aware of the lens moving toward the eye and will feel the touch of the lens.

A novice operator may have difficulty localizing a specific area of interest or identifying the structure visualized. Moreover, longitudinal evaluation requires repositioning of the probe in the same exact location at different times. Therefore, a steep learning curve is likely to be encountered by the IVCM operator. When imaging diseases in which the cornea is very thin or almost perforated (e.g., keratoconus and corneal ulcers), the operator of the instrument must take extra care during scanning. Patients with very painful eyes (e.g., ulcerative keratitis) may not consent to scanning.

18.5 Future Directions and Summary

The technical specifications of IVCM may be improved in the future. For example, the optical and image resolutions may be increased beyond the current standards. Innovations in the optics of scanning may ideally permit noninvasive scanning. The scanning time can be improved if there is some guidance concerning the position of the probe relative to the eye and automatic adjustments of the depth of the scan. With further advancements in technology, an increased field of view and perhaps even higher magnification to analyze minute structures such as CALT will be possible.

There may be new clinical indications for the use of IVCM in ophthalmic clinics. For example, in amoebic infections, the presence of trophozoites and cysts or their relative numbers may give a clue to therapy, such as commencement of steroids. Prescribing steroids can be a critical but difficult decision during amoebic infections. The premature use of steroids before controlling the infection may worsen the outcomes. In the case of pterygium after surgery, the presence of dendritic or inflammatory cells may herald recurrence and warrant more aggressive steroids. These potential indications will require longitudinal studies to support them.

With the increased use of IVCM, both in research and clinical environments, various grading and quantifying systems for ocular parameters such as cell density and cell size have been developed and are likely to be developed in the near future. In conclusion, detailed imaging of the ocular surface structures and associated cell types can be performed using IVCM. This technology will enable in-depth understanding of ocular surface physiology and pathology without the necessity of tissue excisions.

References

Amos, W. B. and J. G. White (2003). How the confocal laser scanning microscope entered biological research. *Biol Cell* 95: 1058–1063.

Ang, J. H. and N. Efron (1990). Corneal hypoxia and hypercapnia during contact lens wear. *Optom Vis Sci* 67(7): 512–521.

Arita, R., K. Itoh, et al. (2008). Noncontact infrared meibography to document age-related changes of the meibomian glands in a normal population. *Ophthalmology* 115(5): 911–915.

Astley, R. A., R. C. Kennedy, et al. (2003). Structural and cellular architecture of conjunctival lymphoid follicles in the baboon (*Papio anubis*). *Exp Eye Res* 76(6): 685–694.

Babu, K. and K. R. Murthy (2007). Combined fungal and acanthamoeba keratitis: Diagnosis by in vivo confocal microscopy. *Eye* 21(2): 271–272.

Berger, S. T., B. J. Mondino, et al. (1990). Successful medical management of acanthamoeba keratitis. *Am J Ophthalmol* 110(4): 395–403.

Bourne, W. M. (2001). Cellular changes in transplanted human corneas. *Cornea* 20(6): 560–569.

Bourne, W. M., L. R. Nelson, et al. (1997). Central corneal endothelial cell changes over a ten-year period. *Invest Ophthalmol Vis Sci* 38(3): 779–782.

Brasnu, E., T. Bourcier, et al. (2007). In vivo confocal microscopy in fungal keratitis. *Br J Ophthalmol* 91(5): 588–591.

Bron, A. J., L. Benjamin, et al. (1991). Meibomian gland disease. Classification and grading of lid changes. *Eye* 5(Pt 4): 395–411.

Bron, A. J. and J. M. Tiffany (2004). The contribution of meibomian disease to dry eye. *Ocul Surf* 2(2): 149–165.

Bron, A. J., J. M. Tiffany, et al. (2004). Functional aspects of the tear film lipid layer. *Exp Eye Res* 78(3): 347–360.

Cairns, J. E. (1968). Trabeculectomy. Preliminary report of a new method. *Am J Ophthalmol* 66(4): 673–679.

Calvillo, M. P., J. W. McLaren, et al. (2004). Corneal reinnervation after LASIK: Prospective 3-year longitudinal study. *Invest Ophthalmol Vis Sci* 45(11): 3991–3996.

Chew, S. J., R. W. Beuerman, et al. (1992). Early diagnosis of infectious keratitis with in vivo real time confocal microscopy. *CLAO J* 18(3): 197–201.

Chiou, A. G., S. C. Kaufman, et al. (1999). Confocal microscopy in cornea guttata and Fuchs' endothelial dystrophy. *Br J Ophthalmol* 83(2): 185–189.

Chiou, A. G., S. C. Kaufman, et al. (2006). Clinical corneal confocal microscopy. *Surv Ophthalmol* 51(5): 482–500.

Ciancaglini, M., P. Carpineto, et al. (2008). Filtering bleb functionality: A clinical, anterior segment optical coherence tomography and in vivo confocal microscopy study. *J Glaucoma* 17(4): 308–317.

Clarke, D. W. and J. Y. Niederkorn (2006). The pathophysiology of acanthamoeba keratitis. *Trends Parasitol* 22(4): 175–180.

Cohen, R. A., S. J. Chew, et al. (1995). Confocal microscopy of corneal graft rejection. *Cornea* 14(5): 467–472.

Connor, C. G. and M. E. Zagrod (1986). Contact lens-induced corneal endothelial polymegathism: Functional significance and possible mechanisms. *Am J Optom Physiol Opt* 63(7): 539–544.

Cotsarelis, G., S. Z. Cheng, et al. (1989). Existence of slow-cycling limbal epithelial basal cells that can be preferentially stimulated to proliferate: Implications on epithelial stem cells. *Cell* 57(2): 201–209.

Czepita, D., W. Kuzna-Grygiel, et al. (2007). *Demodex folliculorum* and *Demodex brevis* as a cause of chronic marginal blepharitis. *Ann Acad Med Stetin* 53(1): 63–67.

Dart, J. K. (1988). Predisposing factors in microbial keratitis: The significance of contact lens wear. *Br J Ophthalmol* 72(12): 926–930.

Darwish, T., A. Brahma, et al. (2007). Subbasal nerve fiber regeneration after LASIK and LASEK assessed by noncontact esthesiometry and in vivo confocal microscopy: Prospective study. *J Cataract Refract Surg* 33(9): 1515–1521.

Davidovits, P. and M. D. Egger (1973). Photomicrography of corneal endothelial cells in vivo. *Nature* 244(5415): 366–367.

De Cilla, S., S. Ranno, et al. (2009). Corneal subbasal nerves changes in patients with diabetic retinopathy: An in vivo confocal study. *Invest Ophthalmol Vis Sci* 50(11): 5155–5158.

Donshik, P. C. and M. Ballow (1983). Tear immunoglobulins in giant papillary conjunctivitis induced by contact lenses. *Am J Ophthalmol* 96(4): 460–466.

Dua, H. S. and A. Azuara-Blanco (1999). Allo-limbal transplantation in patients with limbal stem cell deficiency. *Br J Ophthalmol* 83(4): 414–419.

Dua, H. S., J. S. Saini, et al. (2000). Limbal stem cell deficiency: Concept, aetiology, clinical presentation, diagnosis and management. *Indian J Ophthalmol* 48(2): 83–92.

Duguid, I. G., J. K. Dart, et al. (1997). Outcome of acanthamoeba keratitis treated with polyhexamethyl biguanide and propamidine. *Ophthalmology* 104(10): 1587–1592.

Edwards, M., C. N. McGhee, et al. (2001). The genetics of keratoconus. *Clin Exp Ophthalmol* 29(6): 345–351.

Efron, N. (2007). Contact lens-induced changes in the anterior eye as observed in vivo with the confocal microscope. *Prog Retin Eye Res* 26(4): 398–436.

Erdelyi, B., R. Kraak, et al. (2007). In vivo confocal laser scanning microscopy of the cornea in dry eye. *Graefes Arch Clin Exp Ophthalmol* 245(1): 39–44.

Foulks, G. N. and A. J. Bron (2003). Meibomian gland dysfunction: A clinical scheme for description, diagnosis, classification, and grading. *Ocul Surf* 1(3): 107–126.

Giampani, J. Jr., A. S. Borges-Giampani, et al. (2008). Efficacy and safety of trabeculectomy with mitomycin C for childhood glaucoma: A study of results with long-term follow-up. *Clinics (Sao Paulo)* 63(4): 421–426.

Guthoff, R., T. Klink, et al. (2006). In vivo confocal microscopy of failing and functioning filtering blebs: Results and clinical correlations. *J Glaucoma* 15(6): 552–558.

Guthoff, R. F., A. Zhivov, et al. (2009). In vivo confocal microscopy, an inner vision of the cornea: A major review. *Clin Exp Ophthalmol* 37(1): 100–117.

Hillenaar, T., C. Weenen, et al. (2009). Endothelial involvement in herpes simplex virus keratitis: An in vivo confocal microscopy study. *Ophthalmology* 116(11): 2077–2086.

Holden, B. A., D. F. Sweeney, et al. (1985). Effects of long-term extended contact lens wear on the human cornea. *Invest Ophthalmol Vis Sci* 26(11): 1489–1501.

Holland, E. J. and G. S. Schwartz (1997). Iatrogenic limbal stem cell deficiency. *Trans Am Ophthalmol Soc* 95: 95–107.

Hollingsworth, J. G. and N. Efron (2004). Confocal microscopy of the corneas of long-term rigid contact lens wearers. *Cont Lens Anterior Eye* 27(2): 57–64.

Hollingsworth, J. G., N. Efron, et al. (2005). In vivo corneal confocal microscopy in keratoconus. *Ophthalmic Physiol Opt* 25(3): 254–260.

Houang, E., D. Lam, et al. (2001). Microbial keratitis in Hong Kong: Relationship to climate, environment and contact-lens disinfection. *Trans R Soc Trop Med Hyg* 95(4): 361–367.

Hu, V. H., P. Massae, et al. (2011a). In vivo confocal microscopy of trachoma in relation to normal tarsal conjunctiva. *Ophthalmology* 118(4): 747–754.

Hu, V. H., H. A. Weiss, et al. (2011b). In vivo confocal microscopy in scarring trachoma. *Ophthalmology* 118(11): 2138–2146.

Ibrahim, O. M., Y. Matsumoto, et al. (2010). The efficacy, sensitivity, and specificity of in vivo laser confocal microscopy in the diagnosis of meibomian gland dysfunction. *Ophthalmology* 117(4): 665–672.

Imre, L., M. Resch, et al. (2005). In vivo confocal corneal microscopy after keratoplasty. *Ophthalmologe* 102(2): 140–146.

Inaba, Z. (1982). Long-term results of trabeculectomy in the Japanese: An analysis by life-table method. *Jpn J Ophthalmol* 26(4): 361–373.

Jalbert, I., F. Stapleton, et al. (2003). In vivo confocal microscopy of the human cornea. *Br J Ophthalmol* 87(2): 225–236.

Jie, Y., L. Xu, et al. (2009). Prevalence of dry eye among adult Chinese in the Beijing eye study. *Eye* 23(3): 688–693.

Kanavi, M. R., M. Javadi, et al. (2007). Sensitivity and specificity of confocal scan in the diagnosis of infectious keratitis. *Cornea* 26(7): 782–786.

Kaufman, S. C. and H. E. Kaufman (2006). How has confocal microscopy helped us in refractive surgery? *Curr Opin Ophthalmol* 17(4): 380–388.

Kaye, S. B., C. Lynas, et al. (1991). Evidence for herpes simplex viral latency in the human cornea. *Br J Ophthalmol* 75(4): 195–200.

Keay, L., K. Edwards, et al. (2006). Microbial keratitis predisposing factors and morbidity. *Ophthalmology* 113(1): 109–116.

Knop, E. and N. Knop (2005). The role of eye-associated lymphoid tissue in corneal immune protection. *J Anat* 206(3): 271–285.

Knop, E., N. Knop, et al. (2011a). The international workshop on meibomian gland dysfunction: Report of the subcommittee on anatomy, physiology, and pathophysiology of the meibomian gland. *Invest Ophthalmol Vis Sci* 52(4): 1938–1978.

Knop, E., N. Knop, et al. (2011b). The lid wiper and muco-cutaneous junction anatomy of the human eyelid margins: An in vivo confocal and histological study. *J Anat* 218(4): 449–461.

Knop, N. and E. Knop (2000). Conjunctiva-associated lymphoid tissue in the human eye. *Invest Ophthalmol Vis Sci* 41(6): 1270–1279.

Kobayashi, A., T. Yoshita, et al. (2005). In vivo findings of the bulbar/palpebral conjunctiva and presumed meibomian glands by laser scanning confocal microscopy. *Cornea* 24(8): 985–988.

Kojima, T., R. Ishida, et al. (2011). In vivo evaluation of ocular demodicosis using laser scanning confocal microscopy. *Invest Ophthalmol Vis Sci* 52(1): 565–569.

Korb, D. R., J. P. Herman, et al. (2010). Prevalence of lid wiper epitheliopathy in subjects with dry eye signs and symptoms. *Cornea* 29(4): 377–383.

Krachmer, J. H., R. S. Feder, et al. (1984). Keratoconus and related noninflammatory corneal thinning disorders. *Surv Ophthalmol* 28(4): 293–322.

Ku, J. Y., R. L. Niederer, et al. (2008). Laser scanning in vivo confocal analysis of keratocyte density in keratoconus. *Ophthalmology* 115(5): 845–850.

Kumar, R. L., A. Cruzat, et al. (2010). Current state of in vivo confocal microscopy in management of microbial keratitis. *Semin Ophthalmol* 25(5–6): 166–170.

Labbe, A., B. Dupas, et al. (2005). In vivo confocal microscopy study of blebs after filtering surgery. *Ophthalmology* 112(11): 1979.

Labbe, A., L. Gheck, et al. (2010). An in vivo confocal microscopy and impression cytology evaluation of pterygium activity. *Cornea* 29(4): 392–399.

Lalive, P. H., A. Truffert, et al. (2009). Peripheral autoimmune neuropathy assessed using corneal in vivo confocal microscopy. *Arch Neurol* 66(3): 403–405.

Le, Q. H., W. T. Wang, et al. (2010). An in vivo confocal microscopy and impression cytology analysis of goblet cells in patients with chemical burns. *Invest Ophthalmol Vis Sci* 51(3): 1397–1400.

Lee, S. H., Y. S. Chun, et al. (2010). The relationship between demodex and ocular discomfort. *Invest Ophthalmol Vis Sci* 51(6): 2906–2911.

Lekhanont, K., D. Rojanaporn, et al. (2006). Prevalence of dry eye in Bangkok, Thailand. *Cornea* 25(10): 1162–1167.

Lemp, M. A. (1995). Report of the National Eye Institute/Industry workshop on clinical trials in dry eyes. *CLAO J* 21(4): 221–232.

Lemp, M. A., P. N. Dilly, et al. (1985). Tandem-scanning (confocal) microscopy of the full-thickness cornea. *Cornea* 4(4): 205–209.

Liang, H., C. Baudouin, et al. (2010). Live conjunctiva-associated lymphoid tissue analysis in rabbit under inflammatory stimuli using in vivo confocal microscopy. *Invest Ophthalmol Vis Sci* 51(2): 1008–1015.

Liesegang, T. J. (1997). Contact lens-related microbial keratitis: Part I: Epidemiology. *Cornea* 16(2): 125–131.

Lin, P. Y., S. Y. Tsai, et al. (2003). Prevalence of dry eye among an elderly Chinese population in Taiwan: The Shihpai eye study. *Ophthalmology* 110(6): 1096–1101.

Liu, Z. and S. C. Pflugfelder (2000). The effects of long-term contact lens wear on corneal thickness, curvature, and surface regularity. *Ophthalmology* 107(1): 105–111.

Longo, C., G. Pellacani, et al. (2012). In vivo detection of *Demodex folliculorum* by means of confocal microscopy. *Br J Dermatol* 166(3): 690–692.

Martone, G. M., A. Balestrazzi, G. M. Tosi, P. Pichierri, and A. Caporossi (2009). Pterygium progression detected by in vivo confocal microscopy. Presented at the American Society of Cataract and Refractive Surgery-American Society of Ophthalmic Administration Symposium and Congress. 3–8 April, San Francisco, CA.

Masters, B. R. (1996). *Selected Papers on Confocal Microscopy*. Bellingham: SPIE milestone series.

Masters, B. R. and A. A. Thaer (1994). Real-time scanning slit confocal microscopy of the in vivo human cornea. *Appl Opt* 33(4): 695–701.

Mastropasqua, L., M. Nubile, et al. (2006). Epithelial dendritic cell distribution in normal and inflamed human cornea: In vivo confocal microscopy study. *Am J Ophthalmol* 142(5): 736–744.

Matsumoto, Y., E. A. Sato, et al. (2008). The application of in vivo laser confocal microscopy to the diagnosis and evaluation of meibomian gland dysfunction. *Mol Vis* 14: 1263–1271.

McCarty, C. A., A. K. Bansal, et al. (1998). The epidemiology of dry eye in Melbourne, Australia. *Ophthalmology* 105(6): 1114–1119.

McCarty, C. A., C. L. Fu, et al. (2000). Epidemiology of pterygium in Victoria, Australia. *Br J Ophthalmol* 84(3): 289–292.

Messmer, E. M., M. J. Mackert, et al. (2006). In vivo confocal microscopy of normal conjunctiva and conjunctivitis. *Cornea* 25(7): 781–788.

Miller, D. (1968). Contact lens-induced corneal curvature and thickness changes. *Arch Ophthalmol* 80(4): 430–432.

Millodot, M. (1977). The influence of age on the sensitivity of the cornea. *Invest Ophthalmol Vis Sci* 16(3): 240–242.

Millodot, M. (1978). Effect of long-term wear of hard contact lenses on corneal sensitivity. *Arch Ophthalmol* 96(7): 1225–1227.

Minsky, M. (1961). Microscopy Apparatus. US Patent. 3013467.

Miri, A., T. Alomar, et al. (2012). In vivo confocal microscopic findings in patients with limbal stem cell deficiency. *Br J Ophthalmol* 96(4): 523–529.

Mocan, M. C., P. T. Yilmaz, et al. (2008). In vivo confocal microscopy for the evaluation of corneal microstructure in keratoconus. *Curr Eye Res* 33(11): 933–939.

Moilanen, J. A., M. H. Vesaluoma, et al. (2003). Long-term corneal morphology after PRK by in vivo confocal microscopy. *Invest Ophthalmol Vis Sci* 44(3): 1064–1069.

Murube, J. and L. Rivas (2003). Biopsy of the conjunctiva in dry eye patients establishes a correlation between squamous metaplasia and dry eye clinical severity. *Eur J Ophthalmol* 13(3): 246–256.

Nelson, J. D. and J. C. Wright (1984). Conjunctival goblet cell densities in ocular surface disease. *Arch Ophthalmol* 102(7): 1049–1051.

Nichols, J. J., D. A. Berntsen, et al. (2005). An assessment of grading scales for meibography images. *Cornea* 24(4): 382–388.

Niederer, R. L., D. Perumal, et al. (2007). Age-related differences in the normal human cornea: A laser scanning in vivo confocal microscopy study. *Br J Ophthalmol* 91(9): 1165–1169.

Niederer, R. L., T. Sherwin, et al. (2007). In vivo confocal microscopy of subepithelial infiltrates in human corneal transplant rejection. *Cornea* 26(4): 501–504.

Niederer, R. L., D. Perumal, et al. (2008). Laser scanning in vivo confocal microscopy reveals reduced innervation and reduction in cell density in all layers of the keratoconic cornea. *Invest Ophthalmol Vis Sci* 49(7): 2964–2970.

O'Day, D. M., P. L. Akrabawi, et al. (1979). Laboratory isolation techniques in human and experimental fungal infections. *Am J Ophthalmol* 87(5): 688–693.

Papadia, M., S. Barabino, et al. (2008). In vivo confocal microscopy in a case of pterygium. *Ophthalmic Surg Lasers Imaging* 39(6): 511–513.

Park, S. W., H. Heo, et al. (2009). Comparison of ultrasound biomicroscopic changes after glaucoma triple procedure and trabeculectomy in eyes with primary angle closure glaucoma. *J Glaucoma* 18(4): 311–315.

Parrozzani, R., D. Lazzarini, et al. (2011). In vivo confocal microscopy of ocular surface squamous neoplasia. *Eye* 25(4): 455–460.

Patel, D. V., J. Y. Ku, et al. (2009). Laser scanning in vivo confocal microscopy and quantitative aesthesiometry reveal decreased corneal innervation and sensation in keratoconus. *Eye* 23(3): 586–592.

Patel, D. V., T. Sherwin, et al. (2006). Laser scanning in vivo confocal microscopy of the normal human corneoscleral limbus. *Invest Ophthalmol Vis Sci* 47(7): 2823–2827.

Patel, S. V., J. C. Erie, et al. (2007). Keratocyte density and recovery of subbasal nerves after penetrating keratoplasty and in late endothelial failure. *Arch Ophthalmol* 125(12): 1693–1698.

Patel, S. V., J. W. McLaren, et al. (2002). Confocal microscopy in vivo in corneas of long-term contact lens wearers. *Invest Ophthalmol Vis Sci* 43(4): 995–1003.

Paterson, C. A., R. R. Pfister, et al. (1975). Aqueous humor pH changes after experimental alkali burns. *Am J Ophthalmol* 79(3): 414–419.

Pawley, J. (1995). *Handbook of Biological Confocal Microscopy*. New York: Plenum.

Perez-Gomez, I. and N. Efron (2003). Change to corneal morphology after refractive surgery (myopic laser in situ keratomileusis) as viewed with a confocal microscope. *Optom Vis Sci* 80(10): 690–697.

Petran, M., M. Hadravsky, M. D. Egger, and R. Galambos (1968). Tandem scanning reflected light microscope. *J Opt Soc Am* 58: 661–664.

Pisella, P. J., O. Auzerie, et al. (2001). Evaluation of corneal stromal changes in vivo after laser in situ keratomileusis with confocal microscopy. *Ophthalmology* 108(10): 1744–1750.

Pult, H. (2012). Non-contact meibography in diagnosis and treatment of non-obvious meibomian. *J Optom* 5(5): 2–5.

Pult, H., B. H. Riede-Pult, et al. (2012). Relation between upper and lower lids' meibomian gland morphology, tear film, and dry eye. *Optom Vis Sci* 89(3): E310–315.

Quigley, H. A. (1996). Number of people with glaucoma worldwide. *Br J Ophthalmol* 80(5): 389–393.

Rabinowitz, Y. S. (1998). Keratoconus. *Surv Ophthalmol* 42(4): 297–319.

Radford, C. F., O. J. Lehmann, et al. (1998). Acanthamoeba keratitis: Multicentre survey in England 1992–1996. National Acanthamoeba Keratitis Study Group. *Br J Ophthalmol* 82(12): 1387–1392.

Rock, D. L., A. B. Nesburn, et al. (1987). Detection of latency-related viral RNAs in trigeminal ganglia of rabbits latently infected with herpes simplex virus type 1. *J Virol* 61(12): 3820–3826.

Rosa, R. H. Jr., D. Miller, et al. (1994). The changing spectrum of fungal keratitis in south Florida. *Ophthalmology* 101(6): 1005–1013.

Rosenberg, M. E., T. M. Tervo, et al. (2002). In vivo confocal microscopy after herpes keratitis. *Cornea* 21(3): 265–269.

Roszkowska, A. M., P. Colosi, et al. (2004). Age-related modifications of corneal sensitivity. *Ophthalmologica* 218(5): 350–355.

Saw, S. M., J. Katz, et al. (1996). Epidemiology of myopia. *Epidemiol Rev* 18(2): 175–187.

Schaefer, F., O. Bruttin, et al. (2001). Bacterial keratitis: A prospective clinical and microbiological study. *Br J Ophthalmol* 85(7): 842–847.

Schaumberg, D. A., J. J. Nichols, et al. (2011). The international workshop on meibomian gland dysfunction: Report of the subcommittee on the epidemiology of, and associated risk factors for, MGD. *Invest Ophthalmol Vis Sci* 52(4): 1994–2005.

Sheppard, C. J. and T. Wilson (1979). Effect of spherical aberration on the imaging properties of scanning optical microscopes. *Appl Opt* 18(7): 1058–1063.

Sheppard, C. J. R. and A. Choudhury (1977). Image formation in the scanning microscope. *Opt Acta* 24: 1051–1073.

Sherwin, T., N. H. Brookes, et al. (2002). Cellular incursion into Bowman's membrane in the peripheral cone of the keratoconic cornea. *Exp Eye Res* 74(4): 473–482.

Shimomura, Y. (2008). Herpes simplex virus latency, reactivation, and a new antiviral therapy for herpetic keratitis. *Nihon Ganka Gakkai Zasshi* 112(3): 247–264.

Singh, J., C. O'Brien, et al. (1995). Success rate and complications of intraoperative 0.2 mg/ml mitomycin C in trabeculectomy surgery. *Eye* 9(Pt 4): 460–466.

Smith, G. T. and H. R. Taylor (1991). Epidemiology of corneal blindness in developing countries. *Refract Corneal Surg* 7(6): 436–439.

Smith, J. A., J. Albeitz, et al. (2007). The epidemiology of dry eye disease: Report of the epidemiology subcommittee of the International Dry Eye Workshop (2007). *Ocul Surf* 5(2): 93–107.

Snyder, M. C., J. P. Bergmanson, et al. (1998). Keratocytes: No more the quiet cells. *J Am Optom Assoc* 69(3): 180–187.

Solomon, K. D., L. E. Fernandez de Castro, et al. (2009). LASIK world literature review: Quality of life and patient satisfaction. *Ophthalmology* 116(4): 691–701.

Srinivasan, S., K. Menzies, et al. (2012). Infrared imaging of meibomian gland structure using a novel keratograph. *Optom Vis Sci* 89(5): 788–794.

Stehr-Green, J. K., T. M. Bailey, et al. (1987). Acanthamoeba keratitis in soft contact lens wearers. A case-control study. *JAMA* 258(1): 57–60.

Stehr-Green, J. K., T. M. Bailey, et al. (1989). The epidemiology of acanthamoeba keratitis in the United States. *Am J Ophthalmol* 107(4): 331–336.

Stevens, J. G., A. B. Nesburn, et al. (1972). Latent herpes simplex virus from trigeminal ganglia of rabbits with recurrent eye infection. *Nat New Biol* 235(59): 216–217.

Svishchev, G. M. (1969). Microscope for the study of transparent light scattering objects in incident light. *Opt Spectrosc* 30: 188–911.

Szaflik, J. P., A. Kaminska, et al. (2007). In vivo confocal microscopy of corneal grafts shortly after penetrating keratoplasty. *Eur J Ophthalmol* 17(6): 891–896.

Taylor, K. I. and H. R. Taylor (1999). Distribution of azithromycin for the treatment of trachoma. *Br J Ophthalmol* 83(2): 134–135.

Thakur, A. and M. D. Willcox (2000). Contact lens wear alters the production of certain inflammatory mediators in tears. *Exp Eye Res* 70(3): 255–259.

Thomas, P. A. (2003). Fungal infections of the cornea. *Eye* 17(8): 852–862.

Thylefors, B., C. R. Dawson, et al. (1987). A simple system for the assessment of trachoma and its complications. *Bull World Health Organ* 65(4): 477–483.

Tiffany, J. M. (2003). Tears in health and disease. *Eye* 17(8): 923–926.

Tu, E. Y., C. E. Joslin, et al. (2008). The relative value of confocal microscopy and superficial corneal scrapings in the diagnosis of Acanthamoeba keratitis. *Cornea* 27(7): 764–772.

Tuft, S. J. and A. J. Shortt (2009). Surgical rehabilitation following severe ocular burns. *Eye* 23(10): 1966–1971.

Ucakhan, O. O., A. Kanpolat, et al. (2006). In vivo confocal microscopy findings in keratoconus. *Eye Contact Lens* 32(4): 183–191.

Uchino, M., M. Dogru, et al. (2006). The features of dry eye disease in a Japanese elderly population. *Optom Vis Sci* 83(11): 797–802.

Vaddavalli, P. K., P. Garg, et al. (2006). Confocal microscopy for Nocardia keratitis. *Ophthalmology* 113(9): 1645–1650.

Vaddavalli, P. K., P. Garg, et al. (2011). Role of confocal microscopy in the diagnosis of fungal and acanthamoeba keratitis. *Ophthalmology* 118(1): 29–35.

Vajdic, C., B. A. Holden, et al. (1999). The frequency of ocular symptoms during spectacle and daily soft and rigid contact lens wear. *Optom Vis Sci* 76(10): 705–711.

Vesaluoma, M., J. Perez-Santonja, et al. (2000). Corneal stromal changes induced by myopic LASIK. *Invest Ophthalmol Vis Sci* 41(2): 369–376.

Villani, E., S. Beretta, et al. (2011a). In vivo confocal microscopy of meibomian glands in Sjogren's syndrome. *Invest Ophthalmol Vis Sci* 52(2): 933–939.

Villani, E., G. Ceresara, et al. (2011b). In vivo confocal microscopy of meibomian glands in contact lens wearers. *Invest Ophthalmol Vis Sci* 52(8): 5215–5219.

Viso, E., M. T. Rodriguez-Ares, et al. (2012). Prevalence of asymptomatic and symptomatic meibomian gland dysfunction in the general population of Spain. *Invest Ophthalmol Vis Sci* 53(6): 2601–2606.

Wakamatsu, T. H., M. Dogru, et al. (2008). Tearful relations: Oxidative stress, inflammation and eye diseases. *Arq Bras Oftalmol* 71(6 Suppl): 72–79.

Wakamatsu, T. H., E. A. Sato, et al. (2010). Conjunctival in vivo confocal scanning laser microscopy in patients with Sjogren syndrome. *Invest Ophthalmol Vis Sci* 51(1): 144–150.

Wang, Y., F. Zhao, et al. (2010). In vivo confocal microscopic evaluation of morphologic changes and dendritic cell distribution in pterygium. *Am J Ophthalmol* 150(5): 650–655.

Webb, R. H. (1990). Scanning laser ophthalmoscope. In: Masters, B. R. (ed.), *Noninvasive Techniques in Ophthalmology*, pp. 438–450. New York: Springer-Verlag.

Webb, R. H., G. W. Hughes, et al. (1980). Flying spot TV ophthalmoscope. *Appl Opt* 19(17): 2991–2997.

Webb, R. H., G. W. Hughes, et al. (1987). Confocal scanning laser ophthalmoscope. *Appl Opt* 26(8): 1492–1499.

Weed, K. H., C. J. MacEwen, et al. (2007). Quantitative analysis of corneal microstructure in keratoconus utilising in vivo confocal microscopy. *Eye* 21(5): 614–623.

West-Mays, J. A. and D. J. Dwivedi (2006). The keratocyte: Corneal stromal cell with variable repair phenotypes. *Int J Biochem Cell Biol* 38(10): 1625–1631.

Whitcher, J. P., M. Srinivasan, et al. (2001). Corneal blindness: A global perspective. *Bull World Health Organ* 79(3): 214–221.

Williams, K. A., S. M. Muehlberg, et al. (1997). Long-term outcome in corneal allotransplantation. The Australian corneal graft registry. *Transplant Proc* 29(1–2): 983.

Wilson, T. (1990). *Confocal Microscopy*. London: Academic.

Wright, P. (1982). The chemically injured eye. *Trans Ophthalmol Soc U K* 102(Pt 1): 85–87.

Xiao, G. Q., T. R. Corle, and G. S. Kino (1988). Real-time confocal scanning optical microscope. *Appl Phys Lett* 53: 716–718.

Xiao, G. Q., G. S. Kino, and B. R. Masters (1990). Observation of the rabbit cornea and lens with a new real-time confocal scanning optical microscope. *Scanning* 12: 161–166.

Yeh, D. L., S. S. Stinnett, et al. (2006). Analysis of bacterial cultures in infectious keratitis, 1997–2004. *Am J Ophthalmol* 142(6): 1066–1068.

Yeniad, B., B. Yigit, et al. (2003). Effects of contact lenses on corneal thickness and corneal curvature during usage. *Eye Contact Lens* 29(4): 223–229.

Young, J. Z. and F. Roberts (1951). A flying-spot microscope. *Nature* 167(4241): 231.

Zarei-Ghanavati, S., A. Ramirez-Miranda, et al. (2011). Limbal lacuna: A novel limbal structure detected by in vivo laser scanning confocal microscopy. *Ophthalmic Surg Lasers Imaging* 42(Online): e129–e131.

Zhang, M., J. Chen, et al. (2005). Altered corneal nerves in aqueous tear deficiency viewed by in vivo confocal microscopy. *Cornea* 24(7): 818–824.

Zhivov, A., O. Stachs, et al. (2006). In vivo confocal microscopy of the ocular surface. *Ocul Surf* 4(2): 81–93.

Zhivov, A., J. Stave, et al. (2007). In vivo confocal microscopic evaluation of Langerhans cell density and distribution in the corneal epithelium of healthy volunteers and contact lens wearers. *Cornea* 26(1): 47–54.

19

Computational Modeling of Thermal Damage Induced by Laser in a Choroidal Melanoma

José Duarte da Silva, Alcides Fernandes, Paulo Roberto
Maciel Lyra, and Rita de Cássia Fernandes de Lima

CONTENTS

19.1 Introduction

The medical protocol for treating patients with choroidal melanoma has not yet been fully standardized. Currently, some of the treatment procedures vary in accordance with the tumor's characteristics, such as its dimensions, pigmentation, and location, in addition to the involvement of the surrounding tissues and other organs that may be affected. Among the treatment modalities, there is increasing interest in transpupillary thermotherapy (TTT) with infrared laser, mainly because it is a noninvasive treatment that can be easily applied. During the TTT procedure, the laser radiation crosses the anterior ocular medium, virtually without absorption, reaching the choroidal melanoma where it heats the tumoral tissue. The rise in temperature, with the final temperature ranging from 45°C to 65°C, is responsible for the thermal damage to the tumor cells, which occurs due to the denaturation of the molecules present in the cells and the extracellular fluid. The thermal damage causes changes in the biological tissue, leading to a whitish coloration. This effect is used as an indicator to stop the laser application. Because laser TTT is not yet a standardized procedure for the treatment of ocular melanomas, the value of the thermal damage function can be used to determine the optimal amount of laser radiation needed to treat such tumors.

19.1.1 Choroidal Melanoma

Choroidal melanoma is the most common form of ocular cancer, with an incidence of six cases per million people per year [1]. It primarily affects white patients over the age of 50 years, and it is less common in Africans and Asians. At the time of diagnosis, it can be asymptomatic, but it can also cause vision loss, visual field defects, photopsia, or pain [2]. Choroidal melanomas have the potential to produce metastases, thus leading to death.

Melanomas grow in the choroid, where a large blood flow provides ideal conditions for its growth and the metastases of cancer cells. The typical appearance of a choroidal melanoma consists of a solid tumor, dark brown to a golden color, with a lenticular biconvex shape. In approximately 20% of the cases, the tumor breaks through Bruch's membrane and the retinal pigment epithelium, forming a nodular eruption on the retina. When this eruption occurs, the tumor takes the approximate shape of a round dome or that of a mushroom, which is very characteristic of choroidal melanomas [3,4], as shown in Figure 19.1a and b.

A choroidal melanoma (Figure 19.1b) can be an aggressive tumor, and approximately 30% of patients will die from metastatic disease 2–5 years after their diagnosis [5]. In the early stages, a choroidal melanoma usually does not interfere with the vision and it can be detected during a routine ophthalmoscopic examination. It can cause vision loss from a retinal detachment. A uveal malignant melanoma is rare in patients younger than 30 years of age and appears to be slightly more common in women than in men [6]. Hematogenous dissemination is common and the liver is the preferred locus of metastasis followed by the lungs.

An early diagnosis is important because the cure rate for choroidal melanoma is related to the tumor size. Choroidal melanomas are classified as: small, diameter <10 mm and thickness <3 mm; medium, diameter of 10–15 mm and thickness of 3–5 mm; and large, diameter >15 mm and thickness >5 mm [7,8]. When the tumor is small, laser treatment and the implantation of radioactive materials are effective in saving the eye and the vision. When the tumor is large, the eye should be removed. If the eye is not removed, dissemination can occur to the orbit and to other organs through the bloodstream, causing death.

The choice of treatment for choroidal melanoma is still controversial and the best therapeutic method has not been established. The different therapeutic options include periodic observation, enucleation, exenteration, localized surgical resection, brachytherapy, external beam irradiation of charged particles, photocoagulation, and transpupillary laser

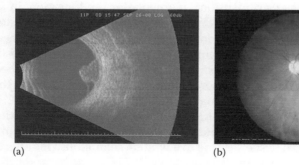

(a)   (b)

FIGURE 19.1
(a) Ultrasound of the human eye with a choroidal melanoma. (b) A red-free fundus photograph of an eye depicting a choroidal melanoma (www.oftalmologiaonline.com.br).

thermotherapy [9]. The surgical removal of the tumor is painful and traumatic, and sometimes it is not effective, so hyperthermic treatment, called laser transpupillary thermotherapy, has been of great interest and presents satisfactory results for certain types of tumors.

19.1.2 Transpupillary Thermotherapy

TTT is a noninvasive treatment method that utilizes a modified diode laser with a wavelength of 810 nm to produce a uniform and localized heat that leads to the obliteration of malformed blood vessels and a reduction in the tumor size [10]. TTT has been shown to be effective in treating small choroidal melanomas, due to the irregular vascular system in tumors, which prevents the optimal distribution of heat, thus heating up the tumor more than the peritumoral tissues.

Oosterhuis et al. [11] and Shields et al. [12] successfully treated small melanomas (up to 4 mm thick) using this method as the sole treatment [13,14]. Irradiation near the infrared spectrum is optimal for TTT because tissue penetration is high and the absorption into the ocular media is minimal [15], such that the laser is almost totally absorbed by the melanin that is present in high concentrations in most melanomas [16]. This absorption causes an increase in the tumor temperature in the range from 45°C to 60°C, resulting in tissue necrosis [17].

Based on the reports of the use of TTT for the treatment of choroidal hemangiomas [18–21], it can be said that, when compared to conventional photocoagulation, the advantage of this procedure is that only a small number of applications are needed to eradicate the lesion. Furthermore, vision recovery is more rapid and effective even in those cases where conventional photocoagulation has been unsuccessful. Reports in the literature show excellent results for patients with circumscribed choroidal hemangioma, and also for retinal detachment treated with TTT [19–21].

Some of the advantages of TTT include immediate necrosis with tumor regression; precision in targeting the laser application; and it is an easy treatment that can be performed under local anesthesia in an outpatient setting. Additionally, TTT causes less damage to the choroid than brachytherapy.

Currently, the length of time of application is a function of the laser power and is determined experimentally by the tissue reaction itself, that is, when a slight change in the color of the melanoma occurs, the treatment is discontinued at this point [22]. This approach is unsatisfactory because it can lead to overtreatment or undertreatment regimens. Therefore, a simulation of these procedures can be important to provide more reliable treatment parameters such as the exposure time and the laser power.

19.2 Mathematical Models

In this study, we used a two-dimensional (2-D) model of the human eye with a choroidal melanoma in order to determine the temperature and the thermal damage in the eye. The model took into account the denaturation front propagation in a biological tissue while being irradiated by a laser source. For the analysis, an ultrasound image of a patient was used, which provided the dimensions of the eye and the melanoma (see Figure 19.2). The modeling and simulation were performed for a patient with a choroidal melanoma, which was treated with infrared laser radiation.

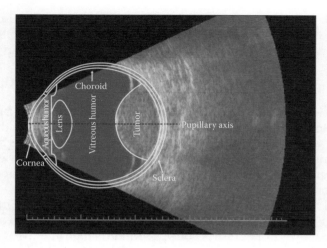

FIGURE 19.2
Scheme for the human eye model with a choroidal melanoma.

19.2.1 Heat Transfer Model

The temperature field was calculated using Pennes' equation. It represents the spatial and temporal temperature distribution in living tissues, and it is known as the bioheat transfer equation (BHTE). It can also be called the "traditional" or "classic" Pennes' bioheat equation. Due to its simplicity, this is the most widely used thermal model for living tissues. The BHTE is a heat transport equation, which includes a source/sink term and takes into account the heat generated by the blood perfusion.

In order to determine the value of the damage function, the Birngruber model was adopted. This model succeeds a more traditional model [23] that was specifically developed for ocular tissues.

To deal with the moving boundary caused by thermal damage, we used a strategy that consists in replacing the values of the physical properties of the tumor (at each point where the value of irreversible damage is reached) by the values of those properties of the vitreous humor.

The referenced BHTE [24] is given by Equation 19.1. This equation was obtained from a balance of energy considering the energy storage, internal energy, heat conduction, and convection inside and outside the control volume, and the local heat generation. The generation of heat due to the chemical reactions and the electrical effects was neglected. The temperature field was obtained by considering a solid, homogeneous, biological medium with isotropic thermophysical properties.

The Cartesian coordinates were used for the 2-D analysis. Therefore, the governing equation was written as

$$\rho_t c_t \frac{\partial T_t}{\partial t} = \frac{\partial}{\partial x}\left(k_t \frac{\partial T_t}{\partial x}\right) + \frac{\partial}{\partial y}\left(k_t \frac{\partial T_t}{\partial y}\right) + Q \quad \text{on} \quad \Omega \times T \qquad (19.1)$$

where:
ρ_t is the tissue density (kg m^{-3})
c_t is the tissue-specific heat (J kg^{-1} K^{-1})
T_t is the tissue temperature (K)

t is time (sec)

k_t is the tissue thermal conductivity (W m^{-1} K^{-1})

Q represents all the terms of the heat source and sink

Ω represents the spatial domain of the problem

$T = [t^i, t^f]$ represents the time interval of interest where t^i is the initial time t^f is the final time

The boundary conditions are shown in Figure 19.3. The first one was imposed to the back surface of the sclera.

$$-k_t \frac{\partial T_t}{\partial \eta} = h_s \left(T_t - T_s \right) \tag{19.2}$$

where:

η is the unit normal vector (m)

h_s is the convection coefficient between the sclera and the body (W m^{-2} K^{-1})

T_s is the sclera temperature (K)

The second boundary condition was applied to the external surface of the cornea. If the temperature of the cornea was higher than that of the environment, the cornea lost heat via three mechanisms: irradiation, convection, and evaporation of the tear film. Then, these cooling mechanisms could be combined in a single heat exchange coefficient, so that

$$-k_t \frac{\partial T_t}{\partial \eta} = h \left(T_t - T_\infty \right) \tag{19.3}$$

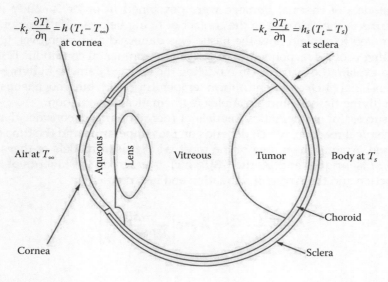

FIGURE 19.3

Computational domain and boundary conditions on the human eye.

where:

$$h = \frac{E + h_{c\infty}\left(T_t - T_\infty\right) + \varepsilon\sigma\left(T_t^4 - T_\infty^4\right)}{T_t - T_\infty} \tag{19.4}$$

E is the energy removal by the evaporation of the tear film (W m^{-2})
$h_{c\infty}$ is the convection coefficient between the cornea and the environment (W m^{-2} K^{-1})
T_∞ is the environment temperature (K)
ε is the emissivity of the cornea (dimensionless)
σ is the Stefan–Boltzmann constant (W m^{-2} K^{-4})

As an initial condition for a transient simulation, the temperature distribution in the human eye under steady-state conditions, obtained previously without the source of heat due to the laser radiation term, was used.

In order to calculate the temperature and the thermal damage in the ocular tissues, the ANSYS-CFX software was used. It is a general-purpose software for computational fluid dynamics (CFD) that combines an advanced solver with powerful pre- and postprocessing tools. Various methods of solution are used in CFD codes. The most common, in which the CFX-ANSYS is based, is known as the finite volume technique. In this technique, the region of interest was divided into smaller subregions, called control volumes. The equation was discretized and solved for each control volume, thereby obtaining an approximate value for each variable at the points of interest within the domain.

19.2.2 Thermal Damage Models

In the present context, thermal damage is defined as irreversible changes caused by the temperature in living biological tissue. This thermal damage can occur when the tissue temperature exceeds the temperature range within the normal physiological processes. Common examples are burns and skin freezing.

The first models of thermal damage were developed in order to study the damage caused by burns to the skin due to the contact of living beings with heat sources. These models attempted to explain how the tissue was damaged and, moreover, to determine how the healing process responded to different environmental conditions [25]. The main arguments to explain the difficulty in modeling the thermal damage in living tissues are: a three-dimensional (3-D) and nonuniform temperature field; inhomogeneous and anisotropic media (living tissues); and a complex mathematical formulation.

The most successful mathematical models of thermal damage consider that a thermal injury is a chemical reaction, which depends on the temperature and the time of exposure to living tissue. Among them, one of the most widely used models of thermal damage is the model of Henriques and Moritz [23], which is based on the kinetics of a first-order chemical reaction and the Arrhenius equation and is expressed by

$$\frac{d\Omega_D\left(r',x,t\right)}{dt} = \bar{A}\exp\left[\frac{-\Delta E}{RT\left(r',x,t\right)}\right] \tag{19.5}$$

where:
Ω_D is the dimensionless indicator of thermal damage
r' is the radial position within the cylindrical beam with radius $\tilde{\sigma}$ (m)

x is the distance from the incidence surface to the absorber layer (m)
$\bar{A}$ is the preexponential constant (sec^{-1})
ΔE is the activation energy for the reaction (J mol^{-1})
R is the universal molar gas constant (J mol^{-1} K^{-1})

The thermal damage is obtained by integrating Equation 19.5:

$$\Omega_D\left(r',x,t\right) = \bar{A} \int_{t_i}^{t_f} \exp\left[\frac{-\Delta E}{RT\left(r',x,t\right)}\right] dt \qquad (19.6)$$

where:
t_i is the starting time of the induced temperature elevation (sec)
t_f is the final time of the temperature elevation (sec)

Based on their experimental work in the porcupine epidermis, Henriques and Moritz [23] selected coefficients such that the complete cell necrosis of the basal epidermal layer was indicated by a value of damage equal to one, $\Omega_D = 1.0$. A value of $\Omega_D = 0.53$ was used by Henriques and Moritz [23] as the threshold of irreversible damage [26], while Diller [27] considered the value of 1.0 for this limit.

The preexponential constant, or frequency factor $\bar{A}$, and the activation energy, or free energy barrier for molecular denaturation, ΔE, depend exclusively on the chemical process involved. The values of $\bar{A}$ and ΔE were obtained by Henriques and Moritz through measurement of the temperature on the skin during a period corresponding to the time of heating, $t_p = t_f - t_i$ [27]. Thus, Equation 19.6 can be approximated as

$$\Omega_D = \bar{A}\, t_p \exp\left(\frac{-\Delta E}{RT}\right) \qquad (19.7)$$

Subsequently, Henriques and Moritz [23] obtained the following coefficients: $\bar{A} = 3.1 \times 10^{98}$ sec^{-1} and $\Delta E = 6.27 \times 10^5$ J mol^{-1}.

Through correlations with histological data, Henriques and Moritz [23] established the following correspondence between the value of the thermal damage function and the degree of the burn:

- First-degree burns: $\Omega_D = 0.53$
- Second-degree burns: $\Omega_D = 1.0$
- Third-degree burns: $\Omega_D = 10,000$

Due to the lack of understanding regarding the physical meaning of Ω_D, other indicators of cell death from thermal damage, such as birefringence and edema formation, have been used [28].

It is important to emphasize that, in the experiments conducted by Henriques and Moritz [23], the thermal damage function was only calculated during the heating process. This model did not consider thermal damage during the cooling period, that is, following the removal of the heat source until the temperature reached its initial value, before the heating process.

Subsequently, Birngruber developed a model to determine the thermal damage to the retina and the choroid from TTT treatment with laser [29]. The model described the effect of heat on the chemical reaction rate and considered the change in the concentration of undamaged molecules, using the Arrhenius law.

The formation rate of the final product reaction, ς_x, was given by

$$\varsigma_x = \frac{RT}{N_a h_p} \exp\left(-\frac{\Delta G}{RT}\right) \tag{19.8}$$

where:

T is the temperature (K)
R is the universal molar gas constant (J mol^{-1} K^{-1})
N_a is Avogadro's number (dimensionless)
h_p is Planck's constant (J sec);
ΔG is Gibbs free energy for process activation (J mol^{-1})

The variation of the undamaged cells concentration can be written as

$$\frac{dC_x}{dt} = -\varsigma_x(T)C_x \tag{19.9}$$

By integrating Equation 19.9, the damage, Ω_D, obtained was

$$\Omega_D = \ln\left(\frac{C_x(0)}{C_x(t)}\right) = \int_0^t \varsigma_x \, dt \tag{19.10}$$

where $C_x(0)$ and $C_x(t)$ were the concentrations of the undamaged cells at the initial and final time, respectively. The Arrhenius integral Ω_D was a positive number, which measured the degree of denaturation of unimolecular proteins. The fraction of molecules that had not been denatured by the heating process, after a time t, was

$$\frac{C_x(t)}{C_x(0)} = e^{-\Omega} \tag{19.11}$$

Therefore, when $\Omega_D = 1.0$, the fraction of nondenatured proteins was equal to 36.8% ($1/e$). This means that 63.2% of the proteins had been damaged or denatured. Henriques and Moritz defined this value as the end point of complete necrosis. Birngruber called this same value the denaturation limit [29].

The Gibbs free energy was given by

$$\Delta G = \Delta E - RT - T \, \Delta S \tag{19.12}$$

where ΔE was the activation energy for the process of denaturation and ΔS was the entropy change during the reaction. The Arrhenius integral, Equation 19.10, was then given by

$$\Omega_D = \frac{R}{N_A h_p} \exp\left(1 + \frac{\Delta S}{R}\right) \int_0^{\tau_{\text{denat}}} T(t) \exp\left(-\frac{\Delta E}{RT(t)}\right) dt \tag{19.13}$$

By considering

$$C = \frac{R}{N_A h_p} \exp\left(1 + \frac{\Delta S}{R}\right)$$ (19.14)

Equation 19.13 becomes

$$\Omega_D = C \int_0^{\tau_{\text{denat}}} T(t) \exp\left(-\frac{\Delta E}{RT(t)}\right) dt$$ (19.15)

Equation 19.15 differs from traditional models in the value of the preexponential constant and the temperature, $T(t)$, which are now part of the integrand of this equation.

An evaluation of the degree of denaturation is a subjective clinical practice and the heating process is interrupted at an arbitrary value of Ω_D. Henriques and Moritz [23], for example, selected $\Omega_D = 1$ as an indicator of irreversible total damage [29]. Birngruber also considered this value, which is characterized by a whitish discoloration of the tissue. According to Birngruber et al., the activation energy for retinal tissue is $\Delta E = 2.9 \times 10^5$ J mol^{-1} and the entropy change is $\Delta S = 595$ J mol^{-1} K^{-1} [29]. These values resulted in a preexponential constant of $C = 6.81 \times 10^{41}$ sec^{-1} [30].

19.3 Analyzed Case

19.3.1 Eye Geometry and Thermophysical Properties

A constructed diagram of the human eye with a choroidal melanoma was based on an ultrasound image (Figure 19.2). For modeling purposes, it was divided into seven regions. The diameter of the eye along the pupillary axis was approximately 24 mm [31]. The back half of the human eye was assumed to be almost spherical [32]. Each region was adopted as homogeneous and the eye was considered symmetric with respect to the pupillary axis once the optic nerve was neglected.

The cornea is the most anterior surface of the eye through which the laser radiation penetrates the ocular globe. Its thickness was assumed to be constant (0.4 mm). The sclera thickness was considered approximately constant (0.53 mm) [33]. The lens of the human eye had a diameter of 8.4 mm and a thickness of 4.3 mm. The tumor dimensions were 14.2 mm (basal diameter) and 7.9 mm (thickness).

One of the major challenges for the construction of mathematical models for biological systems is to find appropriate values for the optical and thermophysical properties involved in the analysis, especially when the model is used in different physiological and environmental conditions [34]. This difficulty stems from the lack of reliable information on the volumetric rate of blood perfusion, especially in neoplasic tissues where it is further complicated by the disorderly growth of the tumor. The values of perfusion rates cannot be accurately measured due to the uncertainty of the calculated temperature values. Moreover, the value and the direction of the blood flow in tumors are not fixed because of the vascular growth in tumors and because of the necrotic process. In general, there is a lack of reliable data on the parameters that are necessary for modeling living tissues.

Most of the data available in the literature were obtained from experiments conducted in animals, especially pigs, rabbits, and monkeys, and were extrapolated to the human case, involving inaccuracies. Therefore, it was assumed that the values of thermal conductivity (k), density (ρ), specific heat (c), blood perfusion (ω), and the absorption coefficient (β) were constant within each region of the eye during the time of the simulation, with the exception of the tumor. These properties can be found in the literature and are described in Table 19.1.

For the points within the melanoma, the thermal conductivity (k), density (ρ), specific heat (c), blood perfusion (ω), and the absorption coefficient (β) were considered as constants and their values were those that corresponded to the values of the tumor. The value of the thermal damage function to these points was less than 1. When the amount of referred damage was equal to or greater than 1, these properties assumed the values corresponding to the vitreous humor. This strategy was used to simulate the advance of the denaturation front into the biological tissue that absorbed the laser radiation.

19.3.2 Simplifying Assumptions

The mathematical modeling was done by considering the following simplifying assumptions:

1. The eye was considered as a solid structure composed of different layers in contact with each other.
2. The incident laser had a pattern "spot," that is, the intensity I_0 was constant and independent of the radial position in relation to the beam center.

TABLE 19.1

Absorption Coefficients, Perfusion Rates, and Thermophysical Properties for the Layers of the Eye and the Melanoma

Ocular Tissue	Density (kg m^{-3})	Specific Heat (J kg^{-1} K^{-1})	Thermal Conductivity (W m^{-1} K^{-1})	Absorption Coefficient[a] (m^{-1})	Perfusion Rate (sec^{-1})
Aqueous humor	1000	3997	0.58	16.82	–
Cornea	1050	4178	0.58	120.52	–
Choroid	1000	4190	0.628	13,128.62	0.012
Lens	1050	3000	0.40	20.26	–
Sclera	1050	4178	0.58	120.52	–
Tumor	1040	3900	0.70	1,377.88	0.00399
Vitreous humor	1000	4178	0.603	7.69	–

Source: Amara, E.H., *Int. J. Heat Mass Transfer.*, 38, 2479–2488, 1995; Cheong, W., Prahl, S.A., Welch, A.J., *J. Quantum Electron.*, 26, 2166–2185, 1990; Niemz, M.H., *Laser–Tissue Interactions—Fundamentals and Applications*, Springer, Berlin, 2004; Rivolta, B., Inzoli, F., Mantero, S., Severini, A., *J. Biomechan. Eng.*, 121, 141–147, 1999; Welch, A.J., *Heat Transfer in Medicine and Biology—Analysis and Applications*, A. Shitzer, R.C. Eberhart, Eds, Plenum, New York, 1985.

[a] Values for the coefficient of absorption of the infrared radiation from the diode laser (810 nm) in the various layers of the eye were obtained by linear interpolation using the data available in the literature. For the cornea, aqueous humor, lens, and vitreous humor, the values have been found in Amara [35] for the wavelengths 694.3 and 1060 nm; for the sclera, the same values were used as those used for the cornea; for the melanoma, the interpolation was made with the values found by Cheong et al. [36] for the wavelengths 630 and 1064 nm; for the choroid, the interpolation was performed with the values found by Niemz [37] for the wavelengths 300 and 730 nm.

3. The laser radiation penetrated into the tissue without scattering.

4. The different tissues were homogeneous and isotropic.

5. The blood temperature was assumed constant and equal to 37°C [39].

6. The generation of metabolic heat was not considered, since it is often less than the amount of heat deposited by laser radiation ($Q_m \ll Q$).

7. The melanoma and retina were considered as one region (tumor) because the retina has a very small thickness and because the largest portion of the infrared radiation is absorbed in the tumoral tissue, which is rich in melanin.

8. The thermophysical properties of the iris and the ciliary body were considered identical to those of the aqueous humor [35]. Therefore, these regions were treated as one region, here called the aqueous humor.

9. The aqueous humor was considered stagnant [34,40,41].

10. The heat transfer within the eye occurred through conduction.

11. The blood perfusions considered were those of the tumor and the choroid. The blood flow within the iris and the ciliary body can also be a heat source inside the eye, but its effect is usually very small when compared to that of the choroid [42].

12. The focusing power of the lens was not accounted for in the present study because of the very small diameter of the laser beam. It reached the cornea in a direction that coincides with the direction of the papillary axis [31].

13. A boundary condition of heat exchange by convection with the body was imposed on the back surface of the sclera.

14. The cornea was considered as the only part of the eye in contact with the external environment. When the temperature of the environment is lower than the temperature of the corneal surface, the eye loses heat by convection, radiation, and evaporation of the tear film. Then, a convective boundary condition is imposed on the corneal surface with a coefficient of heat transfer estimated by Lagendijk [34] using $h = (20 \pm 2)$ W m^{-2} °C^{-1}.

15. The initial temperatures of the different regions of the eye were obtained from a preliminary steady-state simulation of the eye not exposed to radiation and with a uniform initial temperature of 37°C.

16. An infrared diode laser with a continuum wave and a length of 810 nm was used. The laser beam measures 3.0 mm in diameter and the output power is 400 mW [43].

17. The optic nerve is not considered due to its small influence on the temperature distribution in the eye [44].

19.3.3 Numerical Method and Grid Convergence Analysis

In the numerical domain, unstructured meshes were used due to the complex geometry considered. This type of mesh allows local refinements, which can be made to the specific regions of interest.

Figure 19.4 shows a 2-D geometric model of the human eye with a computational mesh generated in the concerned area, which was created using the commercial software GAMBIT. The points of the interfaces that were used to construct the computational mesh were obtained through the computational program Points Acquisition in Digital Images

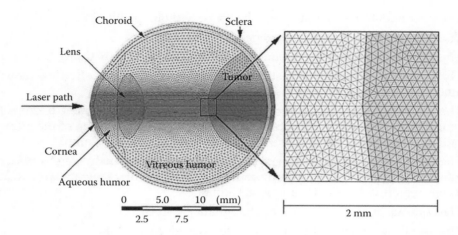

FIGURE 19.4
Domain discretization adopted with a triangular mesh.

(PADI) [45]. Triangular elements were used in the domain with a mesh refinement on the laser radiation path, where the largest and most rapid temperature changes are expected. The commercial program ANSYS-CFX (http://www.ansys.com), which employed the finite-volume method (FVM), was used to calculate the temperatures and the thermal damage caused in the eye and the tumor.

A mesh convergence experiment was conducted to simulate the eye with a choroidal melanoma when exposed to radiation from a laser beam of 3.0 mm in diameter and 56.588 W m^{-2} intensity. The initial temperature profile on the external surface of the cornea was calculated under a steady-state regime, which considered only the blood perfusion in the tumor and the choroid. The body and the blood temperatures were considered to be constant and equal to 37°C. The environment temperature was considered to be 25°C. The temperature values used in this experiment were calculated at five points, all located on the pupillary axis: 3.69×10^{-5} m; 5.20669×10^{-3} m; 1.53196×10^{-2} m; 1.61038×10^{-2} m, and 2.34924×10^{-2} m. These abscissas corresponded to, respectively, the corneal surface (T1), the lens center (T2), the tumor surface (T3), the interior of the tumor (T4), and the interface between the choroid and the sclera (T5). Based on these results, the mesh with 29,388 elements was chosen to conduct all of the numerical simulations analyzed.

Using the same conditions as those used in the mesh convergence tests, some tests were performed to determine the time-step value, which was used in the transient simulations. Based on these results, a time step of five hundredths of a second was selected for the other numerical calculations. Using this time step, the time interval of the whole calculation was 25 min and 19 sec. For a time step of one hundredth of a second, that time interval was extended to 241 min and 12 sec, which was almost ten times greater. Despite these differences, the largest difference in the temperature values was only 0.003°C, which occurred on the surface and inside the tumor.

19.3.4 Validation Studies

The results for the temperatures measured along the pupillary axis when the eye was not irradiated were compared to those of the 2-D model of Scott [34], the 2-D model of Ng and Ooi [38], and the 3-D model of Ng and Ooi [46], using the same boundary conditions and properties. Experiments were conducted under a steady-state regimen using the following parameters: a room temperature of 20°C [34]; a blood temperature of 37°C [47]; a coefficient of heat transfer between the cornea and the environment of 20 W m^{-2} °C^{-1}; a heat transfer coefficient between the sclera and the body of 65 W m^{-2} °C^{-1}; a blood perfusion rate in the choroid of 0012 sec^{-1}; and a blood perfusion rate in the tumor of 0.00399 sec^{-1}. Figure 19.5 shows the temperature profiles along the pupillary axis for the referred models.

Comparing the results obtained with this model to those of the work of Ng and Ooi [45], which is more recent and provides a 3-D approach, there were minor differences in the temperature along the pupillary axis. The maximum difference measured was 0.29°C. These results were used as initial values for the calculations of the transient regime, when laser irradiation commenced on the eye.

19.3.5 Results

The results shown are those of the model used to calculate the temperature and the thermal damage in various ocular tissues, including the damage to the melanoma. Two situations were compared. The first situation used the results for the computed thermal damage without considering the tumor shrinkage. The second situation used the results for the same damage when the thermophysical properties of the tumor were replaced by those of the vitreous humor whenever the local thermal damage reached the value of 1 (i.e., irreversible damage).

Figure 19.6 shows the temperature distribution in the human eye with a choroidal melanoma that was irradiated with a laser of 400 mW power output and a 3.0 mm diameter beam.

Figure 19.6 shows the temperature distribution in a human eye with a choroidal melanoma that was irradiated with a laser of 400 mW power output and a 3.0 mm diameter beam. The left side of the figure shows the results of a numerical simulation that was performed without changing the values of the tumor density, thermal conductivity, specific heat, and the absorption coefficient at points that presented irreversible thermal damage. On the right side of the same figure, the results are those of a numerical simulation in which the values of the thermophysical properties of the tumor were replaced by those corresponding to the humor vitreous, in any location where the thermal damage reached

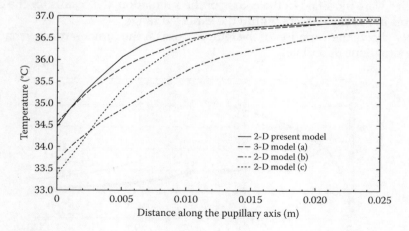

FIGURE 19.5
Steady-state temperature along the pupillary axis for the human eye not exposed to laser radiation. (Data from (a) Ng, E.Y.K. and Ooi, E.H., *Comput. Biol. Med.*, 37, 829–835, 2007; (b) Ng, E.Y.K. and Ooi, E.H., *Comput. Meth. Prog. Biomed.*, 82, 268–276, 2006; (c) Scott, J.A., *Phys. Med. Biol.*, 33, 227–241, 1988.)

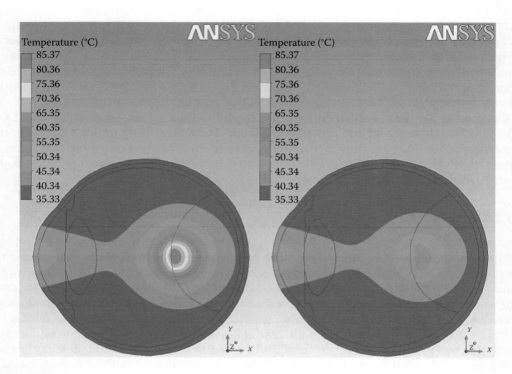

FIGURE 19.6
Color map of the temperature in the eye after 60 sec exposure to laser radiation with a laser having an output power of 400 mW and a beam diameter of 3.0 mm: without changing (*left*) and with changing (*right*) the tumor properties.

values equal to or greater than one. In the first situation, it is evident that the temperature reached values higher than the temperatures reported in the literature [48]. In those experiments, the temperatures varied between 45°C and 65°C. However, when the thermophysical properties were modified in the course of the simulation, the results for the calculated temperatures in the tumor were within the expected range.

Figure 19.7 shows the variation of the temperature on the tumor surface versus time for both of the situations described.

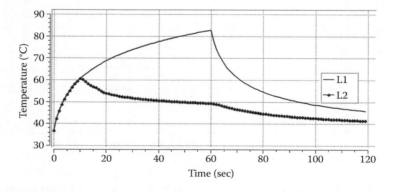

FIGURE 19.7
Temperature on the tumor surface without changing (L1) and with changing (L2) the tumor properties.

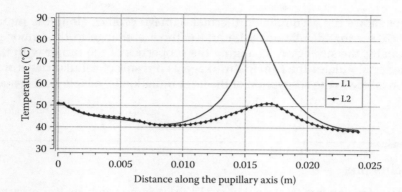

FIGURE 19.8
Temperature profile along the pupillary axis without changing (L1) and with changing (L2) the tumor properties at $t = 60$ sec.

Figure 19.8 shows the temperature profiles along the pupillary axis after 60 sec of exposure to the laser radiation. The dashed curve (L1) represents the temperature profile obtained by a simulation in which the properties of the tumor were kept constant. The solid curve (L2) represents the temperature profile obtained by a simulation in which the tumor properties were replaced by the vitreous humor properties.

In Figure 19.8, the temperature reached the highest values when the properties were held constant. In this case, the maximum temperature reached was 85°C. By changing the tumor property values, the highest temperature reached was approximately 52°C at the same point.

Furthermore, the damage function reached very high values (as high as 4200) when the properties of the tumor were kept constant. However, when the values of the tumor properties were replaced by the vitreous humor properties, the thermal damage accumulated during the TTT procedure reached a maximum value of approximately 2.9 within the tumor (see Figure 19.9). This is about 1450 times lower than the previous value, characterizing a situation closer to reality. The value of thermal damage as high as 4200 did not have a physical meaning, because of tissue loss.

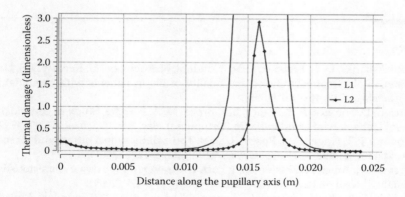

FIGURE 19.9
Thermal damage profile along the pupillary axis obtained by a simulation without changing (L1) and with changing (L2) the tumor properties at $t = 120$ sec.

Figure 19.9 shows the accumulated thermal damage profiles along the pupillary axis, at time $t = 120$ sec for calculations with and without a change to the tumor properties. Computationally, the strategy of changing the properties of the tumor with those of the vitreous humor simulates the tumor shrinkage as a result of cellular denaturation. This denaturation is due to the absorption of the laser radiation by a biological tissue.

19.4 Conclusions

The efficiency of melanoma treatment using TTT depends largely on the amount of energy absorbed by the tumor and the surrounding tissues. The calculation of the amount of energy in heterogeneous tissues is a very complex task mostly due to the lack of accurate information on the coefficients of absorption, the scattering of the laser radiation, and the thermophysical properties of the tissues.

Our model was built with the purpose of calculating the value of thermal damage at various depths within a melanoma. Among other simplifications, the model did not consider the variations of the optical and thermophysical properties of the ocular tissues affected by the temperature or the scattering of the laser radiation penetrating through the eye. However, despite these simplifications, the results are in good agreement with the values reported in the literature. For example, in our model, the damage reached a depth equal to 1.87 mm when the eye was irradiated for 60 sec with a diode laser with the following characteristics: a wavelength equal to 810 nm; an output power of 400 mW; and a beam diameter of 3.0 mm. Although the conditions described by others were not exactly the same as those used in this simulation, values ranging from 0.87 mm [49] to 3.5 mm [11] were reported. Therefore, the strategy of changing the properties' values allowed us to predict the advance of thermal damage within the melanoma and represented an improvement to the currently used strategy, which kept the properties constant throughout the analysis. The methodology presented here can be improved by considering correlations that take into account the variation of the physical properties with the temperature, mainly in melanotic tissues.

References

1. K. J. Cruickshanks, D. G. Fryback, D. M. Nondahl, N. Robinson, U. Keesey, D. S. Dalton, D. M. Robertson, et al., Treatment choice and quality of life in patients with choroidal melanoma, *Arch. Ophthalmol.* **117**, 461–467 (1999).
2. E. S. Arcieri, D. Fonseca, E. T. França, E. F. Braga, M. A. Ferreira, Study of choroidal melanoma at Federal University of Uberlândia (in Portuguese), *Arq. Bras. Oftalmol.* **65**, 89–93 (2002).
3. J. M. Romero, P. T. Finger, R. B. Rosen, R. Iezzi, Three-dimensional ultrasound for measurement of choroidal melanoma, *Arch. Ophthalmol.* **119**(9), 1275–1282 (2001).
4. I. Kaiserman, R. Amer, N. Kaiserman, J. Peer, Ultrasonographic tissue characteristics of mushroom-shaped uveal melanoma, *Curr. Eye Res.* **30**(3), 171–177 (2005).
5. J. A. Shields, C. L. Shields, *Intraocular Tumors: A Text and Atlas*, WB Saunders, Philadelphia, pp. 117–206 (1992).
6. D. C. de A. Cunha, Choroidal Melanoma [in Portuguese], Medstudents: Papers—Ophthalmology Clinic. Clementino Fraga Filho University Hospital (2000).

7. L. E. Zimmerman, I. W. McLean, W. D. Foster, Statistical analysis of follow-up data concerning uveal melanomas, and the influence of enucleation, *Ophthalmology.* **87**, 557–564 (1980).

8. J. A. Shields, C. L. Shields, L. A. Donoso, Management of posterior uveal melanoma, *Surv. Ophthalmol.* **36**, 161–195 (1991).

9. H. G. Valenzuela, Melanoma choroidal: Treatment and medication, Medscape's continually updated clinical reference (2009), http://emedicine. medscape. com, accessed on 05/02/2010.

10. C. L. Shields, J. A. Shields, J. Cater, N. Lois, C. Edelstein, K. Gündüz, G. Mercado, Transpupillary thermotherapy for choroidal melanoma: Tumor control and visual results of 100 consecutive cases, *Ophthalmology.* **105**, 581–590 (1998).

11. J. A. Oosterhuis, H. G. Journee-de Korver, H. M. Kakebeeke-Kemme, J. C. Bleeker, Transpupillary thermotherapy in choroidal melanomas, *Arch. Ophthalmol.* **113**, 315–321 (1995).

12. C. L. Shields, J. A. Shields, P. De Potter, J. Cater, D. Tardio, J. Barrett, Diffuse choroidal melanoma: Clinical features predictive of metastasis, *Arch. Ophthalmol.* **114**, 956–963 (1996).

13. J. G. Journée-de Korver, J. A. Oosterhuis, J. Van Best, J. Fakkel, Xenon-arc phothocoagulator used for transpupillary thermotherapy, *Doc. Ophthalmol.* **78**, 183–187 (1991).

14. J. G. Journée-de Korver, J. A. Oosterhuis, H. M. Kakebeeke-Kemme, D. Wolff-Rouendaal, Transpupillary thermotherapy (TTT) by infrared irradiation of choroidal melanoma, *Doc. Ophthalmol.* **82**(3), 185–191 (1992).

15. L. O. Svaasand, T. Boerslid, M. Oeveraasen, Thermal and optical properties of living tissue: Application to laser-induced hyperthermia, *Laser Surg. Med.* **5**, 589–602 (1985).

16. R. S. B. Newsom, J. C. McAlister, M. Saeed, J. D. A. McHugh, Transpupillary thermotherapy (TTT) for the treatment of choroidal neovascularisation, *Br. J. Ophthalmol.* **85**, 173–178 (2001).

17. B. M. Stoffelns, Primary transpupillary thermotherapy (TTT) for malignant choroidal melanoma, *Acta Ophthalmol. Scand.* **80**, 25–31 (2002).

18. I. S. Othamne, C. L. Shields, J. A. Shields, K. Gündüz, G. Mercado, Circunscribed choroidal hemangiomas managed by transpupillary thermotherapy, *Arch. Ophthalmol.* **117**, 136–137 (1999).

19. J. Garcia-Arumi, L. S. Ramsay, B. C. Guraya, Transpupillary thermotherapy for circumscribed choroidal hemangiomas, *Ophthalmology.* **107**, 351–356 (2000).

20. A. Kamal, A. R. Watts, I. G. Rennie, Indocyanine green enhanced transpupillary thermotherapy of circumscribed choroidal haemangioma, *Eye* **14**(Pt 5), 701–705 (2000).

21. E. Rapizzi, W. S. Grizzard, A. Capone, Transpupillary thermotherapy in the management of circumscribed choroidal hemangiomas, *Am. J. Ophthalmol.* **127**, 481–482 (1999).

22. J. Roizenblatt, A. A. M. Rosa, Transpupillary thermotherapy as a therapeutic option for circumscribed choroidal hemangiomas: A case report (in Portuguese), *Arq. Bras. Oftalmol.* **65**, 257–260 (2002).

23. F. C. Henriques, A. R. Moritz, Studies of thermal injury, I: Conduction of heat to and through the skin and the temperature attained therein. A theoretical and an experimental investigation, *Am. J. Pathol.* **23**, 531–549 (1947).

24. H. H. Pennes, Analysis of tissue and arterial blood temperatures in the resting forearm, *J. Appl. Physiol.* **1**, 93–122 (1948).

25. G. G. Gardner, C. J. Martin, The mathematical modeling of thermal responses of normal subjects and burned patients, *Physiol. Measur.* **15**, 381–400 (1994).

26. A. J. Welch, Laser irradiation of tissue, In *Heat Transfer in Medicine and Biology: Analysis and Applications*, A. Shitzer, R. C. Eberhart, Eds, vol. 2, pp. 135–184, Plenum, New York (1985).

27. K. R. Diller, Modeling of bioheat transfer process, In *Bioengineering Heat Transfer*, Y. I. Cho, Ed., pp. 157–357, Academic Press, Boston, MA (1992).

28. K. R. Diller, J. A. Pearce, Issues in modeling thermal alterations in tissues, *Ann. NY Acad. Sci.* **888**, 153–164 (1999).

29. P. Rol, F. Fankhauser, H. Giger, U. Dürr, S. Kwasniewska, Transpupillar laser phototherapy for retinal and choroidal tumors: A rational approach, *Graefes Arch. Clin. Exp. Ophthalmol.* **238**, 249–272 (2000).

30. R. C. F. Lima, G. S. Holanda, G. M. L. L. Silva, Analysis of thermal damage caused in the eye in refractive surgery for hyperopia: A comparison of different models to simulate thermal burns (in Portuguese), In *Annals of CONEM 2004-National Congress of Mechanical Engineering*, Belém-PA, Brasil (2004).

31. A. Narasimhan, K. K. Jha, L. Gopal, Transient simulations of heat transfer in human eye undergoing laser surgery, *Int. J. Heat Mass Transfer* **53**(1), 482–490 (2009).

32. J. V. Forrester, A. D. Dick, P. McMenamin, W. Lee, *The Eye: Basic Sciences in Practice*, W.B. Saunders, London (2001).

33. M. Cvetković, D. Čavka, D. Poljak, A simple finite element model of heat transfer in the human eye, *International Conference on Software in Telecommunications and Computer Networks*, softCOM, Split pp. 27–31 (2006).

34. J. A. Scott, A finite element model of heat transport in the human eye, *Phys. Med. Biol.* **33**(2), 227–241 (1988).

35. E. H. Amara, Numerical investigation on thermal effects of laser ocular media interaction, *Int. J. Heat Mass Transfer.* **38**, 2479–2488 (1995).

36. W. Cheong, S. A. Prahl, A. J. Welch, A review of the optical properties of biological tissues, *J. Quantum Electron.* **26**, 2166–2185 (1990).

37. M. H. Niemz, *Laser–Tissue Interactions: Fundamentals and Applications*, 3rd edn., Springer, Berlin (2004).

38. B. Rivolta, F. Inzoli, S. Mantero, A. Severini, Evaluation of temperature distribution during hyperthermic treatment in biliary tumors: A computational approach, *J. Biomech. Eng.* **121**(2), 141–147 (1999).

39. E. Y. K. Ng, E. H. Ooi, FEM simulation of the eye structure with bioheat analysis, *Comput. Meth. Prog. Biomed.* **82** (3), 268–276 (2006).

40. A. F. Emery, P. Kramar, A. W. Guy, J. C. Lin, Microwave induced temperature rises in rabbit eye during hyperthermic treatment, *J. Heat Transfer.* **97**, 123–128 (1975).

41. P. Kramar, C. Harris, A. F. Emery, A. W. Guy, Acute microwave irradiation and cataract formation in rabbits and monkeys, *J. Microwave Power* **13**(3), 239–288 (1978).

42. E. H. Ooi, E. Y. K. Ng, Ocular temperature distribution: A mathematical perspective, *J. Mech. Med. Biol.* **9**(2), 199–227 (2009).

43. B. Fuisting, G. Richards, Transpupillary thermotherapy (TTT)—Review of the clinical indication spectrum, *Med. Laser Appl.* **25**, 214–222 (2010).

44. E. H. Ooi, W. T. Ang, E. Y. K. Ng, A boundary element model of the human eye undergoing laser thermokeratoplasty, *Comput. Biol. Med.* **38**, 727–737 (2008).

45. S. K da S. de L. Santos, Developing a tool for acquiring points on digital images for use in calculating temperature through computational modeling (in Portuguese), Master dissertation, Federal University of Pernambuco (2007).

46. E. Y. K. Ng, E. H. Ooi, Ocular surface temperature: A 3D FEM prediction using bioheat equation, *Comput. Biol. Med.* **37**, 829–835 (2007).

47. E. H. Ooi, W. T. Ang, E. Y. K. Ng, Bioheat transfer in the human eye: A boundary element approach, *Eng. Anal. Bound. Elem.* **31**, 494–500 (2007).

48. J. G. Journée-de Korver, J. E. E. Keunen, Thermotherapy in the management of choroidal melanoma, *Prog. Retinal Eye Res.* **21**, 303–317 (2002).

49. M. M. M. Chojniak, T. Guia, F. Uno, C. M. Erwenne, Transpupillary thermotherapy for malignant choroidal melanoma, *Arq. Bras. Oftalmol.* **64**, 133–138 (2001).

Index

For Product Safety Concerns and Information please contact our
EU representative GPSR@taylorandfrancis.com Taylor & Francis
Verlag GmbH, Kaufingerstraße 24, 80331 München, Germany